CORONARY ARTERY ANOMALIES

A Comprehensive Approach

CORONARY ARTERY ANOMALIES

A Comprehensive Approach

Editor

Paolo Angelini, M.D.

Associate Professor
Department of Internal Medicine
Baylor College of Medicine
Houston, Texas

Staff Cardiologist
St. Luke's Episcopal Hospital
Texas Heart Institute
Houston, Texas

Managing Editor

Virginia D. Fairchild, B.A.

Senior Medical Editor
Section of Scientific Publications
Texas Heart Institute
Houston, Texas

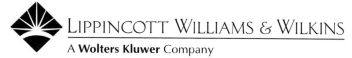

LIPPINCOTT WILLIAMS & WILKINS

A **Wolters Kluwer** Company

Philadelphia · Baltimore · New York · London
Buenos Aires · Hong Kong · Sydney · Tokyo

Editor: Ruth W. Weinberg
Managing Editor: Ellen DiFrancesco
Marketing Manager: Melissa Harris
Production Editor: Kathleen Gilbert
Design Coordinator: Mario Fernández, Jr.

351 West Camden Street
Baltimore, Maryland 21201-2436 USA

227 East Washington Square
Philadelphia, PA 19106

The publisher is not responsible (as a matter of product liability, negligence or otherwise) for any injury resulting from any material contained herein. This publication contains information relating to general principles of medical care which should not be construed as specific instructions for individual patients. Manufacturers' product information and package inserts should be reviewed for current information, including contraindications, dosages and precautions.

Printed in the United States of America

Library of Congress Cataloging-in-Publication Data
Coronary artery anomalies : a comprehensive approach / [edited by]
    Paolo Angelini.
        p.   cm.
    Includes bibliographical references and index.
    ISBN 0-7817-1018-9
    1. Congenital heart disease.   2. Coronary arteries—Abnormalities.
I. Angelini, Paolo.
    [DNLM: 1. Coronary Vessel Anomalies.   2. Coronary Vessels—anatomy
& histology.   WG 300 C81931   1999]
    RC687.C668   1999
    616.1′23043—dc21
    DNLM/DLC
    for Library of Congress   99-10769
                                                                  CIP

The publishers have made every effort to trace the copyright holders for borrowed material. If they have inadvertently overlooked any, they will be pleased to make the necessary arrangements at the first opportunity.

To purchase additional copies of this book, call our customer service department at **(800) 638-3030** or fax orders to **(301) 824-7390**. International customers should call **(301) 714-2324**.

99 00 01 02 03
1 2 3 4 5 6 7 8 9 10

To Mamma Myriam and Papá Sandro

Foreword

Dr. Paolo Angelini has prepared a very scholarly book on coronary artery anomalies. It is the best book on this subject that I have seen. Throughout the years, numerous classification systems for coronary anomalies have been proposed. None of those systems is ideal, but the one proposed by Dr. Angelini is both comprehensive and clinically useful. It shows the thoroughness with which he has penetrated this topic.

Although coronary anomalies are relatively uncommon, lack of knowledge about them can lead to inaccurate diagnoses in the cardiac catheterization laboratory and sometimes to disastrous complications during cardiac operations. One of the most common coronary anomalies is origination of the left circumflex coronary artery from the first portion of the right coronary artery or from the right sinus of Valsalva, with retroaortic coursing to the left atrioventricular sulcus. This anomaly, which may affect as many as 1 in 300 persons, is usually entirely benign. When the left circumflex artery arises directly from the right sinus rather than from the right coronary artery, however, myocardial ischemia can occur during exertion. More rarely, the left main coronary artery arises from the right coronary artery or from the right sinus and follows a retroaortic course to the left side of the heart.

A particularly troublesome coronary anomaly is origination of the left main coronary artery from the right sinus of Valsalva, with coursing of the anomalous artery between the pulmonary trunk and the aorta to the left side of the heart. The typical patient is a young boy who faints during exertion. This anomaly is very dangerous and nearly always requires operative intervention. In contrast, when the right coronary artery arises from the left sinus of Valsalva and courses between the pulmonary trunk and the aorta, it rarely causes any functional disturbance or myocardial ischemia. Except on very rare occasions, this condition can be viewed as a benign anomaly.

Although many coronary anomalies are innocuous, nearly all of them can occasionally lead to problems. A single coronary artery of the right or left type is usually a benign anomaly. In recent years, however, a famous professional basketball player who died suddenly at 40 years of age was found to have a single right coronary artery. By the time it reached the front of the heart, the artery was so small that extensive scarring of the anterior left ventricular wall resulted, followed by sudden death. Origination of both the left anterior descending artery and the left circumflex artery directly from the left sinus (absent left main coronary artery) is always benign. However, at cardiac catheterization, if only one of these arteries is injected with contrast material, a misdiagnosis may occur.

Study of the coronary arteries can teach us a great deal about myocardial ischemia. For example, it has been debated whether myocardial ischemia produces an increase in the myocardial mass. Studies of young children with origination of the left main coronary artery from the pulmonary trunk indicate that these hearts increase in weight considerably by the age of 1 year, when heart failure usually becomes evident. Moreover, because systemic hypertension is so prevalent in adults, it is difficult to prove whether myocardial ischemia resulting from atherosclerotic coronary artery disease produces myocardial hypertrophy. However, this clearly occurs in some coronary anomalies, specifically origination of the left main coronary artery from the pulmonary trunk.

The variability in patient response to a particular coronary anomaly is intriguing. Most patients with origination of the left main coronary artery from the pulmonary trunk die at approximately 1 year of age. Nevertheless, an occasional patient with the same anomaly may live for 50 years and die of a condition totally unrelated to that anomaly. The reason for this extreme variability is a mystery.

Throughout the years, coronary anomalies associated with major congenital malformations of the heart have received considerable attention. Whereas coronary anomalies *not* associated with major congenital cardiovascular anomalies are complex, those *associated* with major congenital cardiovascular anomalies are even more so. Dr. Angelini and his colleagues have done a splendid job in discussing these types of anomalies. I congratulate them for producing a superb book that will be a valuable resource for adult and pediatric cardiologists and for cardiovascular surgeons.

William C. Roberts, M.D.
Editor-in-Chief of *The American Journal of Cardiology*

Preface

This book is designed to offer an updated, comprehensive, and didactic approach to the study of coronary artery anatomy. Coronary anatomy is a highly variable entity. Use of a comprehensive approach is essential for understanding the complexity of this subject, formulating an all-inclusive nosologic scheme, and encompassing the many elements that may be relevant to a detailed study.

An illuminating introduction to coronary anatomy is provided in Chapters 1 and 2 by María V. de la Cruz and coauthors, from the Department of Developmental Biology of the Hospital Infantil in Mexico City and the Texas Heart Institute in Houston. In reviewing the coronary anatomy of different chordates (Chapter 1), these authors point out the critical intrinsic relationship between coronary artery morphology and the evolving anatomy of the myocardial walls (essentially ventricular) and of the respiratory system typology.

Chapter 2 gives an updated description of the critical embryologic stages in the development of the coronary arteries: the precoronary (intertrabecular), the ventriculo-venous, and the end-developmental stage, featuring coronary arteries that originate from the aorta. This chapter cites recent fundamental contributions by different authors regarding the proepicardial organ, which seems to provide the essential components of the epicardial coronary arteries, as well as the cardiac neural crest. It also hints at the major current challenge of clarifying the origin and morphogenesis of the intramyocardial coronary vessels.

In Chapter 3, Valentín Sans-Coma and other biologists at the University of Málaga (Spain) discuss their original findings obtained from a unique experimental model—a family of hamsters selected by means of inbreeding techniques in order to express a high incidence of both anomalous coronary arteries and bicuspid aortic valve. The authors' findings point to the existence of one or more genetic factors that regulate the development of truncal septation and coronary origination from the aortic sinuses, probably by influencing the development of the cardiac neural crest.

Chapter 4 addresses the primary objective of this book by discussing human coronary anomalies in a rational, organized manner. This chapter is based on the experience of the Department of Cardiology at the Texas Heart Institute. The chapter's basic methodology depends on a feature-by-feature description of morphologically normal coronary arteries; once "normality" has been thus defined, coronary anomalies are described as exceptions to the norm. Because normality is hard to define with respect to such a highly variable subject as the anatomy of the coronary arteries, the literature contains no universal definitions of normality. We propose that "normal" be defined as "what is observed in more than 1% of the population" and that this definition be used prospectively to identify coronary anomalies in an otherwise normal population. In the interests of practicality, technical adequacy of description, and clinical relevance, we report the incidence of the different anomalies not on the basis of traditional anatomic descriptions but, rather, on the basis of a prospective analysis of selective coronary angiograms, using the foregoing proposed definition of normality. In attempting to define the essence of each coronary anomaly, this chapter stresses the conceptual approach; however, it also includes an extensive angiographic gallery, which presents examples of most coronary anomalies, along with angiograms and clinical-functional correlations. To provide the latest available information about pathophysiology and clinical relevance, the final section of Chapter 4 discusses all proposed (proven and unproven) pathophysiologic mechanisms and clinical manifestations of coronary anomalies, classifying each anomaly by these parameters.

Whereas coronary anomalies can be surprise findings at angiography (usually when performed in adults for an unrelated clinical reason), they may also produce major clinical manifestations, especially in pediatric patients. In Chapter 5, Thomas Fagan and Michael Nihill, pediatric cardiologists at Baylor College of Medicine and Texas Children's Hospital in Houston, provide a specific clinical discussion that focuses on anomalous origination of the left coronary artery from the pulmonary artery and large coronary fistulas in pediatric patients. In that same chapter, Alexis Palacios-Macedo, Charles Fraser, and Denton Cooley, cardiovascular surgeons at the Texas Heart Institute and Texas Children's Hospital, cover the surgical treatment of these coronary anomalies.

In Chapter 6, Dr. de la Cruz and I summarize the current knowledge about the anatomy of the coronary arteries in certain congenital heart defects that we consider particularly relevant. Interest in this subject is generally stimulated by the following issues: (1) Some congenital heart defects involve abnormal development of the cardiac structures that provide the basic framework for the coronary arteries, that is, the aortic sinuses and left ventricular myocardial mass. It is not surprising that an alteration in the basic framework (congenital heart defect) would lead to an alteration in the morphogenesis of the coronary circulation. Such defects can be viewed as naturally occurring experiments, which could potentially clarify our understanding of normal or abnormal coronary morphogenesis. (2) The surgical approach to some congenital heart defects may be substantially altered by the presence of specific coronary artery patterns (e.g., tetralogy of Fallot, transposition of the great vessels, or pulmonary atresia with an intact ventricular septum).

In Chapter 7, James T. Willerson, Medical Director of the Texas Heart Institute, rounds out the book by presenting some remarks on current and future research into coronary artery anomalies of form and/or function.

This book is being offered to a disparate readership in hopes of stimulating further study and discussion of a complex, poorly organized subject. The recognition, treatment, and prevention of coronary anomalies should be an interdisciplinary effort on the part of primary care physicians, cardiologists, cardiovascular surgeons, public health officials, and specialists in basic biology, among others.

In preparing this book, I have drawn on my 28-year experience at the Texas Heart Institute, the largest cardiovascular center in the world, where thousands of individuals are referred for evaluation and treatment each year. Here, interest in coronary anomalies was initially stimulated by Denton A. Cooley and Grady Hallman, who pioneered numerous operations for correcting congenital disorders in pediatric patients. My own interest in normal and abnormal coronary anatomy was inspired by my proximity to these great surgeons and by the large number of unique coronary variants encountered. These cases aroused intense interest and underlined the need for a more comprehensive approach that could better elucidate the individual nature of a given case.

I wish to acknowledge the kind collaboration of my many cardiology colleagues at the Texas Heart Institute, especially Drs. Bruce E. Barnum, Jaime Benrey, Robert J. Card, Patrick J. Cook, Wayne E. Dear, Carlos M. de Castro, Jr., Sayed Feghali, R. David Fish, Jorge A. Garcia-Gregory, Jorge F. Guttin, Robert J. Hall, Patrick J. Hogan, Zvonimir Krajcer, D. Richard Leachman, Robert D. Leachman (now deceased), Louis Leatherman, Roberto Lufschanowski, Edward K. Massin, Ali Massumi, Virendra S. Mathur, Emerson C. Perin, Donald G. Rochelle, Michele Sartori, Mark J. Schnee, Arthur J. Springer, Eleftherios S. Stamatiou, Neil E. Strickman, Bernardo Treistman, Donald Trillos, Susan Wilansky, James T. Willerson, and Antoine G. Younis, as well as the hundreds of cardiology fellows who have trained at the Institute during the last 28 years. These individuals provided the main source, support, and first audience for the material presented herein.

In addition, I am grateful to the Texas Heart Institute's Section of Scientific Publications for its assistance in the preparation of this book. Specifically, I thank Virginia D. Fairchild for managing and editing this project; Dikombi Gite for typing the manuscript; Christina Chambers for editorial assistance; and Ken Hoge and Melissa J. Mayo for helping with the photographs and illustrations.

Paolo Angelini, M.D.

Contributors

Paolo Angelini, M.D.
Associate Professor
Department of Internal Medicine
Baylor College of Medicine
Houston, Texas
Staff Cardiologist
St. Luke's Episcopal Hospital
Texas Heart Institute
Houston, Texas

José M. Arqué, M.D.
Department of Cardiovascular Surgery
University Hospital "Carlos Haya"
Málaga, Spain

Albert V. Chan, Jr., M.D.
St. Luke's Episcopal Hospital
Texas Heart Institute
Houston, Texas

Denton A. Cooley, M.D.
Surgeon-in-Chief
Texas Heart Institute
Houston, Texas

María V. de la Cruz, M.D., Ph.D.
Head, Department of Developmental Biology
    and Experimental Teratology
Hospital Infantil de Mexico
Mexico City, Mexico

José G. Diez, M.D.
Texas Heart Institute
Houston, Texas

Ana C. Durán, Ph.D.
Department of Animal Biology
Faculty of Science
University of Málaga
Málaga, Spain

Thomas E. Fagan, M.D.
Department of Pediatric Cardiology
Texas Children's Hospital
Houston, Texas

Borja Fernández, Ph.D.
Department of Animal Biology
Faculty of Science
University of Málaga
Málaga, Spain

M. Carmen Fernández, B.S.
Department of Animal Biology
University of Málaga
Málaga, Spain

Charles D. Fraser, Jr., M.D.
Head, Cardiovascular Surgery
Texas Children's Hospital
Houston, Texas

David López, B.S.
Department of Animal Biology
University of Málaga
Málaga, Spain

Ricardo Moreno-Rodriguez, Ph.D.
Department of Developmental Biology
    and Experimental Teratology
Hospital Infantil de Mexico
Mexico City, Mexico

Michael R. Nihill, M.D.
Department of Pediatric Cardiology
Texas Children's Hospital
Senior Cardiologist
Professor of Pediatrics
Baylor College of Medicine
Houston, Texas

Alexis Palacios-Macedo, M.D.
Department of Cardiovascular Surgery
Texas Children's Hospital
Houston, Texas

William C. Roberts, M.D.
Executive Director, Baylor Cardiovascular Institute
Baylor University Medical Center
Dallas, Texas
Editor in Chief
The American Journal of Cardiology

Valentín Sans-Coma, Ph.D.
Head, Department of Animal Biology
Faculty of Science
University of Málaga
Málaga, Spain

Salvador Villason, M.D.
Texas Heart Institute
Houston, Texas

James T. Willerson, M.D.
Medical Director
Director, Cardiology Research
Co-Director, Cullen Cardiovascular Research Laboratories
Editor, Circulation
Texas Heart Institute
Houston, Texas

Contents

Coronary Artery Anomalies: A Comprehensive Approach, edited by P. Angelini.
Lippincott Williams & Wilkins, Philadelphia © 1999.

CHAPTER 1

Phylogeny of the Coronary Arteries

María V. de la Cruz, Ricardo Moreno-Rodriguez, and Paolo Angelini

On the basis of ontogenetic studies in birds and mammals, we believe that the phylogeny of the coronary vessels in the phylum Chordata should be studied in representative classes that have phylogenetic significance. The following characteristics should be studied: (1) the comparative anatomy of the cardiac chambers, (2) the relationship between the architecture of the ventricular walls and the vascular supply, and (3) the spectrum of anatomic origin and distribution of the coronary arteries. The anatomy of the cardiac chambers is important because the topographic distribution of the coronary vessels is closely related to the anatomic features of the ventricles. In addition, the architecture of the ventricles (highly trabeculated with a thin wall, versus compact myocardial with or without trabeculated organization) determines whether the related coronary arteries are absent, sparse, or well developed.

This chapter discusses the three above-mentioned characteristics in the following representatives of phylogenetically significant classes: the shark (*Squalus* spp.) in the class Elasmobranchii; the frog (*Rana* spp.) in Amphibia; the iguana (*Iguana* spp.) in Reptilia; the chick (*Gallus domesticus*) in Aves; and the hamster, pig, dog, deer, and human (*Homo sapiens*) in Mammalia. Because of controversy about the definition and constitution of Reptilia,[4,10,11,15,18,19,23] we chose to study the iguana, which unquestionably belongs to the Reptilia class.

This chapter briefly summarizes our own findings, as well as the pertinent literature regarding this subject. Our findings are based on macro- and microscopic observations of sharks, frogs, iguanas, and chicks. In these studies, india-ink jelly injections allowed optimal visualization of the coronary tree in amphibia, reptilia, and birds.

CLASS ELASMOBRANCHII

The heart of members of the Elasmobranchii class comprises four serial chambers that receive only venous blood; therefore the heart is not organized, as in humans, with side-to-side cavities, but instead is organized in series. In caudal to cephalic order, the chambers are the sinus venosus, a single atrium, a single ventricle, and the bulbus cordis (Fig. 1.1*A*). The sinus venosus and atrium are located dorsally, and the ventricle and bulbus cordis are located ventrally. The sinus venosus, a single, large chamber connected to—but not incorporated into—the atrium, receives systemic venous blood. The atrial chamber is connected to the ventricular chamber. The boundary between these two chambers is called the atrioventricular groove on the external aspect of the heart and the single atrioventricular ring on the internal aspect. The single atrioventricular ring, along with the valve leaflets and chordae tendineae, comprises the single atrioventricular apparatus (Fig. 1.1, *A* and *B*). The ventricular chamber shows no evidence of septation (single ventricle); its wall is thick, compact, and trabeculated. The bulbus cordis, with its thick muscular walls, is continuous with, but not incorporated into, the ventricular chamber. The bulbus cordis has two limits: (1) the proximal bulboventricular groove at the ventricular junction, and (2) the distal boundary constituted by the single arterial trunk or ventral aorta (Fig. 1.1, *A* and *B*). Three strata of semilunar valvular cusps are found in the bulbus cordis: one at the ventricular junction, another in the middle region, and one at the boundary with the arterial trunk or ventral aorta[26] (Fig. 1.1*B*). The ventral aorta continues into the aortic arches at the branchia (Fig. 1.2*A*).

The coronary arteries originate from the fourth branchial efferent artery (hypobranchial, midventral) as two paired (right and left) main trunks.[17] With respect to the coronary pattern in Elasmobranchii, our findings are similar to those reported by Andres and coauthors,[1,3] and we support their choice of nomenclature.[1–3,20] Nevertheless, we believe that the coronary branches that supply the bulbus cordis should

This work was supported by Grant No. 0257-M9107 from the Mexican National Council on Science and Technology (CONACyT) and a grant from Telmex.

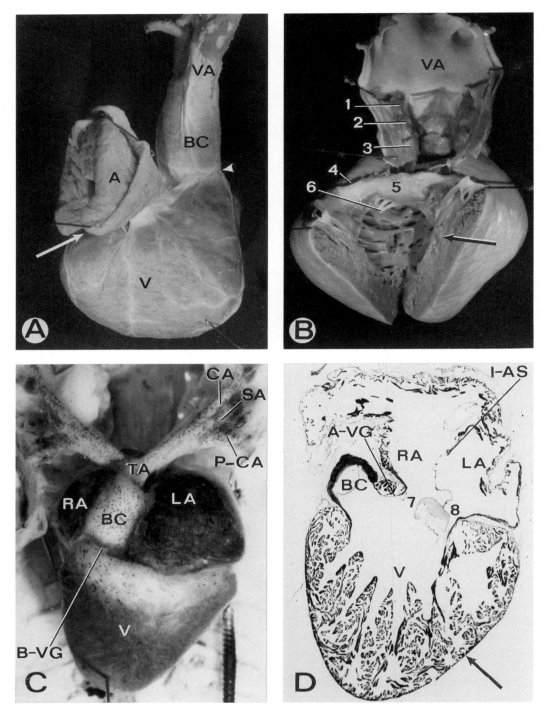

FIGURE 1.1. A. Right lateral view of the heart and ventral aorta of the shark after removal of the sinus venosus. Note the atrioventricular groove (arrow) and the bulboventricular groove (arrowhead). A = atrium (single); BC = bulbus cordis; V = ventricle (single); VA = ventral aorta. **B.** Dorsal view of the shark heart after removal of the atrium and exposure of the inner anatomy. The dorsal walls of the ventral aorta, bulbus cordis, and single ventricle have been opened. Note the three strata (1,2,3) of the sigmoid valves in the bulbus cordis. The single atrioventricular apparatus comprises a lone atrioventricular ring (4), as well as leaflets (5) and chordae tendineae (6). The single ventricle has a thick, compact muscular wall (arrow). VA = ventral aorta. **C.** Ventral view of the frog heart, showing the truncus arteriosus (TA) and the aortic arches. BC = bulbus cordis; B-VG = bulboventricular groove; CA = carotid arch; LA = left atrium; P-CA = pulmo-cutaneous arch; RA = right atrium; SA = systemic arch; V = ventricle (single). **D.** Frontal histologic mid-section of the frog heart, showing the right atrium (RA), left atrium (LA), interatrial septum (I-AS), atrioventricular groove (A-VG), bulbus cordis (BC), and right (7) and left (8) atrioventricular orifices. Also visible are the thin outer wall (arrow), multiple thin trabeculae, and spongy architecture of the single ventricle (V).

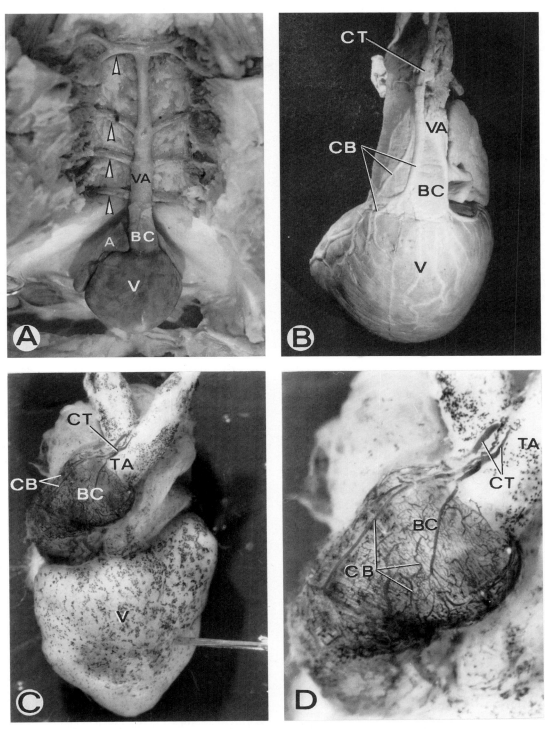

FIGURE 1.2. A. In the shark, the aortic arches (arrowheads) are connected to the ventral aorta (VA). A = atrium (single); BC = bulbus cordis; V = ventricle (single). **B.** Topographic distribution of the coronary main trunks (CT) and the coronary branches (CB) on the ventral surface of the heart and aorta in the shark. BC = bulbus cordis; V = ventricle (single); VA = ventral aorta. **C.** Ventral view of the heart and truncus arteriosus (TA) in the frog, showing the main coronary trunks (CT) on the truncus arteriosus and the coronary branches (CB) on the bulbus cordis (BC). V = ventricle (single). **D.** Higher magnification of Figure 1.2C, showing the two main coronary trunks (CT) and the coronary branches (CB) after injection of india ink. BC = bulbus cordis; TA = truncus arteriosus.

be called bulbar instead of conal, because the bulbus cordis is a mature heart cavity with well-defined anatomic and histologic features (Fig. 1.1B). In contrast, the conus exists only during a period in embryogenesis in which the coronary vessels have not developed. Therefore the term conus should be reserved for indicating a region or segment present only in the embryonic heart.[8,9] Our observations agree with those of other authors,[1–3,20] who reported the presence of coronary trunks on the lateral walls of the ventral aorta; these trunks split into branches located in the subepicardial space of the bulbus cordis and the single ventricular chamber (Fig. 1.1A and 1.2B). According to Andres and associates,[1,3] the location of the coronary trunks may differ among the orders of the Elasmobranchii. The proximal coronary arteries may be dorsal and ventral—or right and left—and the distribution of the distal branches over the bulbus cordis and the ventricular wall may vary.

CLASS AMPHIBIA

The heart of amphibians, as exemplified by the frog, comprises five cardiac chambers: the sinus venosus, two atria (right and left), one common ventricle, and the bulbus cordis. The sinus venosus, a dorsocaudal chamber that receives venous blood, is connected to the right atrium via the sinoatrial orifice. The interatrial septum separates the right atrium from the left atrium (Fig. 1.1D), which receives the pulmonary veins. Each atrium has its own atrioventricular orifice that allows communication with the single ventricular chamber (Fig. 1.1D). On the external aspect of the heart, the atrioventricular orifices correspond to the atrioventricular groove (Fig. 1.1, C and D). The ventricle has a spongelike architecture consisting of a thin, outer, muscular wall and numerous, thin trabeculae within; no interventricular septum is present (Fig. 1.1D). The single ventricular cavity is connected with the bulbus cordis (outlet), and the boundary between these two cavities is identified externally as the bulboventricular groove (Fig. 1.1C). The walls of the bulbus cordis are composed of thick, compact, cardiac muscle (Fig. 1.1D) that contains a complex longitudinal valve called the spiral fold.[17] Also, the bulbus cordis has two strata of semilunar valvular cusps: one stratum at the proximal level of the bulboventricular groove and the other stratum at the distal junction of the bulbus cordis with the truncus arteriosus.[17] The right and left carotid, systemic, and pulmocutaneous arches arise at the cephalic end of the truncus arteriosus in a cephalocaudal direction (Fig. 1.1C).

In most frog hearts, two coronary trunks, which originate from the carotid arch, course along the walls of the truncus arteriosus and spread only over the walls of the bulbus cordis (Fig. 1.2, C and D). No coronary vessels are present on the walls of the ventricle (Fig. 1.2C). This type of ventricular mural architecture is similar to that seen in the chick and human embryo heart before the development of coronary arteries, when metabolic exchanges occur by means of imbibition at the level of the interstitial spaces.

During diastole, the surface of the frog's heart is intensely cyanotic and blue. During systole, however, the color becomes clear pink or whitish, signifying subtotal emptying of the ventricular cavity at the level of the intertrabecular spaces. This phenomenon, even when only grossly observed, suggests that highly effective emptying of the interstitial spaces occurs at each heartbeat. Under these conditions, the effectiveness of metabolic exchanges is obviously related not only to the heart rate but also to the thickness of the myocardial cords/trabeculations. Although no functional study of such a ''coronary-less'' heart model has ever been reported, current information suggests that this model's functional metabolic reserve is quite limited.

CLASS REPTILIA

In the reptilian heart, the venous blood is received by the sinus venosus—a single, dorsal chamber that is connected to, but not incorporated into, the right atrium. An interatrial septum separates the right atrium from the left atrium, which receives the pulmonary veins (Fig. 1.3, A and B). The right and left ventricular chambers are separated by an incomplete interventricular septum (in the iguana). The interventricular foramen adjoins the atrioventricular orifices (Fig. 1.3, A and B), each of which is connected to its corresponding ventricle (Fig. 1.3, A and B).

In the iguana, our findings were not consistent with those of Withers,[26] Lawson,[17] and Burggren,[6] none of whom recognized two separate atrioventricular valves and inlet chambers. In contrast, we observed two separate, complete annuli and small valvular leaflets in both the right and left atrioventricular valvular apparatuses (Fig. 1.3, A and B). In iguanas, the left ventricle lacks a direct outlet, but two aortas and the pulmonary artery (each with semilunar valvular cusps adjacent to the right atrioventricular orifice) originate from the right ventricle.

The reptilian heart lacks a bulbus cordis, as reported by Withers.[26] The arterial blood from the pulmonary veins enters the left atrium and flows into the left ventricle. It then flows across the interventricular foramen into the right ventricle (Fig. 1.3, A and B). Only in the order Crocodylia does one of the aortas emerge directly from the left ventricle and the other aorta, with the pulmonary artery, arise from the right ventricle. Rather than having an interventricular foramen,[26] Crocodylia hearts have a supravalvular orifice known as Panizza's foramen, which communicates between the two aortas. In reptiles, the outer wall of all the ventricular cavities consists of compact myocardium, and the inner wall is highly trabeculated (Fig. 1.3, A and B). In most reptiles, the coronary vessels arise from the aorta that adjoins the interventricular foramen; in the Crocodylia, the coronary vessels arise from the aorta that emerges from the left ventricle. The reptilian coronary vessels spread within the subepicardial space. In the turtle (Chelonia midas)[22] and the iguana, two coronary arteries, one on the anterior wall (Fig. 1.4A) and one on the posterior wall (Fig. 1.4B), are found in the subepicardial

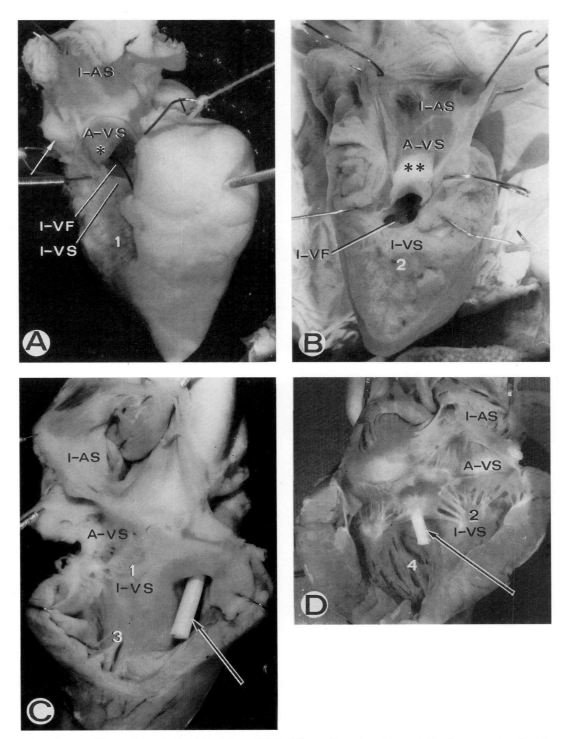

FIGURE 1.3. Dissection of the right **(A)** and left **(B)** cardiac chambers of the iguana, showing the respective right and left aspects of the interatrial septum (I-AS), atrioventricular septum (A-VS), and interventricular septum (I-VS). In the right chamber, the interventricular foramen (I-VF), entered with a wire, is shown in relation to the atrioventricular groove (arrow), right ventricular inlet (1), and right atrioventricular leaflet (*). In the left chamber, note the interventricular foramen (I-VF), left ventricular inlet (2), and left atrioventricular leaflet (**). Dissection of the right **(C)** and left **(D)** cardiac chambers of the chick heart, showing the respective right and left aspects of the interatrial septum (I-AS), atrioventricular septum (A-VS), and interventricular septum (I-VS). Note the right ventricular inlet (1), the left ventricular inlet and the posteromedial papillary muscle of the mitral valve (2), the apical trabeculated region of the right ventricle, and the apical trabeculated region of the left ventricle (4). In views **C** and **D**, a stick has been placed within the right and left ventricular outlets (arrows), respectively.

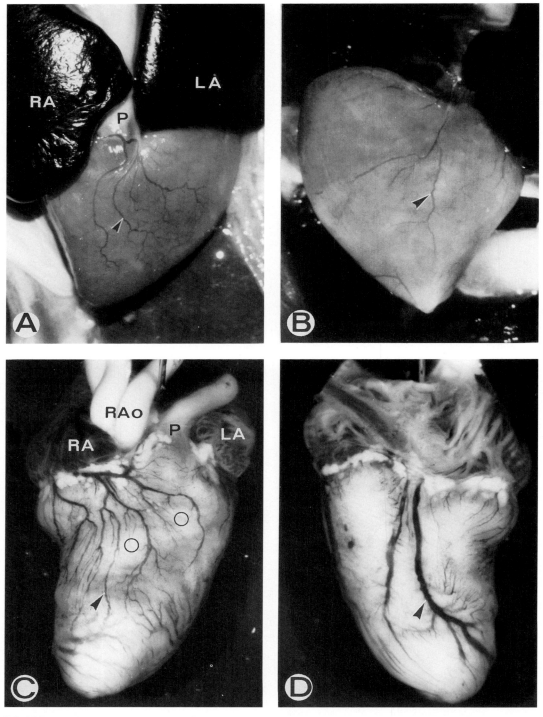

FIGURE 1.4. Hearts of the iguana **(A, B)** and the chick **(C, D)** after injection with india ink. **A.** Ventral view of the iguana heart, showing the absence of a clearly defined left anterior descending coronary artery (arrowhead). Right ventricular branches cross the anterior atrioventricular groove. LA = left atrium; P = pulmonary artery; RA = right atrium. **B.** Dorsal view of the iguana heart, showing the posterior descending coronary artery (arrowhead) and its branches. **C.** Ventral view of the chick heart, showing the absence of the left anterior descending coronary artery. The right coronary artery provides several well-developed anterior right ventricular branches (arrowhead) that cross the interventricular septum (circles). LA = left atrium; P = pulmonary artery; RA = right atrium; RAo = right aortic arch. **D.** Dorsal view of the chick heart, showing a double posterior descending artery, one originating from the right coronary artery (arrowhead), and the other originating from the left circumflex artery.

space. Turtle and iguana hearts have coronary arteries in the atrioventricular grooves, as do bird and mammal hearts.

In the alligator heart, as recently documented by Kohmoto and colleagues[16] in the American alligator, both aortic valves are bicuspid. Only the aorta that arises from the left ventricle (the "left" aorta) has coronary ostia (usually two). The coronary arteries are well developed, and they reach the endocardium, but they are not the only source of myocardial metabolic exchanges. The myocardial architecture is peculiar, because it features (1) a predominantly spongy myocardium that extends 15 mm deep and (2) a thin (2- to 3-mm), compact outer myocardial layer. The alligator heart is unusually small for an animal with such a large body size (typical heart and body weights, 150 g vs 300 kg, respectively). These anatomic features have been regarded as evidence that direct, sinusoidal blood flow contributes functionally to myocardial metabolic exchanges, also resulting from the presence of apparently rich communications between these intertrabecular spaces and the epicardial coronary arteries. Coronarocameral communications probably permit improved runoff of intertrabecular blood during diastole.

In summary, the alligator heart seems to have transitional features that fill the gap between hearts that rely on a purely intertrabecular noncoronary pattern (as seen in the frog) and those that rely predominantly on coronary-mediated metabolic exchanges.

CLASS AVES AND CLASS MAMMALIA

Aves and Mammalia are discussed together because the hearts of birds and mammals are similar. An intact interatrial septum separates the two atria, which are connected to the corresponding ventricles via separate atrioventricular orifices (Fig. 1.3, C and D). In turn, a complete interventricular septum separates the two ventricles. Each ventricle has three regions[12]: (1) an inlet, which has an atrioventricular valve apparatus; (2) a trabeculated apical region; and (3) an outlet, or subarterial segment (Fig. 1.3, C and D). The ventricular walls are thick and compact. The aorta arises from the left ventricle, and the pulmonary artery arises from the right ventricle. The pulmonary veins drain into the left atrium. The main difference between the hearts of birds and mammals involves the position of the sinus venosus: in birds, this structure is connected to—but not incorporated into—the right atrium; in mammals, the sinus venosus forms the dorsal wall of the right atrium. In addition, the aortic arch is located on the right side of the trachea in birds (Fig. 1.4C) and on the left side in mammals.

The study of the basic coronary patterns in birds, mammals, and reptiles requires a brief discussion of the embryologic constitution of the aortas. The specific anatomic features of each of the great arteries are determined in part by the embryologic development of the aortic arches and the septation of the truncus or arterial pole of the heart. The truncus, a tubular embryologic structure, forms the walls of the ascending aorta and main pulmonary trunk. The truncus is limited cephalically by its junction with the fourth and sixth aortic arches and caudally by its junction with the conus. The conus gives rise to the outlet of both ventricles, and its prospective fate is to form cardiac muscle.[8,9] Recent experimental work[13,14,24,25] has shown that migrating cardiac neural crest cells give rise to the aortopulmonary septum, which divides the truncus into the aortic and pulmonary trunks. Initially, six (right-left) pairs of aortic arches are present, but only two—the fourth aortic (or systemic) arch and the sixth aortic (or pulmonary) arch—are connected to the cephalic end of the truncus at the end of embryologic development. The aortic trunk is connected to the right systemic arch in birds and to the left systemic arch (located to the left of the trachea) in mammals. Therefore birds are regarded as having a right aortic arch and mammals as having a left aortic arch. Although frequently used, the terms "right aorta" (instead of right aortic arch) in referring to birds and "left aorta" in referring to mammals are anatomically and embryologically incorrect. In contrast, the truncus of reptiles is divided into two aortic trunks and one pulmonary trunk during septation. Each trunk has independent arterial valves. At the cephalic end of the embryonic truncus, only three aortic arches persist: the sixth (or pulmonary) arch, the right systemic arch, and the left systemic arch. At the end of septation, the right systemic arch is connected to one of the two aortic trunks, and the left systemic arch is connected to the other aortic trunk. Thus the mature reptilian heart has two aortic trunks, each of which connects with a corresponding aortic arch. The pulmonary arterial anatomy is similar in reptiles, birds, and mammals, all three classes having a single pulmonary trunk that divides into right and left branches or arteries. The right pulmonary artery originates from the right proximal segment of the embryologic sixth aortic arch, and the left pulmonary artery originates from the left proximal segment.

In all mammals but the deer, the proximal coronary anatomy is characterized by ostia located in the facing aortic sinuses, adjoining the pulmonary valve. The anterior descending artery and the artery coursing in the left atrioventricular groove usually originate from a common stem, the left coronary main trunk. The anterior interventricular branch (which is usually subepicardial) is well developed only when it gives rise to most of the septal circulation. When a large common septal trunk arises from the proximal anterior interventricular artery (or from the aorta or right coronary artery), the distal anterior subepicardial vessel follows a diagonal course in the anterolateral wall of the left ventricle and does not run along the anterior interventricular groove.

The distribution patterns of distal coronary arteries may vary substantially among individual members of any species, but general rules regarding coronary artery patterns apply to each species or family. The following information may be important to scientists dealing with the coronary circulation or myocardial metabolism in experimental animals.[7]

1. Chick hearts tend to have epicardial main coronary arteries, except for the first septal artery, which is typically a single or double branch that supplies most of the interventricular septum. This branch usually originates from the left main coronary trunk, but it may arise directly from the left or right coronary cusp or from the proximal right coronary artery. The septal branch is entirely intramyocardial. Consequently, a properly defined left anterior descending artery is not usually seen at the anterior interventricular sulcus. The right coronary artery and the circumflex artery are almost identical to those of humans (Fig. 1.4, *C* and *D*).

2. Many mammalian hearts have intramyocardial proximal coronary arteries. Polacek and coauthors[21] classified mammalians into three types according to this parameter. In type A, the proximal coronary arteries are entirely intramyocardial, as in hamsters, squirrels, rats, guinea pigs, and rabbits. In type B, the proximal coronary arteries are predominantly epicardial, with frequent myocardial bridges, as in dogs, cats, goats, sheep, macaques, and humans; in this model the proximal left anterior descending artery is the segment most likely to be intramyocardial. In type C, the proximal coronary arteries are entirely epicardial, as in horses, pigs, and cows. No evidence has ever been reported of any pathologic consequences of a coronary intramyocardial course in animals.

3. In most hamster hearts (see Chapter 3), the coronary arteries are primarily intramural (imbedded in the myocardium from their origin). The interventricular septum is supplied by a large septal artery that originates from the left proximal artery in 70% of cases and from the right proximal artery in 28% of cases. The anterior interventricular sulcus does not have a left anterior descending artery as expected in humans. The left coronary artery branches into the diagonal, obtuse marginal, and posterior arteries of the left ventricle. As explained in Chapter 3, biologists use the term diagonal for the branch of the circumflex artery that supplies the mid free wall of the left ventricle, corresponding to the obtuse marginal-1 artery in humans. Most hamster hearts have a codominant distribution pattern (the right and circumflex arteries provide small branches to the posterior interventricular septum without a well-differentiated posterior descending vessel).

4. The coronary pattern of pig hearts is similar to that of human hearts, with epicardially located main branches that feature terminal circulation (limited collateral circulation between adjacent coronary arteries). The left anterior descending artery is prominent, and either the circumflex artery or the right coronary artery may be dominant. The posterior descending artery is epicardial and may arise from either the circumflex or the right coronary artery.

5. In dog hearts, the gross coronary pattern is similar to that in humans and pigs. The main difference is that dog hearts have well-developed collateral circles between adjacent vessels. Specifically, the left anterior descending artery—a large, prominent epicardial vessel—has visible, functional epicardial collateral vessels between (a) the proximal and distal diagonal branches, (b) the distal anterior descending and circumflex-obtuse marginal branches, and (c) the anterior and posterior descending branches around the cardiac apex. Another unique feature of the dog heart is the presence of moderately large infundibular branches that originate from the proximal left anterior descending artery. These branches do not have a well-developed collateral circulation with the right coronary artery. Ligation of these infundibular branches or of the proximal left anterior descending artery usually leads (also) to a myocardial infarction of the right ventricular infundibulum (outflow tract). The posterior descending artery more often branches from the circumflex artery than from the right coronary artery, but specific large studies of dominance patterns are not available.

6. In the Virginia white-tailed deer, as reported by Bishop and associates[5] on the basis of 962 autopsy cases, the basic coronary pattern is substantially identical to that of humans, but the proximal half of the left anterior descending artery is consistently intramyocardial. Coronary anomalies are apparently frequent, simulating those observed in humans, with an unusually high incidence of an additional ectopic coronary ostium in the right posterior ("noncoronary") cusp. In one case, Bishop and colleagues observed a single coronary artery arising from the right posterior cusp. In the great majority of cases, however, three coronary arteries are present, one arising from each aortic cusp. The circumflex branch originates from the aberrant, posterior ostium, providing circulation to the posterior left ventricles, usually via an atrial intraseptal course. In these coronary patterns, the atrioventricular and sinus node arteries are supplied by the abnormal circumflex branch.

CONCLUSION

In chordates with a single great vessel that emerges from the heart (such as Elasmobranchii and Amphibia), the coronary arteries originate from the branchial arterial system. In contrast, in chordates that have an aorta and a pulmonary artery (such as birds and mammals), the coronary arteries originate from the aortic semilunar valvular sinuses. All reptiles have two aortas and a pulmonary trunk. In reptiles in which both aortas arise from the right ventricle, the coronary arteries are connected to the aortic semilunar valvular sinuses, which are adjacent to the interventricular foramen. In reptiles in which one of the aortas is connected to the left ventricle, the coronary arteries originate from the semilunar valvular sinuses of the aorta, which arises from the left ventricle.

In phylogeny, as in ontogeny, the presence and distribution of the coronary arteries is strictly related to the compactness of the ventricular myocardium, as seen in the members of the Elasmobranchii, Reptilia, Aves, and Mammalia classes that have thick, compact ventricular walls and a rich supply of coronary arteries. In amphibians, coronary arteries are found only on the compact myocardium of the walls of the bulbus cordis; no coronary vessels are seen on the wall of the single ventricle, where the myocardium has a spongy architecture with multiple interstitial spaces that communicate with the ventricular cavity.

The topographic distribution of the coronary vessels is closely related to the number of ventricular chambers. In classes that have two ventricular chambers separated by an interventricular septum (reptiles, birds, and mammals), anterior and posterior descending arteries course along the anterior/posterior interventricular groove—which corresponds internally to the interventricular septum—unless a large proximal septal branch supplies most of the interventricular septum.

REFERENCES

1. Andres AV, Munoz-Chapuli R, Sans-Coma V, et al. Anatomical studies of the coronary system in elasmobranchs. I. Coronary arteries in lamnoid sharks. Anat Rec 1990;187:303.
2. Andres AV, Munoz-Chapuli R, Sans-Coma V. Development of the coronary arteries and cardiac veins in the dogfish (Scyliorhinus canicula). Anat Rec 1993;235:436.
3. Andres AV, Munoz-Chapuli R, Sans-Coma V, et al. Anatomical studies of the coronary system in elasmobranchs. II. Coronary arteries in hexanchoid, squaloid, and carcharhinoid sharks. Anat Rec 1992;233:429.
4. Bakker RT. Dinosaur renaissance. Sci Am 1975;232:58.
5. Bishop MB, Free SL, Davies JNP, et al. The coronary arterial pattern of deer in New York State with special reference to the third (posterior) coronary artery. Am Heart J 1970;70:785.
6. Burggren WW. Cardiac design in lower vertebrates: what can phylogeny reveal about ontogeny? Experientia 1988;44:919.
7. Chase RE, DeGaris CF. Arteriae coronariae (cordis) in the higher primates. Am J Phys Anthropol 1939;24:427.
8. de la Cruz MV, Sanchez-Gomez C, Arteaga M, et al. Experimental study of the development of the truncus and the conus in the chick embryo. J Anat 1977;123:661.
9. de la Cruz MV, Sanchez-Gomez C, Palomino MA. The primitive cardiac regions in the straight tube heart (stage 9) and their anatomical expression in the mature heart: an experimental study in the chick embryo. J Anat 1989;165:121.
10. Gaffney ES. Phylogenetic relationships of the major groups of Amniotes. In: Panchen AL, ed. Systematics Association Special Volume 15. The terrestrial environment and the origin of land vertebrates. New York: Academic Press, 1980:593.
11. Gauthier JA, Kluge AG, Rowe T. The early evolution of Amniota. In: Benton MJ, ed. The phylogeny and classification of the tetrapods. Vol. 1. Amphibians, reptiles, and birds. Oxford (UK): Systematics Association Publications, 1988:103.
12. Goor DA, Lillehei CW. Congenital malformations of the heart: embryology, anatomy and operative considerations. New York: Grune & Stratton, 1975:1–37.
13. Kirby ML, Kirby LT, Hays BM. Characterization of conotruncal malformations following ablation of "cardiac" neural crest. Anat Rec 1985;213:87.
14. Kirby ML, Waldo KL. Neural crest and cardiovascular patterning. Circ Res 1995;77:211.
15. Kluge AG. On the special treatment of fossils and taxonomics. Burden: a response to Loconte. Cladistics 1990;6:191.
16. Kohmoto T, Argenziana M, Yamamoto N, et al. Assessment of transmyocardial perfusion in alligator hearts. Circulation 1997;95:1585.
17. Lawson R. The comparative anatomy of the circulatory system. In: Wake MH, ed. Hyman's comparative vertebrate anatomy. 3rd ed. Chicago: The University of Chicago Press, 1992:448–554.
18. Loconte H. Cladistic classification of Amniota: a response to Gauthier et al. Cladistics 1990;6:187.
19. Lovtrup S. On the classification of the taxon tetrapoda. Systa Zool 1985;34:463.
20. Munoz-Chapuli R, Macias D, Ramos C et al. Cardiac development in the dogfish (Scyliorhinus canicula): a model for the study of vertebrate cardiogenesis. Cardioscience 1994;5:245.
21. Polacek P, Zechmeister A. The occurrence and significance of myocardial bridges and loops on coronary arteries. Opuscola Cardiologica. Acta Facultatis Medicae Universitatis Brunensis, Brno, Czech Republic, 1968.
22. Quesada R, Madriz LF. Vascularizacion coronaria de la tortuga marina (Chelonia mydas). Rev Biol Trop 1986;34:253.
23. Villela OF, Navarro SAG. Clasificacion actual de los Amniota. Ciencias 1993;7:63.
24. Waldo KL, Kirby ML. Cardiac neural crest contribution to the pulmonary artery and sixth aortic arch artery complex in chick embryos aged 6 to 18 days. Anat Rec 1993;237:385.
25. Waldo KL, Kirby ML. Development of the great arteries. In: de la Cruz MV, Markwald RR, eds. Living morphogenesis of the heart. Boston: Birkhauser Publishing, 1998.
26. Withers PC. Circulation: chordate circulatory system. In: Withers PC, ed. Comparative animal physiology. Philadelphia: Saunders, 1992: 693–715.

Coronary Artery Anomalies: A Comprehensive Approach, edited by P. Angelini.
Lippincott Williams & Wilkins, Philadelphia © 1999.

CHAPTER 2

Ontogeny of the Coronary Vessels

María V. de la Cruz, Ricardo Moreno-Rodriguez, and Paolo Angelini

Several key studies have contributed to our understanding of the morphogenesis of the coronary vascular system.[15,16,19,26] Manasek[19] was the first to show that the epicardium is derived from extracardiac tissue. In studies of the quail heart, Viragh and coauthors[26] described the proepicardial organ. In studies of the neural crest, Le Lievre and Le Douarin[16] and Kirby and associates[15] provided valuable information about the embryologic development of the great arteries. Furthermore, the development of "in vivo" techniques has furthered the study of embryogenesis. Development of the heart and the coronary vasculature is a dynamic process that involves a progressive, sequential, uninterrupted, and irreversible series of events.

In this chapter, we will summarize our current understanding of the morphogenesis of the coronary arteries. Embryologic development of the coronary vascular system may be divided into four sections: (1) origin of the stem cells that will form the coronary vascular system, (2) appearance of the primitive coronary vessels, their fate, and the onset of coronary venous circulation, (3) connection of the primitive coronary vessels with the aorta, and (4) establishment of the basic coronary distribution patterns and their anatomic relationship to the heart.

ORIGIN OF THE STEM CELLS THAT WILL FORM THE CORONARY VASCULAR SYSTEM

In 1969, in studies of the chick embryo, Manasek[19] used transmission electron microscopy to show that the epicardium originates at Hamburger-Hamilton[11] (HH) stage 14 from extracardiac cells found in the dorsal wall of the sinus venosus; this fact negated the previous supposition of a myoepicardial mantle, as described by Mollier[22] in 1905 and accepted by others.[8] In 1989, Hiruma and Hirakow[13] re-

ported findings similar to those of Manasek. In studying chick embryos at stage 14, Hiruma and Hirakow used transmission electron microscopy, scanning electron microscopy, and computer-generated reconstruction models to describe the migration of epicardial cells from a mesothelial protrusion on the right ventral wall of the sinus venosus. Furthermore, they reported that these protrusions eventually form "villous processes" that extend along the dorsal wall of the heart in the atrioventricular groove and into the inner curvature of the cardiac tube. By stage 23, this epicardial layer covers the dorsal and ventral walls of the ventricles. Viragh and coworkers[26] called these protrusions of the sinus venosus the "proepicardial organ" (Fig. 2.1).

The contributions of Manasek[19] and Hiruma and Hirakow[13] regarding the extracardiac origin of the epicardium were the basis for hypothesizing that the vascular subepicardial network is also of extracardiac origin. Viragh and coauthors[26] used anti-QH-1 endothelial antibodies to study the cellular composition of the proepicardial organ in chick-quail chimera embryos. They found that the endothelial cells of the coronary vessels are derived from the proepicardial organ located in the region of the sinus venosus, from which stem cells migrate inside the subepicardial space in the regions corresponding to the atrioventricular and interventricular grooves. In the adult heart, these grooves correspond to the location of the left anterior descending, circumflex, and right coronary artery main trunks (coronary vascular rings). In more recent studies of chick embryos at stages 17 to 18, Mikawa and Gourdie,[21] using retroviral labeling, confirmed that cells from the proepicardial organ give rise to both the definitive epicardial layer and the endothelium of the coronary vessels. In addition, these authors reported that the medial smooth muscle and the connective tissue of the definitive coronary vessels also originate from the proepicardial organ.

The contribution of the neural crest to the developing heart has been studied in chimeric quail and chick embryos. In 1975, Le Lievre and Le Douarin[16] suggested that the cardiac

This work was supported by Grant No. 0257-M9107 from the Mexican National Council on Science and Technology (CONACyT) and a grant from Telmex.

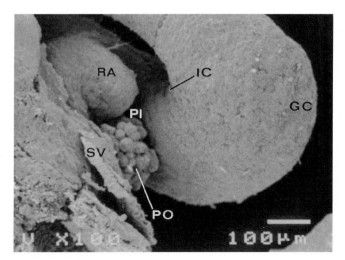

FIGURE 2.1. Scanning electron micrograph of the right external surface of the chick embryo heart at stage 14. Notice the developing proepicardial organ caudal to the right atrium in the ventral wall of the sinus venosus. GC = great curvature; IC = inner curvature; PI = primitive inlet; PO = proepicardial organ; RA = right atrium; SV = sinus venosus.

neural crest gives rise to the smooth muscle and connective tissue of the tunica media of the great arteries (the ascending aorta and the main pulmonary artery). Furthermore, the cardiac neural crest is important in septation of the truncal segment. Whether the neural crest is the only contributor to the aortic media is unknown. Moreover, whether the aortic media would develop in the absence of the neural crest is also unknown. Formation of the facing (adjacent) valve sinuses of the aortic and pulmonary trunks is related to truncal septation, but the contribution of the neural crest to this event has not been studied. In chick-quail chimera experiments, Waldo and colleagues[27] substituted quail cardiac neural crest in the chick embryo; the tunica media of the coronary arteries of the chick did not contain quail cells. The foregoing studies[16,27] indicate that the cardiac neural crest gives rise to the smooth muscle of the aortic tunica media but not to the smooth muscle of the coronary artery media.

APPEARANCE OF THE PRIMITIVE CORONARY VESSELS, THEIR FATE, AND THE ONSET OF CORONARY VENOUS CIRCULATION

The initial, highly trabeculated pattern of the ventricular myocardium evolves into a compact configuration. During this fundamental change in the architecture of the myocardium, the subepicardial primitive coronary vessels first appear as vascular lakes or cellular aggregates that eventually transform into arteries and veins.

Many studies have been published regarding the development of the subepicardial coronary vascular network in the human embryo. According to early studies by Licata,[17] subepicardial vessels first appear in humans during the sixth week of development. More recently, in studying human embryos at Streeter's horizon XIV (28 to 30 days), Hirakow[12] reported that the coronary vessels first appear in situ, in the subepicardial space, as endothelial tubes without a tunica media. Conte and Pellegrini[6] described the first appearance of coronary vessels at horizon XV (31 to 32 days). In addition, at horizon XIV (28 to 30 days), they observed isolated groups of cells in the subepicardial space at the atrioventricular and interventricular grooves and in other portions of the ventricular wall. The authors suggested that these cell populations would give rise to the coronary vessels. Cardiac septation is considerably advanced at the stages of development at which all of these investigators studied the coronary vessels. Licata[17] described the essential features of the main coronary arteries, as seen in the mature heart, as already defined in the 9-week embryo.

In studying chick embryos, Hiruma and Hirakow[13] observed that the coronary vessels first appear in the subepicardial space at stage 23. In addition, these authors reported that the early coronary vessels are composed of endothelium only, without a tunica media, and that groups of subepicardial cells precede the appearance of the coronary vessels, confirming the findings of Conte and Pellegrini[6] in human embryos. In studying quail embryos, Viragh and coworkers[26] described the first appearance, at stage 19, of similar coronary vessels in the subepicardial space. Furthermore, these authors observed prominent angiogenesis in the dorsal region of the atrioventricular, interventricular, and sinoatrial grooves at stages 25 to 26.[26] In the chick and the quail, the coronary vessels first appear when cardiac septation (truncal and ventricular) is advanced, as they do in human development.

In summary, the first coronary vessels in human, chick, and quail embryos are constituted exclusively of endothelial cells without a tunica media, yet they will eventually give rise to both coronary arteries and veins. Thus we propose that these vessels be called primitive coronary vessels (Fig. 2.2, A–D). The factors that determine development of these vessels into typical coronary arteries and veins are unknown. Hemodynamic factors are probably important, as are the primitive vessels' eventual connections (i.e., to the sinus venosus versus the aorta).

Conte and Pellegrini[6] found that, in the human embryo, the primitive coronary vessels connect with the sinus venosus or with the aorta at horizon XV; consequently the future coronary arteries and veins would appear simultaneously. In the human embryo, Hirakow[12] observed that the primitive coronary vessels connect initially with the sinus venosus (horizon XVII), whereas their connection with the aortic root takes place afterward (horizon XVIII–XIX). Also in human embryos, Hutchins and associates[14] observed connection of the primitive coronary vessels with the sinus venosus at horizons XV to XVII and with the aorta at horizon XVIII. The studies of Hirakow[12] and of Hutchins and colleagues[14] indicate that the first primitive coronary vessels to define themselves are the future coronary veins. In the chick embryo, Waldo and

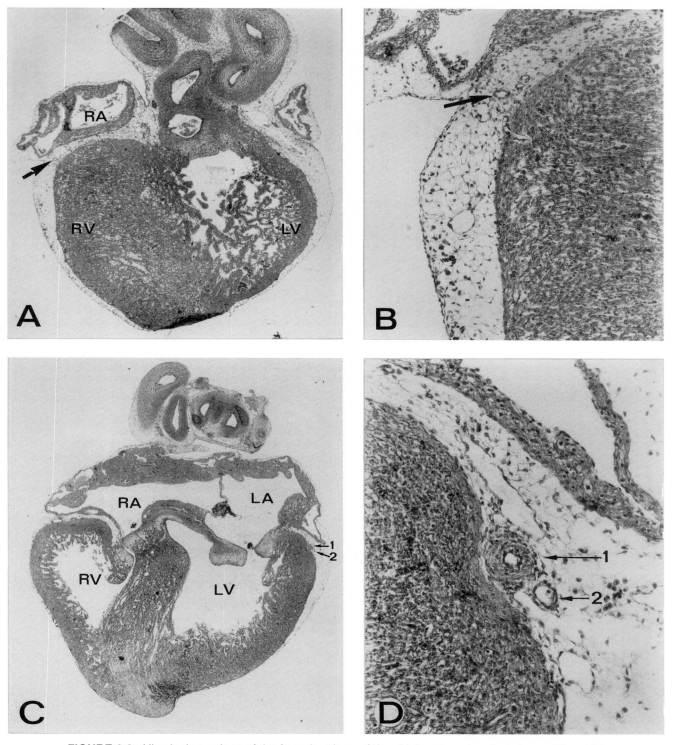

FIGURE 2.2. Histologic sections of the four chambers of the chick embryo heart at stages 30 and 36.
A. The chick heart at stage 30, showing the primitive coronary vessels (arrow). **B.** Enlarged view of
Figure 2.2A, showing absence of a tunica media in the vessel walls (arrow). **C.** Histologic section of
the heart at stage 36, showing differentiation of the walls of a coronary artery (1) and vein (2). LA =
left atrium; LV = left ventricle; RA = right atrium; RV = right ventricle. **D.** Enlarged view of Figure
2.2C, showing the same artery (1) and vein (2).

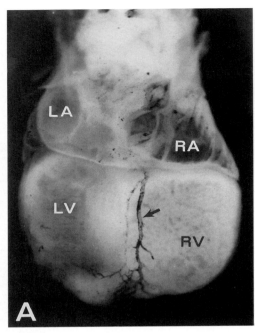 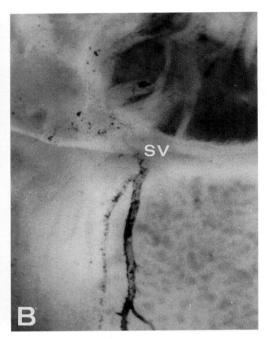

FIGURE 2.3. Dorsal view of the chick embryo heart at stage 30, showing the coronary vessels draining into the sinus venosus after injection of india ink into the right ventricular cavity. At this stage of development, organization of the coronary arteries is not established. **A.** The future posterior descending vein (arrow) drains into the sinus venosus. LA = left atrium; LV = left ventricle; RA = right atrium; RV = right ventricle. **B.** Enlarged view of Figure 2.3*A.* SV = sinus venosus.

coworkers[28] observed, by means of india-ink injections, that the primitive coronary vessels connected with the sinus venosus on day 6 and with the aorta on day 7.5. We recently confirmed this observation in our laboratory. We ligated the base of the great arteries in chick embryos (stage 30) and occluded the right or left atrioventricular orifice with a glass rod that had a ball tip. We then injected gelatin india ink into the right ventricular cavity and observed the staining of vessels in the atrioventricular groove, which drained into the sinus venosus (Fig. 2.3, *A* and *B*). We also injected the left ventricle. In both cavities, we observed subepicardial vessels draining into the sinus venosus at a stage when the coronary arteries were not yet connected with the aorta. Studies in chick[25] and rat[23] embryos suggest that connections between the sinusoidal intertrabecular spaces and subepicardial vessels persist up to the late prenatal period, but they tend to disappear soon thereafter.

The nature of the epithelial cells that cover the cardiac sinusoidal intertrabecular spaces (which probably contribute to formation of the intramural coronary arteries) has recently been studied. In mesoderm explant experiments in the quail embryo, Linask and Lash[18] studied the distribution of premyocardial and preendocardial cells in the formative regions of the heart (cardiogenic areas). Using immunostaining techniques with anti–N-cadherin and anti–QH-1 antibodies, these investigators identified three populations of cells: those expressing the N-cadherin antigen, those expressing the QH-1 antigen, and those expressing both antigens. They concluded that endocardial and myocardial cells originate from a common precursor cell type that expresses both antigens. The endocardial cells eventually lose the cadherin antigen. Similarly, Markwald[20] concluded that the endoderm induces the precardiac mesoderm to differentiate into preendocardial and premyocardial cells. Together, these studies indicate that endocardial cells originating in the precardiac mesoderm cover the cardiac sinusoidal intertrabecular spaces.

CONNECTION OF THE PRIMITIVE CORONARY VESSELS WITH THE AORTA

Two hypotheses[2,4] have been proposed concerning the aortic endothelium's role in connecting the subepicardial primitive coronary network to the aorta. According to one hypothesis, the aortic endothelium actively participates in this connection by forming "coronary buds" at the level of the primordial semilunar valve cusps. According to the other hypothesis, the aortic endothelium is "passively" entered by prongs of the subepicardial primitive coronary network.

The first hypothesis is based on early studies done in chick[1] and human[6,7,12] embryos. In these embryos, hollow sprouts of endothelial cells, which appeared in the root of the aorta, at the future sinuses of Valsalva, connected with the subepicardial primitive coronary vessels. According to the second hypothesis, however, which is supported by more recent studies by Bogers and colleagues,[4] the aortic endothelium does not actively participate in this connection. These researchers did not find hollow sprouts or endothelial evaginations off the aortic wall in microscopic studies in rat and human embryos or in transmission electron microscopy studies in rat embryos. Using anti–QH-1 antibodies in quail embryos, Bogers and coauthors[3] showed that coronary vessels penetrated the tunica media of the aorta at a time when the intima of the aorta seemed to be unaffected. It is important to remember that, at the time of the aortic-coronary connection, the walls of the coronary vessels are composed only of endothelium.[24,28] In addition, the coronary arteries tend to connect consistently only with the facing sinuses of Valsalva (adjacent to the pulmonary artery). In the chick embryo, Waldo and associates[28] observed that multiple channels from the primitive coronary vessels were initially present near the facing and nonfacing aortic sinuses, but only two channels persisted—one in each facing sinus. More recently, in chick-quail chimera embryos, Poelmann and coworkers[24] observed findings similar to those of Waldo and associates[28] but described ''strands'' instead of channels meeting the aortic wall.

In india-ink angiographic studies of chick embryos, we found that the primitive coronary vessels in the area of the future left coronary artery connect with the aorta at stage 32 and that the right coronary primitive vessels connect with the aorta at stage 34 (Fig. 2.4, *A* and *B*).

The factors that determine the specific site of penetration of the coronary vessels on the aortic wall are still unknown. However, the finding that the two facing sinuses (the aortic and pulmonary) are formed by the truncal septum, whereas the nonfacing sinuses are formed by the intercalated truncal swellings, may be of fundamental importance. Furthermore, observation of the abundance of cardiac neural crest cells in the truncal septum[27] may be important to our understanding of the mechanisms involved in the appearance of coronary artery connections with the aorta.

ESTABLISHMENT OF THE BASIC CORONARY PATTERNS AND THEIR ANATOMIC RELATIONSHIP TO THE HEART

Morphogenesis of the coronary arteries occurs during two chronologic periods. During the first period, the topographic distribution of the primitive coronary vessels is defined in relation to the established architecture of the heart, particularly the compact ventricular myocardial masses. During the second period, specific coronary-aortic connections are established by a process of vascular interaction.[1,3,5,28]

As previously mentioned, Viragh and associates[26] reported that the cells in the subepicardial space that give rise to the coronary vessels are initially organized in linear strands or tubular structures. At this stage, the first cardiac septum (the figure-of-8–shaped septum)[9,10] has developed, transforming the single-chambered heart into an organ with four cavities. The first cardiac septum is composed of the septum primum (at the atrial level) and the superior and inferior cushions of the atrioventricular canal and the primi-

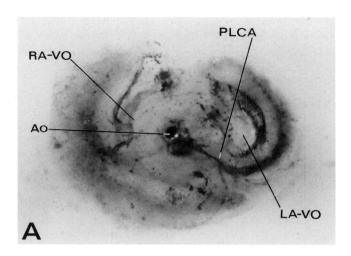

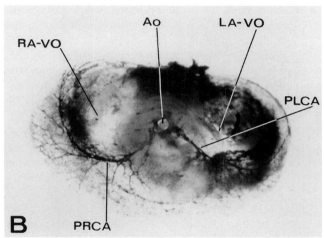

FIGURE 2.4. Transverse sections of the chick heart (stages 32 and 34) at the level of the atrioventricular orifices and the great arteries. The left and right coronary arteries have been injected with gelatin-india ink. **A.** The primitive left coronary artery (PLCA) is connected with the aorta (Ao) at stage 32. **B.** The primitive right coronary artery (PRCA) is connected with the aorta (Ao) at stage 34. LA-VO = left atrioventricular orifice; RA-VO = right atrioventricular orifice.

tive interventricular septum (at the ventricular level).[9,10] Furthermore, the external surface of the heart develops two grooves: the atrioventricular groove and the interventricular groove. Eventually, two vascular rings tend to develop during angiogenesis[1,6,7,12]: the coronary ''atrioventricular ring'' (right coronary and left circumflex arteries) appears at the atrioventricular groove, and the coronary ''interventricular ring'' (anterior and posterior descending branches) appears at the interventricular groove.

The final coronary arterial pattern is further defined by two factors: interruption of what initially seem to be complete coronary rings and development of the dependent myocardial masses. Interruption of the coronary rings probably occurs simultaneously with establishment of the aortic origination of the coronary arterial circulation and its drainage into the coronary venous system. The diameter of the coronary arteries is closely influenced by the amount of blood flow throughout embryogenesis. The specific mechanisms that determine coronary patterns and size are unknown.

CONCLUSIONS

1. The cells that form the walls of the main (extramural) coronary arteries and veins are extracardiac in origin and arise from the proepicardial organ.
2. The walls of the cardiac ''sinusoidal'' intertrabecular spaces are composed of endothelial cells, which seemingly result from differentiation of cells derived from the primitive cardiogenic areas. The intertrabecular spaces may evolve into parts of the intramyocardial coronary network.
3. Because the walls of the primitive subepicardial coronary vessels are composed exclusively of endothelial cells, the distinction between coronary arteries and veins is based on their eventual connections; the arteries connect to the aorta, the veins to the sinus venosus. The morphogenetic factors that determine whether a primitive coronary vessel becomes an artery or a vein are unknown.
4. Primitive coronary vessels tend to connect selectively with the facing aortic cusps but not with the pulmonic or the nonfacing aortic cusps. We do not yet know what factors determine where in the aortic sinuses the coronary vessels penetrate.
5. The basic coronary pattern seems to be intimately related to the anatomy of the ventricular myocardial masses, as suggested by the fact that the primitive coronary arteries organize along the interventricular and atrioventricular grooves, where compact myocardium first appears. The luminal diameter of each coronary artery is closely related to the dependent myocardial mass.

ACKNOWLEDGMENT

The authors thank Dr. Jorge Espino Vela for his kind assistance in translating this manuscript into English.

REFERENCES

1. Aikawa E, Kawano J. Formation of coronary arteries sprouting from the primitive aortic sinus wall of the chick embryo. Experientia 1982; 38:816.
2. Angelini P. Normal and anomalous coronary arteries: definitions and classifications. Am Heart J 1989;117:418.
3. Bogers AJ, Gittenberger-de Groot AC, Dubbeldam JA, et al. Scanning electron microscopy substantiates histology in showing the inadequacy of the existing theories on the development of the coronary arteries and their connections with the arterial trunks. Acta Morphol Neerl Scand 1988;26:225.
4. Bogers AJ, Gittenberger-de Groot AC, Dubbeldam JA, et al. The inadequacy of the existing theories on development of the proximal coronary arteries and their connexions with the arterial trunks. Int J Cardiol 1988; 20:225.
5. Bogers AJ, Gittenberger-de Groot AC, Poelmann RE, et al. Development of the origin of the coronary arteries, a matter of ingrowth or outgrowth? Anat Embryol (Berl) 1989;180:437.
6. Conte G, Pellegrini A. On the development of the coronary arteries in human embryos, stage 14–19. Anat Embryol 1984;169:209.
7. Corone P, Corone A, Dor X, et al. Les arteres coronaires et leurs variations, une explication embriologique. C R Acad Sc III 1984;299:451.
8. Davis CL. Development of the human heart from its first appearance to the stage found in embryos of twenty paired somites. Contrib Embryol 1927;19:245.
9. de la Cruz MV, Castillo MM, Villavicencio L, et al. The primitive interventricular septum, its primordium, and its contribution in the definitive interventricular septum. ''In vivo'' labeling study in the chick embryo heart. Anat Rec 1997;247:512.
10. de la Cruz MV, Gimenez-Ribotta M, Saravalli O, et al. The contribution of the inferior endocardial cushion of the atrioventricular canal to cardiac septation and to the development of the atrioventricular valves: study in the chick embryo. Am J Anat 1983;166:63.
11. Hamburger V, Hamilton H. A series of normal stages in the development of the chick embryo. J Morphol 1951;88:49.
12. Hirakow R. Development of the cardiac blood vessels in staged human embryos. Acta Anat 1983;115:220.
13. Hiruma T, Hirakow R. Epicardial formation in embryonic chick heart: computer-aided reconstruction, scanning and transmission electron microscopic studies. Am J Anat 1989;184:129.
14. Hutchins GM, Kessler HA, Moose GW. Development of the coronary arteries in the embryonic human heart. Circulation 1988;77:1250.
15. Kirby ML, Gale TF, Stewart DE. Neural crest cells contribute to aorticopulmonary septation. Science 1983;220:1059.
16. Le Lievre CS, Le Douarin NM. Mesenchymal derivatives of the neural crest: analysis of chimeric quail and chick embryos. J Embryol Exp Morphol 1975;34:125.
17. Licata RH. The human embryonic heart in the ninth week. Am J Anat 1954;94:73.
18. Linask KK, Lash J. Early heart development: dynamics of endocardial cell sorting suggests a common origin with cardiomyocytes. Dev Dyn 1993;195:62.
19. Manasek FI. Embryonic development of the heart. II. Formation of the epicardium. J Embryol Exp Morphol 1969;22:333.
20. Markwald RR. Overview: formation and early morphogenesis of the primary heart tube. In Clark EB, Markwald RR, Takao A, eds. Developmental mechanisms of heart disease. Armonk, New York: Futura, 1995: 149–168.
21. Mikawa T, Gourdie RG. Pericardial mesoderm generates a population of coronary smooth muscle cells migrating into the heart along with ingrowth of the epicardial organ. Dev Biol 1996;174:221.
22. Mollier S. Die erste Anlage des Herzens bei den Wirbeltieren. In Hertwig O, ed. Handbuch der Vergleichenden und Experimentellen Entwicklungslehre der Wirbeltiere. Jena: Fisher, 1906:1026.
23. Ostadal B, Schiebler TH, Rychter Z. Relations between the development of the capillary wall and myoarchitecture of the rat heart. Adv Exp Med Biol 1971;19:31.
24. Poelmann RE, Gittenberger-de Groot AC, Mentink MMT, et al. Development of the cardiac coronary vascular endothelium, studied with antiendothelial antibodies, in chicken-quail chimeras. Circ Res 1993; 73:559.
25. Rychter Z, Ostadal B. Fate of sinusoidal intertrabecular spaces of the cardiac wall after development of the coronary vascular bed in chick embryo. Folia Morphol (Prague) 1971;19:31.
26. Viragh S, Gittenberger-de Groot AC, Poelmann RE, et al. Early development of quail heart epicardium and associated vascular and glandular structures. Anat Embryol 1993;188:381.
27. Waldo KL, Kumiski DH, Kirby MD. Association of cardiac neural crest with development of the coronary arteries in the chick embryo. Anat Rec 1994;239:315.
28. Waldo KL, Willner W, Kirby MD. Origin of the proximal coronary artery stems and a review of ventricular vascularization in the chick embryo. Am J Anat 1990;188:109.

Coronary Artery Anomalies: A Comprehensive Approach, edited by P. Angelini.
Lippincott Williams & Wilkins, Philadelphia © 1999.

CHAPTER 3

Coronary Artery Anomalies and Bicuspid Aortic Valve

Valentín Sans-Coma, Ana C. Durán, Borja Fernández, M. Carmen Fernández, David López, and José M. Arqué

More than 50 years ago, Roberts and Loube[26] reported that the presence of a single coronary artery was often associated with a bicuspid aortic valve. In 1971, Hillestad and Eie[14] published similar statements. However, findings from both studies were based on a limited number of cases. In fact, the presence of an anomaly of the coronary artery in association with a bicuspid aortic valve is uncommon. Both types of congenital anomalies are usually reported as independent traits. Left dominance of the coronary artery system[13,16,17,20,23,34] is the only coronary feature frequently found in patients with bicuspid aortic valve. In contrast, recent research in the Syrian hamster has indicated a significant association between bicuspid aortic valve and anomalous origin of the left coronary artery.[5,6,29] We will discuss this association because we believe that this information will be useful in studying the etiologic factors involved in the development of both bicuspid aortic valve and anomalous origin of the coronary arteries.

THE AORTIC VALVE IN THE SYRIAN HAMSTER

In the Syrian hamster (*Mesocricetus auratus*), the normal aortic valve is tricuspid (Fig. 3.1),[31-33] consisting of three aortic sinuses—the right, left, and dorsal (the posterior or noncoronary sinus in humans)—and three leaflets (Table 3.1). From the ventricular view, a fibrous interleaflet triangle can be seen between each adjacent sinus; thus three interleaflet triangles are present in the subaortic outflow tract. The interleaflet triangles are located in the right-dorsal, left-dorsal, and ventral positions.

Congenital bicuspid aortic valve in the Syrian hamster (Fig. 3.2) is similar to the anteroposterior type of bicuspid aortic valve seen in humans. The valve has two aortic sinuses (ventral and dorsal), two leaflets, and two interleaflet triangles.[31-33]

In some hamsters with a bicuspid aortic valve, a more or less developed raphe is located in the ventral aortic sinus (Fig. 3.2).[31,33] Varying in size, the raphe may encroach on the leaflet or may be confined to the aortic wall. On histologic examination, the raphe is similar to a true commissure.[31] In animals with a raphe, the distance between the two commissures is usually longer on the ventral side than on the dorsal side (Fig. 3.2), and the interleaflet triangles are located in the right-dorsal and left-dorsal positions. In contrast, in hamsters that have a bicuspid aortic valve without a raphe, the distance between the two commissures is similar, and the two interleaflet triangles are located on the right and left.

Anatomic and histologic studies in the Syrian hamster[31,33] have shown a continuous phenotypic spectrum of aortic valve morphology. At one end of the spectrum is the tricuspid aortic valve with no commissural fusion; at the other end is the bicuspid aortic valve with no raphe. The intermediate stages are represented by (1) tricuspid aortic valves with more-extensive or less-extensive fusion of the ventral commissure and a ventral interleaflet triangle that is decreased in size according to the degree of fusion, and (2) bicuspid aortic valves with a more-developed or less-developed raphe. Embryologic studies[33] have revealed that all variants of this valvular morphologic spectrum develop from three mesenchymal valve cushions—the right, left, and dorsal cushions. Furthermore, fusion of the right and left cushions at the beginning of valvulogenesis is a key factor in the formation of bicuspid aortic valves and tricuspid aortic valves with fusion of the ventral commissure. In addition, studies based on crossing experiments have shown that the phenotypic spectrum of aortic valve morphology is subject to a quantitative mode of inheritance.[31]

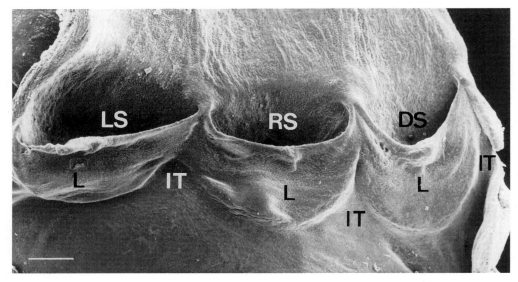

FIGURE 3.1. Scanning electron photomicrograph of a normal, tricuspid aortic valve from a Syrian hamster displayed in an open-cut view. DS = dorsal aortic sinus; IT = interleaflet triangle; L = leaflet; LS = left aortic sinus; RS = right aortic sinus. Scale bar = 300 μm.

TABLE 3.1. *Nomenclature of the semilunar valve sinuses and leaflets: Syrian hamsters versus humans*

Syrian hamsters	Humans
Aortic valve	
Right	Right anterior
Left	Left posterior
Dorsal	Right posterior
Pulmonary valve	
Right	Right posterior
Left	Left posterior
Ventral	Left anterior

NORMAL CORONARY ARTERY ANATOMY IN THE SYRIAN HAMSTER

The heart of the Syrian hamster has no interventricular grooves, and the coronary arteries enter the myocardium shortly after arising from the aorta. Two coronary arteries are present (Fig. 3.3, *A–E*); the right coronary artery arises from the right aortic sinus, and the left coronary artery arises from the left sinus.[30] When the aortic valve is bicuspid, the right and left coronary arteries originate from the right and left sides of the ventral aortic sinus, respectively.[29]

The right coronary artery (Fig. 3.3*A*) supplies the right

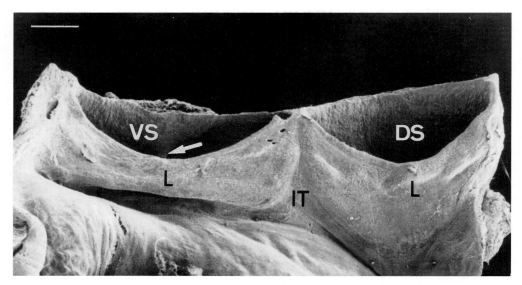

FIGURE 3.2. Scanning electron photomicrograph of a bicuspid aortic valve from a Syrian hamster displayed in an open-cut view. A raphe (arrow) is located in the ventral aortic sinus. DS = dorsal aortic sinus; IT = interleaflet triangle; L = leaflet; VS = ventral aortic sinus. Scale bar = 300 μm.

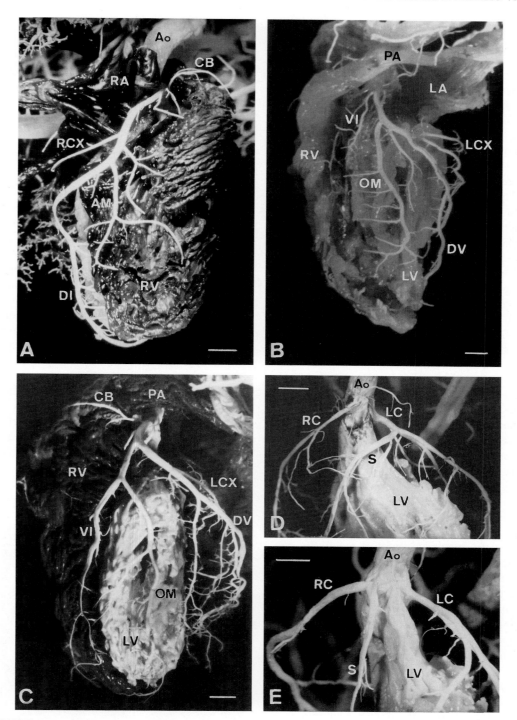

FIGURE 3.3. Internal casts of the heart, great arterial vessels, and coronary arteries of the Syrian hamster, showing a normal coronary artery pattern. **A.** Course and branching of the right coronary artery. **B.** Course and branching of the left coronary artery. **C.** Course and branching of a left coronary artery with a well-developed ventral interventricular branch. **D.** Septal artery arising from the left coronary artery. **E.** Septal artery arising from the right coronary artery. AM = acute marginal branch; Ao = aorta; CB = conal branch; DI = dorsal interventricular branch; DV = dorsal ventricular branch; LA = left atrium; LC = left coronary artery; LCX = left circumflex branch; LV = left ventricle; OM = obtuse marginal branch; PA = pulmonary artery; RA = right atrium; RC = right coronary artery; RCX = right circumflex branch; RV = right ventricle; S = septal artery; VI = ventral interventricular branch. Scale bars = 1 mm. (Reprinted from Sans-Coma V, Arqué JM, Durán AC, et al. The coronary arteries of the Syrian hamster, *Mesocricetus auratus* (Waterhouse, 1839). Ann Anat 1993;175:53 with the permission of Gustav Fischer Verlag).

side of the heart.[30] The right main coronary trunk runs parallel to the right atrioventricular sulcus and sends branches to the right atrium and the ventral wall of the right ventricle. The main trunk usually has a well-developed conal branch and an acute marginal branch whose course varies toward the apex of the heart. Having reached the acute margin of the heart, the main trunk bifurcates into two principal branches that supply the dorsal wall of the right ventricle: the right circumflex branch and the dorsal interventricular branch.

The left coronary artery (Fig. 3.3*B*) supplies the left side of the heart.[30] The left main coronary trunk passes dorsally around the pulmonary trunk and then enters the myocardium. Before reaching the obtuse margin of the heart, the main trunk sends branches to the left atrium. In some cases, the conal branch arises from the left, not the right, main coronary trunk.

The branching of the left main coronary trunk varies.[30] The trunk usually bifurcates at the obtuse margin of the heart (Fig. 3.3*B*). One of the resulting vessels is the obtuse marginal branch, which supplies the ventral aspect of the left ventricle. The other vessel at the bifurcation soon divides into the left circumflex branch and the dorsal ventricular branch, which supply the dorsal wall of the left ventricle. In a few hearts, the left main coronary trunk divides in a fanlike manner, giving rise to the obtuse marginal branch, the left circumflex branch, and the dorsal ventricular branch.

In some hearts, a ventral interventricular branch arises from the left coronary main trunk. This branch does not usually extend past the proximal third of the ventral interventricular limit (Fig. 3.3*B*). However, in some cases the vessel is well developed and extends to the apex of the heart (Fig. 3.3*C*). In such cases, the ventral interventricular branch usually gives rise to the obtuse marginal branch.

The interventricular septum is supplied mainly by one septal artery or, occasionally, two septal arteries.[10,30] In 70% of hearts, a single septal artery originates from the left coronary artery (Fig. 3.3*D*). In 28% of hearts, the vessel arises from the right coronary artery (Fig. 3.3*E*). In the remaining 2% of hearts, two septal arteries are found; one originates from the right coronary artery, the other from the left. Although the branching of the septal artery varies, the vessel always sends perpendicular and oblique branches that supply most of the ventral and dorsal septal surfaces. In addition, the septum is supplied by thinner penetrating vessels from the right and left coronary arteries. The presence of one or two well-developed septal arteries is the most constant feature of intramyocardial coronary arteries in mammals.[10,11]

CORONARY ARTERY ANOMALIES IN THE SYRIAN HAMSTER

Two coronary ostia—right and left—are usually seen in the Syrian hamster; however, the presence of a third ostium, although infrequent, is considered normal and is not re-

garded as an anomaly.[30] The third ostium is the result of the separate origin of either the septal artery or the conal branch. The following coronary artery anomalies have been described in the Syrian hamster: a solitary right coronary ostium in the aorta; a solitary left coronary ostium in the aorta; a left coronary artery originating from the pulmonary artery; a left coronary artery arising from the dorsal aortic sinus; and a third, accessory coronary artery arising from the pulmonary artery.

Solitary Right Coronary Ostium in the Aorta

The most common coronary artery anomaly in the Syrian hamster is a solitary right coronary ostium (Fig. 3.4).[1,28,29] Two variants of this type of anomaly are found: anomalous origin of the left coronary artery from the right coronary artery (86% of cases) and a single right coronary artery (14% of cases). In hamsters in which the left coronary artery originates from the right coronary artery, the right coronary artery is normal and originates from the right aortic sinus when the aortic valve is tricuspid (Fig. 3.4) or from the right side of the ventral aortic sinus when the valve is bicuspid. In addition, a true left coronary artery is present.[28] The left main coronary trunk arises either from the right coronary artery (Fig. 3.4), close to its origin from the aorta (79% of cases), or from the septal artery, which is a branch of the right coronary artery (21% of cases). The left main coronary trunk usually crosses the infundibular septum to reach the left margin of the subpulmonary infundibulum, then divides to form the obtuse marginal branch, the left circumflex branch, and the dorsal ventricular branch. In some hearts,

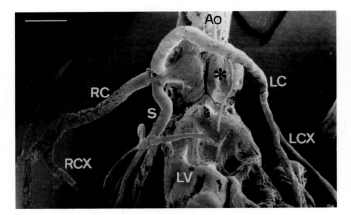

FIGURE 3.4. Scanning electron photomicrograph of an internal cast of the left ventricle, aorta, and coronary arteries of a Syrian hamster with a single right coronary ostium in the aorta. The aortic valve is tricuspid. The right coronary artery arises from the right aortic sinus, and the left coronary artery originates from the main stem of the right coronary artery. The asterisk indicates the left aortic sinus of Valsalva, from which no coronary artery arises. Ao = aorta; LC = left main coronary artery; LCX = left circumflex branch; LV = left ventricle; RC = right coronary artery; RCX = right circumflex branch; S = septal artery. Scale bar = 1 mm.

however, the left main coronary trunk runs anterior to the right ventricular outflow tract within the ventricular wall and divides at the left margin of the heart into the normal left coronary artery branches (Fig. 3.4). Occasionally, no circumflex branch can be seen arising from the left main coronary trunk. In such cases, the right circumflex branch is larger than normal and supplies the dorsal wall of the left ventricle.

In hamsters with a single right coronary artery, only one coronary artery arises from the right aortic sinus. This vessel is larger and branches more than a normal right coronary artery. The single right coronary artery originates from the right aortic sinus when the aortic valve is tricuspid and from the right side of the ventral aortic sinus when the valve is bicuspid. There is no true left coronary artery; in some cases, however, a left circumflex branch, an obtuse marginal branch, or both, may be found arising from the right coronary artery. Usually, the left ventricle is supplied mainly by branches from both the right coronary artery and the septal artery.[28]

Solitary Left Coronary Ostium in the Aorta

This type of anomaly is unusual in the Syrian hamster.[1,28] In fact, only 17 cases have been reported, and all have been associated with a tricuspid aortic valve. In these hearts, the left coronary artery arises from the left aortic sinus, and the septal artery originates from the left coronary artery main trunk. In addition, a right coronary artery with a fairly normal branching pattern is present. In most cases (92%), the right coronary artery arises from the septal artery; however, in a few cases (8%), the right coronary artery arises directly from the left main coronary trunk and crosses the interventricular septum to the right side of the heart.

Left Coronary Artery Originating From the Pulmonary Artery

Anomalous origin of the left coronary artery from the pulmonary artery (Figs. 3.5 and 3.6) is the second most common coronary artery anomaly found in the Syrian hamster.[1,5,27,28] In hamsters with this anomaly, two coronary arteries are present. The right coronary artery originates from the right aortic sinus when the aortic valve is normal and from the right side of the ventral aortic sinus when the valve is bicuspid. The left coronary artery arises from the left pulmonary sinus (Fig. 3.6). The branching of the dilated and tortuous right coronary artery varies; however, several branches of the vessel invariably supply the left ventricle. The left coronary artery is smaller and has fewer branches. Although the arrangement of anastomoses between the two coronary arteries varies, one or several branches of the right coronary artery extend toward the left ventricle to connect with the left coronary artery (Fig. 3.5). In all hearts with

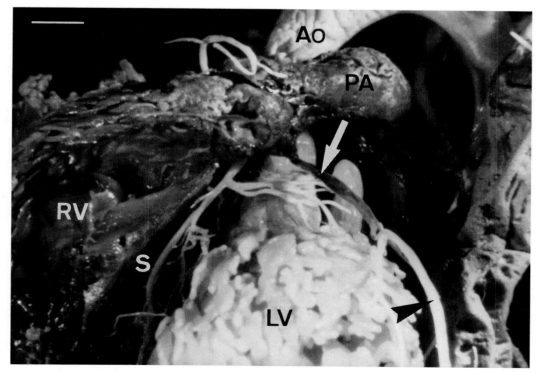

FIGURE 3.5. Internal cast of the ventricles, aorta, and coronary arteries of a Syrian hamster with a left coronary artery originating from the pulmonary artery. The arrowhead shows a branch of the right coronary artery that anastomoses with the left coronary artery (arrow). Ao = aorta; LV = left ventricle; PA = pulmonary artery; RV = right ventricle; S = septal artery. Scale bar = 1 mm.

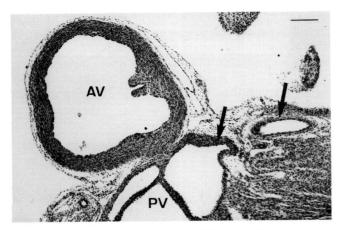

FIGURE 3.6. Transverse section of the heart from a young Syrian hamster, at the distal level of the aortic valve. The left coronary artery (arrows) originates from the left pulmonary sinus. AV = aortic valve; PV = pulmonary valve. Hematoxylin and eosin. Scale bar = 150 μm.

this type of anomaly, the interventricular septum is supplied mainly by a well-developed septal artery (Fig. 3.5), which originates from the right coronary artery or from a separate ostium in the aorta. Syrian hamsters with this anomaly usually survive without difficulty and usually succeed in reproducing.

Left Coronary Artery Arising From the Dorsal Aortic Sinus

The third most common coronary artery anomaly in the Syrian hamster is anomalous origin of the left coronary artery from the dorsal aortic sinus (Fig. 3.7). This anomaly can be classified into two principal types.[2,6] In one type, a right and a left coronary artery with normal branches are present. In the second type, both the obtuse marginal and the dorsal ventricular branches arise from the right coronary artery, and the left circumflex branch arises independently. In both types of anomalous hearts, the right coronary artery originates from the right aortic sinus when the aortic valve is tricuspid and from the right side of the ventral aortic sinus when the valve is bicuspid (Fig. 3.7). Depending on the case, the left main coronary artery or the left circumflex branch arises from the center of the dorsal aortic sinus when the aortic valve is tricuspid or from the center of the dorsal aortic sinus (or close to the left commissure) when the valve is bicuspid. The coronary vessel that proceeds from the dorsal aortic sinus always originates at an acute angle with respect to the aortic wall (Fig. 3.7). The septal artery usually originates from the right coronary artery (94% of cases[2]); however, in a small percentage of cases, it arises either from a separate ostium in the aorta (3%) or from the left main coronary trunk (3%).

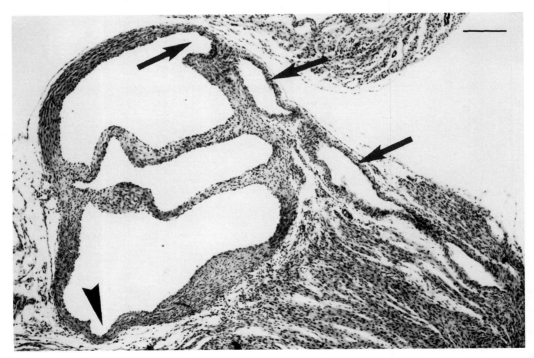

FIGURE 3.7. Transverse section of the aortic valve from an adult Syrian hamster. The aortic valve is bicuspid. The left coronary artery (arrows) originates from the dorsal aortic sinus, forming an acute angle with the aortic wall. The arrowhead shows the origin of the right coronary artery. Hematoxylin and eosin. Scale bar = 150 μm.

TABLE 3.2. *Relationship between coronary artery patterns and aortic valve condition in the 1633 Syrian hamsters examined*

| Aortic valve | Normal | Solitary coronary ostium | | Anomalous origin of LCA from | | Accessory coronary[a] |
		Left	Right	Pulmonary artery	Dorsal aortic sinus	
Tricuspid (n = 933)	754 (80.8)	3 (0.3)	115 (12.3)	34 (3.7)	25 (2.7)	2 (0.2)
Bicuspid (n = 700)	379 (54.1)	0 (0)	203 (29.0)	67 (9.6)	51 (7.3)	0 (0)

[a] Arising from the pulmonary artery.

Accessory Coronary Artery Arising From the Pulmonary Artery

Only two cases of a third, accessory coronary artery originating from the pulmonary artery have been observed in the Syrian hamster; both hearts had tricuspid aortic valves.[7,10] In this anomaly, the right coronary artery branches normally, but the right circumflex branch passes the dorsal interventricular boundary to supply the dorsal wall of the left ventricle. The left coronary artery arises from the left aortic sinus and extends along the ventricular septum as a true septal artery. The accessory coronary artery is smaller than the left coronary artery, and anastomoses occur between the two vessels.

ASSOCIATION BETWEEN CORONARY ARTERY ANOMALIES AND BICUSPID AORTIC VALVE IN THE SYRIAN HAMSTER

Our knowledge regarding the association between coronary artery anomalies and bicuspid aortic valve comes from studies of a single inbred family of Syrian hamsters.[29,32,33] The family originated from an unrelated pair of hamsters with normal coronary arteries and tricuspid aortic valves and is perpetuated by systematic breeding of siblings or, occasionally, offspring of siblings. We have produced 28 inbred generations with more than 1700 hamsters. In these inbred hamsters, the mean frequency of coronary artery anomalies is almost 31%, and that of bicuspid aortic valves is 43%.

We have assessed the arrangement of the coronary arteries and the condition of the aortic valve in 1633 inbred Syrian hamsters (Table 3.2). We pooled data from male and female hamsters, because we found no statistical difference between the sexes with respect to the occurrence of coronary artery anomalies or bicuspid aortic valve. To test for an association between anomalous coronary patterns and the morphology of the aortic valve, we performed a chi-square contingency test (Table 3.3) under the null hypothesis that they are independent events. We excluded two coronary anomalies, single left coronary ostium and accessory coronary artery arising from the pulmonary artery, because of limited data. Our results show that the simultaneous occurrence of a coronary artery anomaly and a bicuspid aortic valve is not a random event. However, these anomalies do occur independently; therefore, the two events are not morphogenetically dependent. Rather, some other cause predisposes to the concurrent presence of coronary artery anomalies and a bicuspid aortic valve. In the Syrian hamster all congenital coronary artery anomalies that are significantly associated with the presence of a bicuspid aortic valve are characterized by anomalous origin of the left coronary artery or the absence of a true left coronary artery. This finding strongly suggests that abnormalities of the coronary arteries and aortic valve result from

TABLE 3.3. *Contingency test of coronary artery patterns versus aortic valve condition[a]*

| Aortic valve | Normal | Solitary right coronary ostium | Anomalous origin of LCA[b] from: | | $\Sigma\chi^2$ |
			Pulmonary artery	Dorsal aortic sinus	
Tricuspid (n = 928)	754 (645.8)	115 (181.3)	34 (57.6)	25 (43.3)	—
χ^2	18.13	24.25	9.67	7.73	59.78[c]
Bicuspid (n = 700)	379 (487.2)	203 (136.6)	67 (43.4)	51 (32.7)	—
χ^2	24.03	32.16	12.83	10.24	79.26[c]
TOTAL (n = 1628)	1133	318	101	76	—
$\Sigma\chi^2$	45.16[c]	56.40[c]	22.50[c]	17.98[c]	139.04[c]

[a] Expected values are shown in parentheses.
[b] Left coronary artery.
[c] $P < .001$.

a common underlying morphogenetic defect, which is expressed as (1) a bicuspid aortic valve, (2) anomalous origin or absence of the left coronary artery, or (3) both of these abnormalities.

FINAL COMMENTS

According to the classic theory regarding the formation of the coronary vasculature, the proximal coronary arteries develop as coronary artery buds that hollow out from the aorta to connect with the peritruncal plexus of capillaries in the subepicardial layer of the developing heart.[37] However, results from studies of quail[4] and chick[40] embryos have contradicted this classic theory. These embryo studies have shown that the proximal coronary arteries grow *into* the aorta, not *out from* the aorta. Endothelial cells penetrate into the media of the aorta from the peritruncal ring of coronary artery vasculature to form the proximal coronary arteries. In studies of quail-chick chimeras,[25] the quail endothelial cells grow into the aorta at several sites, but the capillaries coalesce to form coronary arteries at only two of these sites. Therefore, in an embryologic sense, a left coronary artery that arises from the pulmonary artery is considered to be connected to the pulmonary artery in the same way as a left coronary artery that arises from the dorsal aortic sinus is connected to that sinus. Moreover, a solitary coronary ostium in the aorta results from a sole successful penetration of the peritruncal plexus of capillaries into the aorta.

In studies of the chick, Hood and Rosenquist[15] showed that ablating the cardiac neural crest results in anomalies of the coronary arteries. These authors concluded that all the anatomic features that characterize the normal site of origin of the proximal coronary arteries depend on, or are influenced by, the neural crest. The absence of cells from the neural crest causes a spatial disorder of the development of the proximal coronary arteries, resulting in a wide spectrum of coronary artery abnormalities. In more recent chick studies, Waldo and associates[39] have shown that the tunica media of the coronary arteries and the aortic sinuses does not contain cardiac neural crest cells; therefore, neural crest cells do not appear to induce capillary penetration directly. However, the same authors have shown an exclusive association between parasympathetic ganglia and nerves derived from the cardiac neural crest and the persisting coronary arteries. This finding suggests that the presence of parasympathetic ganglia is required for survival of the definitive coronary arteries.

In the Syrian hamster, bicuspid aortic valve does not result from improper development of the conotruncal ridges or from conotruncal malseptation, valve cushion agenesis, or lesions acquired after normal valvulogenesis, as proposed in several classic studies. The fusion of the right and left valve cushions at the beginning of valvulogenesis is a key factor in the formation of bicuspid aortic valve[33]; therefore we have hypothesized that fusion of the valve cushions is the result of anomalous behavior of the cardiac neural crest cells.[33]

This statement is based on three facts. First, the cardiac neural crest gives rise to ectomesenchyme, which supports the development of the aortic arch arteries and of the aorticopulmonary septum that divides the cardiac outflow tract into the aortic and pulmonary tracts.[3,12,19,24] Second, in quail-chick chimera embryos, ectomesenchymal cells from the cardiac neural crest colonize the aortic and pulmonary valve primordia.[35,36] This observation indicates that neural crest cells are involved in the formation of the cardiac semilunar valves.[35,36] Finally, bicuspid aortic valve in humans is significantly associated with congenital malformations of the aortic arch and other systems derived from the neural crest.[8,9,18,21,22,38]

Together, these observations suggest that defects of the neural crest cells may be the common cause of the anomalies of the coronary arteries and aortic valve seen in the Syrian hamster. Further studies are necessary to verify this hypothesis.

ACKNOWLEDGMENT

The present work was supported by grants PB89-0577, PB92-0413, and PB95-0475 from the DGICyT (Ministerio de Educación y Ciencia, Madrid) and the Consejeria Educación y Ciencia (Junta de Andalucía). The authors thank Lic. M. Cardo (Málaga) and Dr. J. Cubo (Barcelona) for their valuable collaboration; and G. Martín, J. J. Canca, and L. Vida (Málaga) for their technical assistance.

REFERENCES

1. Arqué JM, Sans-Coma V, Durán AC, et al. Origen anómalo de la arteria coronaria izquierda en el tronco pulmonar y su relación con otras anomalías coronarias primarias: estudio experimental. Rev Esp Cardiol 1989;42:399.
2. Arqué JM, Thiene G, Cardo M, et al. Anomalous origin of the left coronary artery from the nonfacing aortic sinus: a study in the Syrian hamster. Cardiovasc Pathol 1993;2:35.
3. Bockman D, Redmond M, Waldo KL, et al. Effect of neural crest ablation on development of the heart and arch arteries in the chick. Am J Anat 1987;180:433.
4. Bogers AJJC, Gittenberger-de Groot AC, Poelmann RE, et al. Development of the origin of the coronary arteries, a matter of ingrowth or outgrowth? Anat Embryol 1989;180:437.
5. Cardo M, Fernández B, Durán AC, et al. Anomalous origin of the left coronary artery from the pulmonary trunk and its relationship with the morphology of the cardiac semilunar valves in Syrian hamsters. Basic Res Cardiol 1994;89:94.
6. Cardo M, Fernández B, Durán AC, et al. Anomalous origin of the left coronary artery from the dorsal aortic sinus and its relationship with aortic valve morphology in Syrian hamsters. J Comp Pathol 1995;112: 373.
7. Durán AC, Arqué JM, Cardo M, et al. Descripcion morfológica de una nueva anomalía arterial coronaria en el hámster sirio, *Mesocricetus auratus* (Waterhouse, 1839); su interpretación genética y filogenética. Misc Zool 1988;12:329.
8. Durán AC, Daliento L, Frescura C, et al. Unicommissural aortic valve and its association with other congenital heart disease. Cardiol Young 1995;5:132.
9. Durán AC, Frescura C, Sans-Coma V, et al. Bicuspid aortic valves in hearts with other congenital heart disease. J Heart Valve Dis 1995;4: 581.
10. Durán AC, Sans-Coma V, Arqué JM, et al. Blood supply to the interventricular septum of the heart in rodents with intramyocardial coronary arteries. Acta Zool-Stockholm 1992;73:223.
11. Durán AC, Sans-Coma V, Cardo M, et al. The blood supply to the

interventricular septum of the heart in Soricoidea (Mammalia). Zool Anz 1991;227:279.

12. Fukiishi Y, Morris-Kay GM. Migration of cranial neural crest cells to the pharyngeal arches and heart in rat embryos. Cell Tissue Res 1992; 268:1.

13. Higgins CB, Wexler L. Reversal of dominance of the coronary arterial system in isolated aortic stenosis and bicuspid aortic valve. Circulation 1975;52:292.

14. Hillestad L, Eie H. Single coronary artery. Acta Med Scand 1971;189: 409.

15. Hood LC, Rosenquist TH. Coronary artery development in the chick: origin and deployment of smooth muscle cells, and the effects of neural crest ablation. Anat Rec 1992;234:291.

16. Hutchins GM, Nazarian IH, Bulkley BH. Association of left dominant coronary arterial system with congenital bicuspid aortic valve. Am J Cardiol 1978;42:57.

17. Johnson AD, Detwiler JH, Higgins CB. Left coronary artery anatomy in patients with bicuspid aortic valves. Br Heart J 1978;40:489.

18. Kappetein AP, Gittenberger-de Groot AC, Zwinderman AH, et al. The neural crest as a possible pathogenetic factor in coarctation of the aorta and bicuspid aortic valve. J Thorac Cardiovasc Surg 1991;102:830.

19. Kirby ML, Gale TF, Stewart DE. Neural crest cells contribute to normal aorticopulmonary septation. Science 1983:220:1059.

20. Lerer PK, Edwards W. Coronary arterial anatomy in bicuspid aortic valve. Necropsy study of 100 hearts. Br Heart J 1981;45:142.

21. Miyabara S, Suzumori K, Uemura Y, et al. Fetal cystic hygroma in sibs: developmental analysis of coexisting cardiovascular malformations relevant to pathogenesis. Birth Defects, Original Article Series 1993;29:303.

22. Miyabara S, Suzumori K, Winking H, et al. Structural defects of the vascular system in 45,X fetuses: integrated interpretation of the pathogenesis. In: Hibi I, Takano K, eds. Basic and clinical approach to Turner syndrome. New York: Elsevier Science Publishing, 1993:61–68.

23. Murphy ES, Rosch J, Rahimtoola SH. Frequency and significance of coronary arterial dominance in isolated aortic stenosis. Am J Cardiol 1977;33:505.

24. Nishibatake M, Kirby ML, Van Mierop L. Pathogenesis of persistent truncus arteriosus and dextroposed aorta in the chick embryo after neural crest ablation. Circulation 1987;75:255.

25. Poelmann RE, Gittenberger-de Groot AC, Metink MMT, et al. Development of the cardiac vascular endothelium studied with anti-endothelial antibodies in chicken-quail chimeras. Circ Res 1993,73:559.

26. Roberts JT, Loube SD. Congenital single coronary artery in man. Am Heart J 1947;34:188.

27. Sans-Coma V, Arqué JM, Durán AC, et al. Origin of the left main coronary artery from the pulmonary trunk in the Syrian hamster. Am J Cardiol 1988;62:159.

28. Sans-Coma V, Arqué JM, Durán AC, et al. Anomalous origin of the coronary arteries in mammals. Zool Anz 1989;223:254.

29. Sans-Coma V, Arqué JM, Durán AC, et al. Coronary artery anomalies and bicuspid aortic valves in the Syrian hamster. Basic Res Cardiol 1991;86:148.

30. Sans-Coma V, Arqué JM, Durán AC, et al. The coronary arteries of the Syrian hamster, *Mesocricetus auratus* (Waterhouse, 1839). Ann Anat 1993;175:53.

31. Sans-Coma V, Cardo M, Durán AC, et al. Evidence for a quantitative genetic influence on the formation of aortic valves with two leaflets in the Syrian hamster. Cardiol Young 1993;3:132.

32. Sans-Coma V, Cardo M, Thiene G, et al. Bicuspid aortic and pulmonary valves in the Syrian hamster. Int J Cardiol 1992;34:249.

33. Sans-Coma V, Fernández B, Durán AC, et al. Fusion of valve cushions as a key factor in the formation of congenital bicuspid aortic valves in Syrian hamsters. Anat Rec 1996;244:490.

34. Scholz DG, Lynch JA, Willerscheidt AB, et al. Coronary arterial dominance associated with congenital aortic valve. Arch Pathol Lab Med 1980;104:417.

35. Sumida H, Akimoto N, Nakamura H. Distribution of the neural crest cells in the heart of birds: a three dimensional analysis. Anat Embryol 1989;180:29.

36. Takamura K, Okishima T, Ohdo S, et al. Association of cephalic neural crest cells with cardiovascular development, particularly that of the semilunar valves. Anat Embryol 1990;182:263.

37. Tomanek RJ. Formation of the coronary vasculature: a brief review. Cardiovasc Res 1996;31:E46.

38. Van Mierop LHS, Kutsche LM. Cardiovascular anomalies in DiGeorge syndrome and importance of neural crest as possible pathogenetic factor. Am J Cardiol 1986;58:133.

39. Waldo KL, Kumiski DH, Kirby ML. Association of the cardiac neural crest with the development of the coronary arteries in the chick embryo. Anat Rec 1994;239:315.

40. Waldo KL, Willner W, Kirby ML. Origin of the proximal coronary artery system and review of ventricular vascularization in the chick embryo. Am J Cardiol 1990;188:109.

Coronary Artery Anomalies: A Comprehensive Approach, edited by P. Angelini.
Lippincott Williams & Wilkins, Philadelphia © 1999.

CHAPTER 4

Normal and Anomalous Coronary Arteries in Humans

Paolo Angelini, Salvador Villason, Albert V. Chan, Jr., and José G. Diez

Part I
HISTORICAL BACKGROUND

Interest in coronary anatomy and the nature of the coronary vessels was cautiously aroused in the 16th century, when inquisitive Renaissance scholars began to perform anatomic investigations in the early European medical schools. Until then, anatomic knowledge had been heavily influenced by the philosophical and theological teachings of the ancient, rediscovered masters of the Greek and Arabic schools. Aristotle (384–322 BC), the philosophical interpreter of nature, and Galen of Pergamum (129–199 AD), the great physician, were the main authorities whose theories continued to dominate the medical schools of Salerno, Bologna, Padua, and eventually Louvain, Paris, and London during the Renaissance.

Leonardo da Vinci (1452–1519), a lone, ingenious spirit, examined a few animal hearts (probably of oxen) and also briefly touched on coronary anatomy while exploring the arcane viscera of the chest.[531] His main interest seemed to be in applying the principles of hydraulic physics to cardiovascular function. Leonardo tended to rely on instinctive curiosity rather than organized, formal methods. He left us only brief notes, accompanied by precise, faithful sketches of the coronary anatomy, including the aortic trifoliate valve, the right and left coronary ostia, and the proximal course of the right and left coronary arteries (Fig. 4.1). He noted that the coronary arteries become progressively smaller as they progress toward the cardiac apex.[531] He also accurately described the coronary veins and the coronary sinus; his observation of the arrangement of these structures supported his assumption that an artery is always accompanied by a vein.[531] Leonardo's approach exemplified the new method of critical, direct observation, which a little more than a century later would allow better-trained, more-disciplined scientists to understand how the circulation works.[531]

The presence of a pulmonary circulation organized in series with the systemic circulation had been postulated by isolated early researchers: Ibn-na-Nafis, a 13th-century Arab physician working in Damascus; Miguel Serveto, a passionate 16th-century Spanish theologian; and Cesalpino, a 16th-century anatomist from Padua, who coined the term "pulmonary circulation."[526] Nevertheless, it was not until 1628 that William Harvey (1578–1657), a physician trained in Padua but later active in London, and Cambridge, propounded a clear, complete, organized concept of the circulation, thereby founding the discipline of physiologic anatomy. Discovery of the systemic capillary network awaited the introduction of the microscope. It was Marcello Malpighi (1628–1694), operating mainly in Bologna, who first described the circulation of blood through the peripheral capillary network.[526]

Regarding the coronary arteries in particular, the founder of descriptive anatomy, the great Flemish anatomist Andreas Vesalius (1514–1564), produced a series of fundamental *tabulae anatomicae* (Venice, 1538), that were followed by his comprehensive treatise "De Humani Corporis Fabrica Libri Septem" (Basel, 1543), which became the basic textbook of anatomy for generations of physicians throughout Europe. Interestingly, one famous *tabula anatomica* showed the right coronary artery (RCA) originating from the left coronary artery (LCA) and coursing anterior to the pulmonary outflow tract (Fig. 4.2). Similarly, a single coronary ostium was mentioned by Fallopius (Venice, 1562).[508] Not until 1761, did G. P. Morgagni accurately and definitively describe the two main coronary vessels.[508] During the ensuing centuries, various investigators published occasional descriptions of peculiar or unusual coronary anatomic features: the work of A. C. Thebesius and R. Vieussens was especially noteworthy.[508]

With the advent of the 20th century, physicians became increasingly aware of the complexity and variability of the coronary anatomy. In 1926, this concept was reinforced and put into a biologic prospective by Grant and Regnier,[146] who

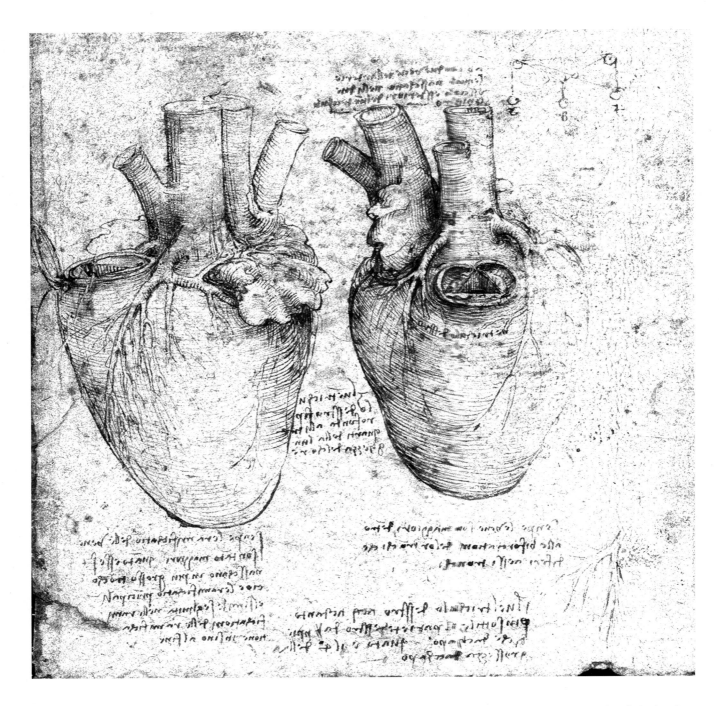

FIGURE 4.1. Leonardo da Vinci's drawings of the heart after removal of the pulmonary trunk above the valve (left drawing: lateral view; right drawing: frontal view). The two coronary arteries are clearly represented, one coursing on each side of the pulmonary outflow tract. The pulmonary sinuses are also precisely and correctly drawn in relation to the aortopulmonary contact point. (Courtesy of The Royal Collection©, Her Majesty Queen Elizabeth II.)

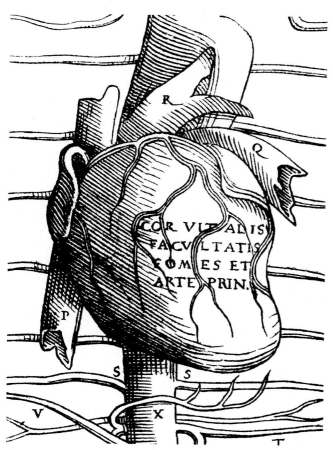

FIGURE 4.2. The coronary vessels (detail), as drawn in the "Six Tables" of Vesalius and Kalkar, from which Vesalius taught during his early years as professor of anatomy in Padua (see text). (Literary source, Vesalius A, Kalkar JS [1538]. Tabulae Anatomica, P.D. Bernard, Venice. Photo courtesy of the Blocker History of Medicine Collections, Moody Medical Library, The University of Texas Medical Branch, Galveston, TX.)

described the comparative anatomy of the coronary vessels in the different animal species. During the middle decades of the 20th century, several anatomists and surgeons made valuable contributions to the descriptive anatomy of the coronary arteries in humans. Particularly notable contributions were made by M. J. Schlesinger, J. E. Edwards, G. Baroldi, T. N. James, and W. C. Roberts.

The explosive popularization of selective angiography, as introduced by Mason Sones[370] in 1962, made cardiac specialists highly aware of the great variability of the coronary anatomy, even in the normal heart. Since then, thousands of short series and individual cases of coronary anomalies have been reported in the literature, eliciting not only widespread interest but also great frustration because of the complexity of the subject matter.

In 1967, Baroldi and Scomazzoni presented an excellent monograph summarizing the current knowledge of normal coronary anatomy.[508] During the 1960s, other investigators at the Armed Forces Institute of Pathology, in Washington

DC, undertook the pioneering project of describing congenital coronary anomalies in a coordinated, conceptual form.[42] Because their approach was based on clinical significance, they proposed to use the terms "minor and major" as organizing parameters in referring to coronary anomalies.[42] They further noted that some anomalies (such as seen in pulmonary atresia with intact ventricular septum and aortic atresia) were secondary consequences of congenital heart defects. This classification system became popular with several later authors, who simply added data from individual centers or unusual new cases to the same nosologic scheme. Another style that the Armed Forces group inaugurated (or indulged in) was to elaborate an embryogenetic theory based on anatomic observations of coronary anomalies. This theory assumed that the early embryonic coronary arteries were already present in the common undivided truncus, before any subdivision occurred, and that abnormal spiral septation of the truncus would cause ectopic origination.[42] Today we know that both assumptions (coronary origination from the undivided truncus and abnormal spiral subdivision of the truncus in cases of coronary anomalies) are erroneous, but the basic intuition that congenital anomalies have an embryogenic relevance was essentially correct and important. Unfortunately, as later authors came to realize, a morphogenetic explanation may not be so conveniently available in the absence of basic facts of normal descriptive embryology.[28]

An alternative classification device was introduced by Ogden,[285,286] who proposed to organize coronary anomalies according to anatomic morphologic parameters: anomalies of origin, course, and termination. Obviously, this approach was more comprehensive and rational than a system based only on clinical relevance, which depended on the evolution of medical opinion and practice.

Major contributions to the nosologic interpretation of coronary anomalies came from the most experienced centers and the most active pathologists, including J. E. Edwards, William C. Roberts, S. Bahrati, H. N. Neufeld, R. Virmani, and Hugh A. McAllister, Jr. More recent progress in the field of coronary artery interpretation has resulted from a more pointed approach aimed at (1) identifying the clinical relevance of certain apparently innocent morphologic variants by studying large populations, especially young persons dying suddenly of unclear causes, and (2) objectively documenting the claim of myocardial ischemia, especially by means of nuclear myocardial perfusion studies and provocation tests in the catheterization laboratory.

CORONARY ARTERY ANATOMY: WHAT IS NORMAL?

The only branches of the ascending aorta are the coronary arteries. They supply the heart and are two in number, right and left, arising near the commencement of the aorta immediately above the free margin of the semilunar valves. . . . The right coronary artery runs along its posterior surface as far as the posterior interventricular groove, where it divides into two branches, one of which (transverse) continues onward in the groove between the left auricle and ventricle. . . . The other (descending) courses along the posterior interventricular furrow. *(Gray's Anatomy, 1901 edition[509])*

Since the beginning of this century, when the preceding passage was published in a leading textbook of human anatomy, there has been a continuously expanding awareness of the great variability of the coronary anatomy and the difficulty of defining normal coronary arteries. This expanding awareness has mainly been the result of the introduction of selective coronary angiography, coronary bypass surgery, and catheter-based angioplasty. A growing number of coronary features have become clinically relevant, and an increasing number of variants have become apparent. Today, discussions of this subject are far more detailed than would have been considered relevant just a few decades ago. Moreover, as further developments occur, discussions can be expected to become even more complex in the future.

So far, the rich literature on coronary anomalies has been marred by a recurrent, inconclusive debate about the definition of coronary normality: What is normal (or unusual but normal) as opposed to atypical, abnormal, aberrant,[234,235,505] anomalous, accessory, ectopic, incidental,[19] a variant,[414] or a less common variant? What is a major or minor[42,115] anomaly or a clinically[29,412] or hemodynamically[20,97,231] significant anomaly? At a time when confusion still governs the terminology and concepts related to coronary anomalies, we would like to propose a method of study and a discipline that may promote a more rational organization of the subject matter. In this method, *coronary anomalies are defined by exclusion, on the basis of a description of the normal coronary anatomic features.* This fundamental organizational concept, which one of us (PA) proposed in 1989,[480] seems to have been widely validated since that time.[82,105,302] Only by means of a feature-by-feature description of the normal coronary anatomy can coronary anomalies be defined. Some features, such as the presence or absence of a common main trunk of the left coronary artery (LCA), are dichotomous; in these cases, normal is easily defined ("normal is to have a common trunk"). Other features are better described on the basis of a continuous spectrum of quantitative data, which can be assessed with a normal, or Gaussian, distribution curve observed in large populations. In such cases, *"normal" should probably be defined as the interval between two standard deviations from the mean value,* as commonly used in biologic studies. Additionally, the terminology used to distinguish normal and abnormal coronary arteries should be based solely on morphologic grounds and should avoid the issue of clinical relevance. Clinical or functional repercussions of coronary anomalies are obviously important, and they will be discussed at the end of this chapter (see Pathophysiologic Mechanisms and Clinical Implications of Coronary Anomalies). Unfortunately, some questions cannot yet be resolved on the basis of currently available knowledge; in these cases, one can only propose certain criteria to be tested in further studies or certain empir-

ical solutions to be temporarily adopted by common agreement.

METHODS FOR STUDYING CORONARY MORPHOLOGY

Traditional descriptions of coronary morphology are based on anatomic observations in necropsy specimens. The primary tools are gross inspection and fine dissection with the aid of magnifying loupes. Injection/corrosion methods involve both injection of a semisolid gelatin mass or of chemical fibers (which tend to solidify in response to changes in temperature) and corrosion induced by changes in the chemical environment. Injection of radiopaque media, followed by radiography, is also a well-established method for evaluating autopsy specimens. Each of these observational methodologies has its indications, advantages, and limitations.

Gross Anatomic Inspection

Gross anatomic inspection—obviously the simplest, most readily available method for examining autopsy specimens—is often quite adequate. It is preferred for studying the coronary ostial anatomy, because it is well suited for describing the location of the ostia with respect to aortic root reference structures (the semilunar leaflets, commissures, and sinotubular junction). Gross anatomic inspection (sometimes with the aid of magnifying lenses) is also preferred for describing the intrinsic anatomic features of the proximal coronary anatomy (for example, slitlike ostial ridges in coronary arteries that originate tangentially with respect to the aortic wall). For evaluating a coronary artery's course, distal distribution, and termination (as in cases of small anomalous fistulous communications), the gross anatomic approach is less appropriate: it is not as precise as injection-corrosion or radiographic methods.

The great value of gross anatomic inspection lies in its convenience and negligible cost. Its most obvious limitation is its reliance on necropsy material. Indeed, because of the widespread clinical introduction of precise diagnostic imaging methods (such as computerized axial tomography, nuclear magnetic imaging, echocardiography, and angiography), necropsy studies are currently performed with decreased frequency.

Injection-Corrosion Techniques

Injection-corrosion techniques are quite satisfactory for showing coronary distribution patterns.[192,351,508] At their most sophisticated level of execution, these techniques can allow visualization of even the finest collateral network. However, because this approach depends on corrosion techniques to better delineate the coronary luminal spaces, it is inadequate for determining the relationship between coronary arteries and their adjacent structures (such as the dependent myocardial segments). Moreover, injection-corrosion techniques are delicate, time-consuming, and expensive, requiring special technical knowledge on the part of the investigator. In recent decades, these techniques have largely been replaced by radiologic methods.

Radiologic Visualization

Radiology may be performed in vivo, as well as in cadaveric specimens. In recent decades, in vivo selective coronary angiography has become an unparalleled tool for studying coronary anatomy.[2,48,122,186,355,370,442] Because of this method's safety, its capacity for precise stereoscopic imaging (achieved by combining multiple simultaneous or sequential projections), and its excellent rendition of coronary anatomic details in motion (by means of enhanced radiologic techniques, digital enhancement, and electronic magnification), it is currently used in some 2 million patients per year worldwide. Moreover, it has been used in the great majority of recent investigational studies of coronary anatomy.

In cadavers, radiologic single-plane coronary angiography introduces a serious artifact, related to superimposition of the different planes (the cardiac free walls, septa, atria, and ventricles). This artifact tends to negate the advantage of greater detail during visualization of the fine coronary anatomy in a nonbeating heart. To overcome this technical problem, Schlesinger[351] proposed an "unrolling technique" by which the ventricular septum and both atrial walls are eliminated, transforming the cadaver heart into a flat surface. Obviously, this technique introduces other artifacts and precludes examination of certain relevant cardiac structures. Nevertheless, it is an expedient means of studying, for example, coronary dominance.

Newer Imaging Techniques

Because of its high cost, coronary angiography is not appropriate as a primary screening test for ruling out coronary anomalies. For this purpose, noninvasive clinical imaging techniques are safer, more convenient for the patient, and more cost-efficient—particularly echocardiography[6,123,131,331] but also nuclear magnetic resonance imaging[99,107,222,412,460,462,463] and computerized axial tomography at rapid rates of image acquisition. These methods can document the presence of a coronary anomaly or at least greatly raise the level of suspicion. For providing a thorough anatomic description, however, they are inferior to coronary angiography, not only because of their intrinsic physical characteristics but also because their basic approach is tomographic (whereas the coronary arteries do not lie in a single plane). Doppler signal interrogation can greatly enhance ultrasonographic imaging by facilitating vessel identification and providing flow velocity data. Echocardiography, magnetic resonance imaging, and computerized axial tomography can frequently allow diagnosis of the larger coronary fistulas and anomalous origination of a coronary artery from the pulmonary artery. Orig-

ination of a coronary artery from an anomalous aortic location or from the anomalous course of a proximal coronary artery can also be reliably identified with echocardiography,[456] especially using the transesophageal approach.[449,482] On the contrary, the distal coronary anatomy cannot be adequately visualized with these methods.[519,521]

Questions related to myocardial perfusion, especially those aimed at ruling out myocardial ischemia in the presence of coronary anomalies, can best be resolved by nuclear myocardial perfusion scintigraphy coupled with exercise or pharmacologic stress testing or by metabolic radioactive tracers coupled with positron emission tomography. In the near future, these testing modalities will become more relevant: they will be used to definitively and categorically establish the clinical relevance of certain coronary anomalies that are still unclear and to guide the management of individual patients, based on objective evidence of reversible segmental ischemia.

NORMAL CORONARY ARTERIES IN HUMANS: DESCRIPTIONS AND DEFINITIONS

A coronary artery is defined as any artery or arterial branch that carries blood to cardiac parenchyma (i.e., any structure located within the pericardial cavity). The cardiac parenchyma includes not only the myocardium but also the semilunar and atrioventricular valves, the great vessels (the proximal aorta, the pulmonary trunk, and a short segment of the superior vena cava), and the visceral pericardium or epicardium. The parietal pericardium should not be included, so the pericardial arteries should not be considered coronary.

The name and nature of a coronary artery or branch is defined by that vessel's distal vascularization territory, not by its origin. A coronary artery that arises from the right anterior sinus of Valsalva and that branches into the left anterior descending (LAD) and circumflex territories is not a right coronary artery (RCA) but, rather, a left main trunk with an ectopic origin. Similarly, *the different sinuses of Valsalva are identified not by the coronary arteries that originate from them but, rather, by their own topographic location.*

When considering the spectrum of coronary morphologies, *"normal" should mean "what is commonly observed,"* [394,480] and the terms *abnormal or anomalous* should be used for any form *observed in less than 1% of the general human population.*[480] This criterion is proposed as the dividing line between (1) normality, which would include the more frequent variations *(normal variants),* and (2) abnormality, which would consist of relatively infrequent variations *(anomalies).*

In essence, a useful convention is all that, on purely anatomic grounds, distinguishes a normal coronary artery pattern from an abnormal variant. Only certain anomalies (such as a coronary aneurysm) predispose the patient to a morbid state, and very few anomalies (such as anomalous origination of a coronary artery from the pulmonary artery) constitute, in themselves, a disease state. Pathophysiologic and clinical considerations should be clearly distinguished from, and subordinate to, anatomic description.

With respect to its basic reference framework, the coronary artery anatomy should be related to the aortic sinuses at one extreme and the dependent myocardium at the other. The essential reference for describing the origination of the coronary arteries is the aortic root. *Anatomically, the aortic root consists of three equal-sized[507] semilunar leaflets, three intercuspal spaces,* and *three sinuses of Valsalva,* as well as *the sinotubular junction,* which separates the aortic root from the ascending aorta (Fig. 4.3). In a normal human heart, the aortic valve is situated posterior to—and slightly to the right

of—the pulmonary valve, just anterior to the recess between the tricuspid and mitral annuli (Fig. 4.4). The posterior wall of the aortic root is the anterior wall of the sinus transversus pericardii, a liquid-filled pericardial space that separates the aorta from the right and left atria (Fig. 4.4).

The aortic and pulmonary valves have a single adjacent contact point, which is the consistent remnant of the embryologic aortopulmonary septum (Fig. 4.4). This point is a useful reference for describing the semilunar cusps and sinuses. Indeed, the circumference of each semilunar valve is normally divided into three equal 120° sectors, and *the aortopulmonary contact point* is easily and consistently locatable and helps identify the site of one *(joining or adja-*

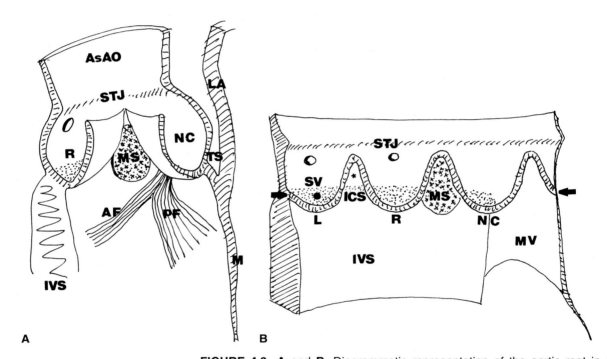

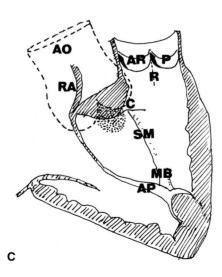

FIGURE 4.3. A and **B.** Diagrammatic representation of the aortic root in cross-section (grossly sagittal, view **A**) and in rectified form (unrolled root, view **B**), after excision of the semilunar cusps to reveal the implantation line of the cusps (view **B**, arrows). The aortic root is limited distally by the sinotubular junction. The sinuses of Valsalva are limited distally by the sinotubular junction and proximally by the implantation line of the cusps. The bottom section of each cusp is shadowed to indicate the underlying muscular septum (view **B**, solid circle). The intercuspal triangles or spaces (view **B**, asterisk), have different wall constituents depending on the specific location. View **A:** AF = anterior fascicle of the bundle of His; AsAO = ascending aorta; IVS = interventricular septum; LA = left atrial wall; M = section of mitral valve; MS = membranous septum; NC = so-called noncoronary sinus; PF = posterior fascicle of the bundle of His; R = right sinus; STJ = sinotubular junction; TS = transverse septum. View **B:** ICS = intercuspal space or triangle; IVS = interventricular septum; L = left sinus; MS = membranous septum; MV = anterior leaflet of the mitral valve; NC = so-called noncoronary sinus; R = right sinus; STJ = sinotubular junction; SV = sinus of Valsalva. **C.** Relationship between the aortic root and the right ventricular cavity. AO = aorta; AP = anterior papillary muscle of the tricuspid valve; AR = anterior right pulmonary cusp; C = crista supraventricularis; MB = moderator band; P = posterior pulmonary cusp; R = raphe of the right ventricular outflow tract (a residual sign of the fusion line between the embryologic conal ridges); RA = right atrial anterior wall; SM = crista septo-marginalis. Shaded area = membranous ventricular septum.

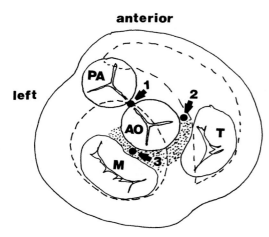

FIGURE 4.4. Schematic representation of the base of the heart (coronal plane) after removal of the atrial walls and the ascending aorta/pulmonary artery. At site 1 the pulmonary annulus is adjacent to the aortic annulus, representing a remnant of the aortopulmonary embryologic septum: This is the consistent site of the anterior commissure of the aortic valve and the posterior commissure of the pulmonary valve. Site 2 indicates the position of the membranous septum. Site 3 shows the relationship between the aortic annulus and the mitral and tricuspid annulus, as well as mitral-aortic continuity. The interrupted lines indicate the approximate positions of the left and right ventricular cavities. AO = aorta; M = mitral valve; PA = pulmonary valve; T = tricuspid. The shaded area represents the sinus transversus pericardii.

cent) *aortic and pulmonary commissure* (Fig. 4.4). In the normal aortic valve, this commissure is termed anterior or left anterior; in the pulmonary valve, however, the adjacent commissure is called posterior or right posterior.

The two aortic sinuses that adjoin the aortopulmonary contact point are the site of origin for the great majority of the coronary arteries, whether their anatomy is normal or abnormal. The right and left anterior sinuses are called the *"facing sinuses,"* because they face the pulmonary artery. According to traditional teaching, coronary arteries never originate from the sinus opposite the aortopulmonary contact point (the nonadjacent, nonfacing, or right posterior sinus). Therefore, this aortic sinus is also referred to as "noncoronary." In reality, however, coronary origination from the noncoronary sinus has been observed in a few rare cases (see page 46), some of which have been reported in the literature.

The three aortic valve cusps and sinuses have been variably labeled. In Nomina Anatomica (1989),[530] the aortic valve leaflets and sinuses are called *posterior, right, and left.* However, the terms *noncoronary, right (coronary), and left (coronary),* are in widespread clinical use. We encourage the use of topographic descriptive terminology: *right posterior, right anterior, left anterior, and right posterior* (so-called noncoronary). In this approach, the relative location of the cusps is determined with respect to the orthogonal planes, in the coronal plane of the heart (Fig. 4.4). Especially when

describing the coronary anatomy by means of angiography, one would also consider the vertical (superoinferior) axis. In this orientation, the aortic sinuses are not all located at the same level; instead, the left anterior sinus is slightly higher than the others, and the right posterior sinus is slightly lower. Indeed, the anterior commissure of the aorta (which adjoins the aortopulmonary contact point) is the highest point of the aortic valve annulus (Fig. 4.5). The (embryologically conjoined) planes of the aortic and pulmonary valves are slightly different, and they are oriented not horizontally but obliquely, with an anterior lift that causes the pulmonary valve to be slightly higher (more cephalad) than the aortic valve (Fig. 4.5). In any given case, the anatomy of the aortic root should be specifically analyzed and mentioned, never just assumed to be normal, especially when one is describing a coronary anomaly.[141,165,176,194,202,227,348,390,440]

The compact myocardium, which forms during initial embryologic development, from an earlier myocardial structure characterized by a mostly trabecular spongy architecture, cannot grow and function in the absence of a coronary artery system (see Chapter 2). On full development, each myocardial fiber is surrounded by a close network of arteriolar and capillary branches.[499] In the normal human heart, most of the myocardial mass belongs to the left ventricle, and both coronary arteries (left and right) primarily serve the left ventricular mass. Myocardial organization is the fundamental determinant of the anatomy of the distal coronary artery tree. In any coronary anatomic pattern, the potentially modifiable features generally relate to the *proximal coronary segments* (which have a *conductive function*) rather than the *arteriolar segments* (which have a *resistance-modulating function*) or the *capillary segments* (which have a *nutritive function*). For this reason, the following discussion deals essentially with the conductive segments.

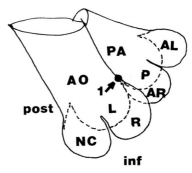

FIGURE 4.5. Relationships between the aortic sinuses and the pulmonary sinuses, as seen in the right anterior oblique projection. The aortic valve annulus is oriented obliquely (tilted anteriorly and superiorly), as is the pulmonary annulus. 1 = the contact point between the aortic and pulmonary sinuses. The left aortic sinus (L) is higher than the right (R) and the noncoronary (NC) sinuses. The antero-left (AL, nonadjacent) pulmonary sinus is located at a higher level than the anterior right (AR) and posterior (P) pulmonary sinuses (the adjacent or facing sinuses). AO = aorta; inf = inferior; PA = pulmonary artery; post = posterior.

Origination of the Coronary Ostia

Normally (i.e., in more than 1% of individuals), *the human coronary arteries have two or three coronary ostia.*[421] Whereas two ostia (the right and left) are typically present, it is also normal to see a separate aortic ostium for a conal or infundibular branch, or third coronary artery,[350] which is present in 23 to 51% of normal hearts.[191,351,508] Less frequently, separate origination of the LAD and circumflex arteries from the aorta, in the absence of a common left main trunk, produces a third (or fourth) coronary ostium. This condition was studied by several anatomists, and the reported frequency of absent left main trunk varied from 0.4 to 8.0%, depending on the criteria used by the different investigators.[94,192,351,391,413,508] If the defining criterion is minimal evidence of a common left main trunk, however rudimentary, like a common aortic niche, the lower estimates are correct. In contrast, if the criterion is absence of a clearly individualized common trunk, the higher estimates are correct. The question of whether an absent left main trunk is an anomaly or a normal variant will be discussed again later in this chapter.

The coronary ostia are normally located in the middle of the right anterior and left anterior sinuses, just above the upper free margin of the semilunar leaflets (in the open position) and just below the sinotubular junction. This general rule applies to cases involving two, three, or even four coronary ostia. As already suggested in the literature,[19,23,227,413,480] a specific, detailed anatomic study needs to be undertaken with the aim of establishing, in a large human population with normal hearts, the spectrum of coronary ostial distribution in both the horizontal plane (oriented along the circumference of the aortic annulus) and the vertical plane (oriented along the longitudinal axis of the ascending aorta). Only after a precise description becomes available can the standard deviations in the two axes be determined and anomalies be exactly defined (Fig. 4.6).

Normally, *the proximal segment of a coronary artery arises at a nearly orthogonal angle from the aortic wall*

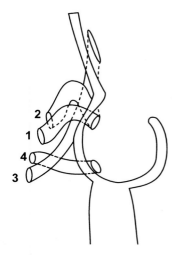

FIGURE 4.7. Cross-sectional view of the right coronary cusp, showing four examples of variant coronary origination: 1, normal, grossly orthogonal to the aortic wall; 2, uplifted; 3, downward with a tangential path (in a case of ectopic origination from the ascending aorta); 4, horizontal (in a case of low, ectopic origination).

(Fig. 4.7). This angle has never been precisely studied in a large population, and the normal range has never been established, but it is important that distinctly unusual angles of coronary origination be recognized, especially during selective catheterization in clinical studies. Coronary ostia that originate ectopically are consistently associated with *acute ("tangential") arterial origination* from the aortic wall, and only rarely does acute angulation occur in the context of a normal ostial location.

In size, *the coronary ostia are typically equal to, or larger than, the proximal segment of the related coronary artery.*[301] As *the coronary arteries* produce side branches and progress downstream, they *gradually decrease (but never increase) in diameter.*

The course of the coronary arteries is mostly epicardial, at least in humans, although the *proximal LAD* is intramural in 5 to 25% of cases, producing a systolic narrowing or milking effect when observed angiographically (see Intramural Coronary Artery). *The coronary arteries normally terminate in the capillary network* via arteriolar segments, which are responsible for most of the coronary tree's hemodynamic resistance (see Overview of Coronary Physiology). Direct coronary artery communications with the cardiac cavities or with veins are considered generically abnormal (see Anomalies of Termination: Coronary Fistulas).

Although an *ideal "coronary luminal size/dependent myocardial mass ratio"* no doubt exists, its normal range has been difficult to define.[175,205,230,233,247,281,301,408,428,499] It is important that this ratio be clarified, however, to better elucidate anomalies such as coronary ectasia, coronary aneurysm, coronary hypoplasia, or absent coronary artery. The current open debate about how to define these entities stems from the lack of universally accepted parameters of normal

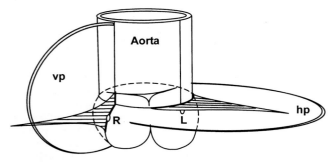

FIGURE 4.6. Schematic representation of the aortic root and the ascending aorta, showing the conceptual pattern of distribution of the right (R) and left (L) coronary ostia in the vertical (for the right) and horizontal (for the left) planes (vp and hp, respectively). See text.

coronary size. Indeed, the absolute coronary artery diameter increases with age[247] and is greatly influenced by the pattern of "coronary dominance." Use of the criterion of relative diameter ratio (>150% of the diameter of the neighboring "normal" segment of the same artery[371]) to define coronary ectasia presupposes that a normal segment is present and recognized, which is not always true in a given case.[230] A more practical, acceptable approach to defining normal coronary size may be based on measurements of coronary flow velocity at rest and after maximum vasodilation, since it is clinically impractical or impossible to obtain an anatomic quantitative description of the distal capillary bed. Gould[145] proposed that a given flow velocity at rest and a maximal flow reserve (ability to increase blood flow with maximal vasodilation) of x4 to x5 with respect to baseline is evidence of normal epicardial coronary size (flow velocity) and arteriolar vasodilatory capacity (functional reserve), respectively. Before valid general statements can be made, however, larger studies must be performed in this regard. Gould's approach would imply that a coronary segment with a decreased flow velocity suggests coronary ectasia, while an increased flow velocity would suggest either a localized stenosis or a hypoplastic segment (congenital stenosis?). Mild forms of coronary hypoplasia (at any level), involving a diminished maximal flow reserve (but a normal flow at rest), may indeed exist as a substrate accounting for some cases of the poorly defined entity known as syndrome X (myocardial ischemia without coronary stenosis). A similar mismatch has been proposed as the mechanism for cardiomyopathy in an experimental model of chronic ventricular overload.[14] Definitive studies need to be undertaken in this regard (see also Coronary Hypoplasia). Generally, we can state that *it is normal for all myocardial segments to have a congenitally adequate arterial circulation with respect to basal and exercise requirements,* and any apparent deviations (such as "absent" coronary artery) should generally have an alternative cause—either ectopic origination of a vessel, which can be difficult to demonstrate angiographically, or acquired vascular occlusion in the absence of demonstrable collaterals (see Absent Coronary Artery).

The normal anatomic features of each coronary artery and its main branches are detailed in the following pages.

Right Coronary Artery

Normally, *the RCA arises from an ostium located just below the sinotubular junction, in the middle of the right anterior sinus of Valsalva, and courses into the right atrioventricular groove.* If the right anterior cusp has more than one ostium, the additional ostium—and there may be more than one[508]—is related to a conal (or more precisely, infundibular) branch. In terms of a *minimal identifying descriptor, the RCA is defined as that vessel which courses in the right atrioventricular groove and provides nutrient branches to the right ventricular free wall.* (In cases of congenital atrioventricular discordance or situs inversus, the right atrioven-

tricular groove is the groove related to the anatomic right ventricle). In the absence of preexisting literature on this subject, we propose that the artery in the right atrioventricular groove be named the RCA *if it reaches the acute margin of the heart.* On the other hand, if it produces only a few anterior right ventricular branches and does not reach the acute margin of the heart, the lone right-anterior-cusp artery should be called the *infundibular* (or conal) *branch.* Such a condition is usually associated with a large left coronary system, in which the left circumflex artery reaches the acute margin from the posterior aspect of the heart and provides the coronary circulation for most of the heart. In this case, one is dealing with a single coronary artery originating from the left anterior sinus, with the RCA arising ectopically from the distal circumflex artery and an independent conal or infundibular branch originating from the right coronary cusp (see Single Coronary Artery).

In defining the essence of the RCA in these terms, one cannot expect to exhaust the subject of its anatomic variance: this artery may stop at the acute margin of the heart or may continue to the crux or the left atrioventricular groove, ending in the posterolateral left ventricular branch or even the ramus medianus or the diagonal branch and occasionally extending up to the LAD. What is the "normal" maximal extension of the RCA? Because of a lack of prospective ad hoc studies in large populations, *a "very dominant" RCA, terminating in a left posterolateral branch short of the obtuse margin of the heart should be considered the extreme (largest normal) variant.* An RCA that provides branches to the obtuse margin (and beyond) should be considered abnormal, and this condition should be called "anomalous origination of the circumflex artery from the distal RCA." It is also normal for an RCA to provide a posterior descending branch that follows the posterior atrioventricular groove as far as the apex of the heart but not beyond.

In summary, the dependent territory of the normal RCA may vary: at one extreme, the artery may just reach the acute margin of the right ventricle; at the other extreme, the artery may stop just short of providing an obtuse marginal branch (Fig. 4.8).

Descriptions of the right and circumflex arterial patterns have usually been limited to defining the dominant versus nondominant variants, depending on the origin of the posterior descending branch. Indeed, in classifying normal RCA patterns, Baroldi and Scamazzoni[508] included a "type-II" pattern, in which the RCA produces not only the posterior descending but also the obtuse marginal branch. Unfortunately, these authors failed to define the circumflex artery, leaving room for inconsistency. Currently, it would seem crude and inadequate to describe the RCA anatomic spectrum in terms of simple dominance alone, especially in light of practical considerations related to anatomic-physiologic correlations (using echocardiography and nuclear myocardial scintigraphy) and therapeutic interventions (bypass surgery and catheter angioplasty). Ideally, a map of the left ventricular myocardial mass, including the interventricular

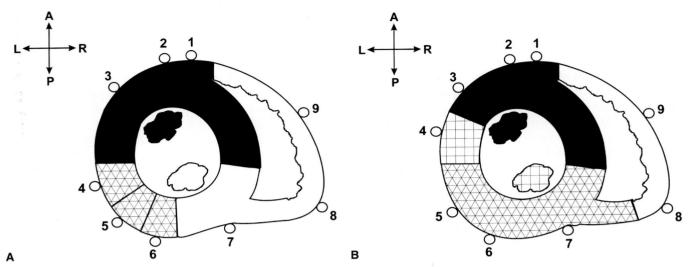

FIGURE 4.8. Horizontal cross section of the heart showing the myocardial segments supplied by the LAD (black), RCA (white), circumflex (triangles), and ramus medianus (squares) in cases of dominant RCA **(A)** and dominant circumflex **(B)**. The numbered circles around the sections represent the location of individual coronary branches: 1 = LAD; 2 = second diagonal; 3 = first diagonal; 4 = obtuse marginal (case **A**) or ramus (case **B**); 5,6 = further obtuse marginal branches; 7 = posterior descending artery; 8 = acute marginal; 9 = anterior right ventricular branch. The section of the papillary muscles is shown inside the left ventricular cavity.

septum, should be constructed to indicate the respective territories of the RCA, LAD, and circumflex artery (Fig. 4.8). For clinical angiographic purposes, we support the policy of describing the coronary artery patterns and distributions, including detailed mention of the main secondary branches (as small as about 1.5 mm in diameter), according to their territorial distribution (Fig. 4.8). In most cases (about 90% in humans), the RCA is ''dominant,'' meaning that it generates a posterior descending branch, which provides blood flow mainly to the posteroseptal left ventricular myocardium, past the proximal, predominantly conductive section of this vessel, which gives off only small branches to the free wall of the right ventricle. One of the RCA's terminal branches, which originates at the crux of the heart, provides nutrient flow to the atrioventricular node. That terminal branch may facilitate angiographic location of the interventricular septum, as the atrioventricular node is situated in the cephalad, posterobasal portion of the interventricular septum, just underneath—and in front of—the coronary sinus's opening into the right atrium (Eustachian valve).

Normally, *the RCA does not provide branches that cross the anterior interventricular sulcus* into the left ventricular territory. A small septal (interventricular) branch may originate from the proximal RCA or directly from the right anterior cusp by means of an independent ostium.

Of the multiple small, highly variable atrial branches that may arise from the RCA, the sinus node artery is the one most commonly recognized. Nevertheless, its origin and course vary widely. In 50% of cases, the sinus node artery arises from the proximal RCA. In the remaining cases, it branches from the proximal circumflex or mid RCA.[192,508]

The other atrial branches have a highly variable, unpredictable morphology. Individually, they are generally considered unimportant for clinical purposes, with the possible exception of a branch that follows the crista terminalis (the line of separation between the smooth posterior section of the right atrium and the highly trabeculated anterior portion).

Left Coronary Artery

The LCA originates from the middle portion of the left anterior sinus of Valsalva, just above the level of the free edge of the open aortic cusp and just below the sinotubular junction. The exact site of the left coronary ostium varies. Specific studies should be undertaken to identify the value of two standard deviations in the distribution curve of the left coronary ostial site, as proposed in the case of the RCA (Fig. 4.6). *The left coronary ostium is usually single,* so it is normal to see a common LCA trunk. In an ad hoc review of 1950 consecutive selective coronary angiograms (see pages 38–43), the authors documented absence of a left main coronary trunk (with double orifices, and separate origination of the circumflex and LAD arteries) in less than 1% of cases, a finding that defines this condition as a coronary anomaly. A proximal coronary vessel originating from the left ostium is called the left main stem or trunk only if it gives rise to both the LAD and the circumflex artery. In anomalous cases, in which one of these arteries does not originate from the LCA, the trunk that arises from the left anterior sinus should be called not the left main but the proximal LAD or circumflex artery, whichever is appropriate.

Because the left main coronary trunk arises orthogonally

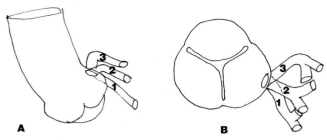

FIGURE 4.9. Schematic views of left coronary variants, in the frontal **(A)** and horizontal **(B)** planes, showing different orientations of the left main trunk: in **A**, inferior tilt (A1), normal orthogonal tilt (A2), and superior tilt (A3); in **B**, anterior tilt (B1), normal orthogonal tilt (B2), and posterior tilt (B3).

from the aortic sinus, it usually lies in the coronal plane of the heart. Occasionally, the left main trunk may be oriented more anteriorly or posteriorly, superiorly or inferiorly (Fig. 4.9). Again, specific studies are needed with regard to the spectrum of normal variation in left main trunk orientation.

Because the left main trunk is only a short (conductive) arterial segment, from which the circumflex and LAD arteries normally spring, and because the latter vessels are the two main nutrient components of the LCA, some experts have proposed that *the LAD and circumflex be termed "arteries"* and that the farther, *secondary ramifications,* such as the diagonal or medians, be called *branches or rami.*[508]

Despite the great variability in the morphology of the LCA system, the following fairly consistent rules may be set forth.

- *The LAD courses in the anterior interventricular groove, the circumflex artery in the left atrioventricular groove.*
- The LAD gives off branches to both the septum and the anterolateral wall of the left ventricle, including the anterolateral papillary muscle, and the circumflex artery produces branches to the posterolateral wall of the left ventricle, usually including the posteromedial papillary muscle (Fig. 4.8).
- The LAD terminates *at* the cardiac apex, or 1 to 2 cm *before or after* the apex.
- The anterior septal branches (perforators) originate from the LAD, at the anterior interventricular sulcus, at a grossly perpendicular angle with respect to the cardiac surface; these branches immediately become intramural, coursing within the ventricular septum.
- The LAD seldom produces sizable branches (i.e., large enough for bypass surgery or angioplasty) that extend to the free wall of the right ventricle, but it does frequently produce smaller branches, which are directed toward the anterior wall of the right ventricle. These branches may become more prominent if collateral circuits are established between the LAD and RCA, involving both the proximal segment (Vieussens' circle) and the distal segment of the LAD. In the latter case, the collaterals connect the anterior ventricular or acute marginal branches of the RCA with the distal LAD.[349–351]

- The diagonal branches, which, in human adults have a luminal diameter of >1.5 mm, consist of one to three independent vessels that arise from the LAD at variable downward angles and course over the anterolateral free wall of the left ventricle. Anatomists and angiographers customarily call "first diagonal" the first branch that arises from the LAD in its downstream course. Conversely, surgeons prefer to use the term "Diag-1" for the first branch encountered lateral to the LAD and "Diag-2" for the next branch, which has a more lateral course (Fig. 4.10). In the future, this nomenclature should be rendered uniform by a universal agreement.
- The terms "ramus medianus," "intermedius," or "intermediate branch" refer to a coronary branch that covers a variable extent of the free wall of the left ventricle, posterior to the territory of the diagonal artery and anterior to the first obtuse marginal branch of the circumflex artery. Therefore, the "ramus medianus" is defined as the intermediate vessel between the first diagonal and first obtuse marginal branches. In some hearts, no sizable vessel fits this definition. The origination site does not define the nature of the ramus medianus, because this vessel may occasionally arise from the proximal LAD or directly from the left main or proximal circumflex artery. The obtuse margin of the heart is neither a precise anatomic feature (Fig. 4.8) nor an angiographically recognizable entity but a useful approximate term for identifying a point or line in the free wall of the left ventricle. Moreover, unlike the anterior or posterior interventricular groove, the obtuse margin is not a consistent site for a large epicardial coronary branch. Therefore, one occasionally has trouble determining which branch to call the ramus medianus, and in a sizeable number of cases (30%?), experienced observers will agree that this vessel is missing.

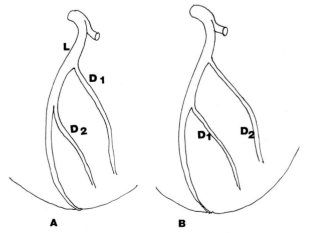

FIGURE 4.10. The alternative nomenclatures generally used by angiographers and anatomists **(A)** or by surgeons **(B)**. See text. D_1 = first diagonal branch; D_2 = second diagonal branch; L = LAD.

- The circumflex artery runs along the left atrioventricular groove, descends beneath the left atrial appendage, and courses downward toward the crux of the heart for a variable distance. *An LCA that has a circumflex artery that does not reach the crux of the heart is customarily called "nondominant." An LCA that has a circumflex artery that reaches the crux and produces the posterior descending branch,* along the posterior interventricular groove (Fig. 4.8), *is called "dominant."* In reality, however, "right and left dominance" is a poor term because, as James[192] noted, the LCA is larger than the RCA in most normal hearts, even when the RCA provides the posterior descending branch. Current terminology referring to dominance should be replaced by nomenclature that describes the posterior interventricular septum's blood supply or its distribution, avoiding any reference to literal "dominance." In addition, it is important to realize that the circumflex artery and the RCA are not the only arteries that can participate in vascularizing the posterior third of the interventricular septum; another possible participant is the LAD, which may not end at the apex but, rather, may turn around it and then follow the posterior interventricular groove for a variable length. For further discussion of this point, see page 58.
- It is probably useful to define *the "minimal circumflex artery"* as that vessel which *provides at least one branch to the territory of the obtuse margin.* In cases in which the LCA's territory does not extend to the obtuse margin, one would expect the circumflex artery to originate ectopically (usually from the RCA), and the LCA would be considered an LAD in the absence of a common left main trunk.
- Atrial branches commonly originate from the circumflex artery (especially those branches directed to the left atrium, but sometimes also those directed at the right atrium and the sinus node's territory). Such branches less frequently arise from the left main trunk, and they never arise from the LAD. In some 40% of normal hearts, the artery to the sinus node originates from the proximal circumflex artery.[192,508] The atrioventricular node artery may originate from the circumflex artery, but only if the latter artery reaches the cardiac crux, usually with a dominant pattern.

In considering the wide spectrum of epicardial coronary artery patterns in normal human hearts, one can arrive at the following basic conclusion: in all hearts, any left ventricular myocardial segment has essentially the same amount of arterial supply (measured by capillary density) as any other segment, but the proximal arterial vessels can be organized into a great number of alternative patterns. A proper, uniform, widely accepted system of nomenclature must be established to promote reliable interobserver communication, which is especially important from the clinical standpoint.

INCIDENCE OF CORONARY ANOMALIES: ANGIOGRAPHIC ANALYSIS OF 1950 CASES

The recent literature contains several reports about the incidence of coronary anomalies, either in the general patient population or in patients with clinical evidence of myocardial ischemia. These reports involve both angiographic and autopsy series. Some of them specifically concern the incidence of coronary anomalies in young persons,[85,106,241] athletes,[254,514–518,534] soldiers,[245] patients recovering from an acute myocardial infarction,[37,143,424] those suffering sudden death,[393,513,520] or those studied by angiography for suspected coronary artery disease.[21a,76,77,196,197,206,406,430,437] Unfortunately, the entry criteria and methodology used by the different investigators are poorly described and variably defined, yielding unreliable figures that are not strictly comparable.

A higher incidence of coronary anomalies has been consistently observed in young victims of sudden death than in adults undergoing routine autopsy examination (incidence: 4 to 15% versus about 1%, respectively). The medical community still hesitates to accept these differences at face value, however, because the reporting centers tend to have a particular, well-recognized interest in congenital coronary anomalies; therefore, the incidence of these rare entities is probably artifactually heightened because of a referral bias. In addition, the results depend on whether certain relatively common entities such as muscular bridges are specifically investigated and counted as coronary anomalies.

To help clarify the incidence of coronary anomalies, our group at the Texas Heart Institute evaluated selective coronary angiograms obtained from 1950 consecutive patients with documented or suspected coronary artery obstructive disease and otherwise normal hearts.

Patients and Methods

Materials and Techniques

Coronary angiograms performed in 2000 consecutive cases between January and May 1989 were retrieved from the archives of St. Luke's Episcopal Hospital's cardiac catheterization laboratories and were prospectively reviewed according to the criteria described herein. Fifty angiograms were excluded because they either were nonselective or did not adequately show all of the expected coronary vessels. The remaining 1950 angiograms were technically satisfactory and, therefore, were included in the study. The population included adult patients (1369 men and 581 women) with an average age of 56.7 years (Table 4.1).

In the great majority of cases, multiple projections had been obtained by means of the Judkins technique, using preformed right and left coronary catheters. In a minority of cases, alternative catheters (mainly the Multipurpose or Am-

TABLE 4.1. *Demographics of the patient population (Total n = 1950)*

Patient group	Number	Percentage
Patients with coronary artery disease	1290/1950	66
Patients without coronary artery disease	660/1950	33
Men	1369/1950	79
Women	581/1950	21
Men with coronary artery disease	1019/1369	74.4
Women with coronary artery disease	271/581	46.6

platz right or left coronary preformed curves) were used after the primary catheters failed to allow selective catheterization. Such failure occurred with greatly increased frequency in cases of coronary anomalies, especially when the coronary ostium was juxta-commissural or tangentially oriented with respect to the aortic wall. Although the brachial approach entailed less frequent need for a secondary catheter, even in the presence of anomalous coronary origination, this approach was used in less than 10% of cases.

In almost all cases, Renografin® or Hypaque-76® was injected as a contrast medium. Unlike the currently more popular low-osmolar media, Renografin and Hypaque have slightly better contrast characteristics. They cause more severe transient bradycardia, allowing better definition of the myocardial blush phase of coronary angiography and, therefore, better definition of the dependent myocardial territory.[224]

Criteria for Describing the Angiographic Anatomy of the Coronary Tree (Fig. 4.11)

We specifically and systematically studied the following coronary angiographic features:

Origin

To elucidate the relationship between the coronary ostia and the aortic sinuses, we examined the morphology of the coronary sinuses (best seen in the right anterior oblique orientation with a 30° cranial tilt or in the left anterior oblique orientation with a 30° caudal tilt); the vertical level of the coronary ostia in the aortic root, with respect to the bottom of the aortic sinus and to the sinotubular junction or ridge; and the orientation of the proximal coronary stems (variants: normal, tangential). To adequately describe these features angiographically, it was often greatly advantageous to dispose of nonselective injections at the cusp. (Such injections are not routinely performed in clinical studies.) In most cases of coronary anomalies, however, some nonselective contrast injections were necessary because of the initial difficulty of selectively cannulating unusual, unexpected ostia with routine preformed angiographic catheters.

Proximal Coronary Trunks

When the proximal trunks of the RCA, LAD, and/or circumflex artery were combined into a single vessel, they were called mixed trunks and were labeled as follows: RCA-circumflex, RCA-LAD, RCA-LAD-circumflex, LAD-RCA, or LAD-RCA-circumflex.

Course

In describing anomalies of origination, the proximal course of a coronary artery is frequently an open question. Therefore, the relationship between the coronary arteries and other cardiac structures (mainly the atrioventricular and semilunar valves) was studied by inference, and the coronary courses were observed in different angiographic projections to reconstruct their tridimensional anatomy.[185] In some cases, a catheter was positioned in the pulmonary artery for reference. In complex cases, simultaneous right and left ventriculography, or at least biplane aortography, was available.

Coronary Patterns

The myocardial territories of distribution of the coronary branches were studied by inference. The examination focused on the following main features:

1. Left main trunk. The presence or absence of a left main trunk was defined by the presence or lack of visualization of the circumflex or LAD during injection of the ostium of the opposite artery (the LAD or circumflex, respectively). Angiograms were excluded if they involved excessive subselective positioning of the catheter in any of the two left branches. Some reflow in the aortic sinus was necessary to rule out artifactual studies.

2. The LAD branch was identified by its anterior course and multiple septal penetrating branches, not necessarily by its diagonal branches. The diagonal arteries were defined as secondary branches that typically, but not necessarily, originated from the proximal segment of the LAD and spread over the anterior and lateral wall of the left ventricle, next to the anterior interventricular groove artery (the LAD). The diagonal artery may also have originated from the left main trunk, the circumflex, or the ramus medianus.

3. The posterior descending branch was identified on the basis of its multiple posterior septal penetrating branches.

4. The atrioventricular node artery was noted as an indicator for the posteroinferior edge of the interventricular septum (the location of the atrioventricular node). By itself, however, this branch was not considered capable of identifying the dominant artery, which was assumed to be the vessel(s) that supplied the posterior descending arteries with their posterior septal branches (Fig. 4.12).

5. Specific attention was dedicated to the blood supply of the intraventricular septum during the late phase of

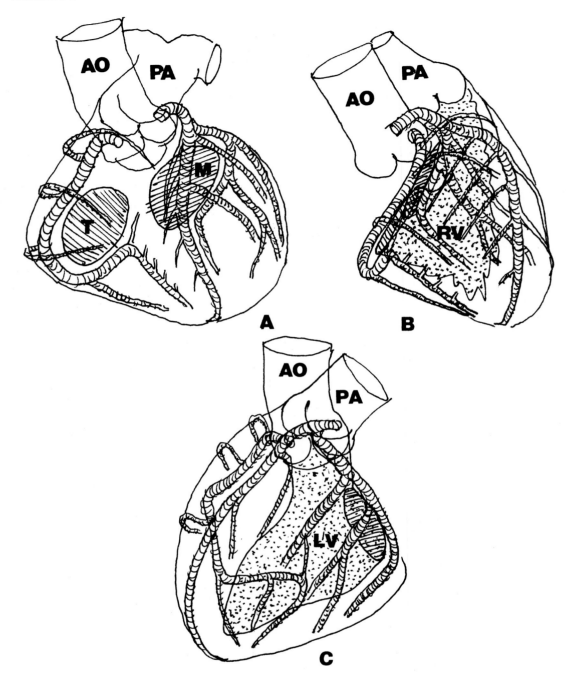

FIGURE 4.11. Relationship between coronary arteries and cardiac structures as seen in the frontal **(A),** right anterior oblique **(B),** and left anterior oblique **(C)** projections. AO = aorta; LV = left ventricle; M = mitral valve; PA = pulmonary artery; RV = right ventricle; T = tricuspid valve.

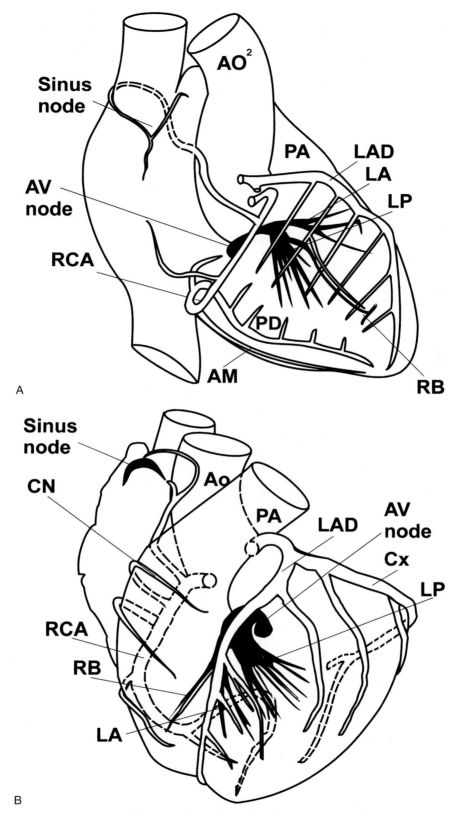

FIGURE 4.12. Right **(A)** and left **(B)** anterior oblique views of the main coronary branches and related cardiac structures. Abbreviations: AM = acute marginal artery; Ao = aorta; AV = atrioventricular; CN = conal branch; Cx = circumflex artery; LA = left anterior fascicle of the left bundle branch; LAD = left anterior descending artery; LP = left posterior fascicle of the left bundle branch; PD = posterior descending branch; PA = pulmonary artery; RB = right bundle; RCA = right coronary artery; SN = sinus node.

41

coronary angiography, when myocardial blushing is frequently seen, especially in the left anterior oblique projection, during angiography of both the LCA and the RCA.

6. The obtuse margin of the heart (left ventricle) was identified by recognizing the border of the heart in the left anterior oblique projection (at about 45°; see Figures 4.8 and 4.11). The circumflex artery was identified as the vessel that coursed in the left atrioventricular groove, crossing the obtuse margin of the heart. The larger lateral wall branches, starting from the obtuse margin and moving posteriorly toward the posterior descending artery, were labeled the obtuse marginal 1 (OM1), obtuse marginal 2 (OM2), and obtuse marginal 3 (OM3).

7. Right coronary branches. We used the following nomenclature for right coronary branches:

   a. "Infundibular (or conal) branch" (Fig. 4.12) was used to designate branches that serve the anterior free wall of the right ventricular outflow tract (grossly the 3- to 5-cm segment of myocardial territory below the pulmonary valve). These branches may have direct independent aortic origination. Because infundibular branches that originate separately are usually smaller than the tip of the diagnostic catheter, selective catheterization of such independent branches was rarely observed.

   b. "Right ventricular branch" was used to designate branches that serve the free wall of the inlet and the apical portion of the right ventricle. We tried only to identify the acute marginal branch as the artery that lies closest to the acute margin of the heart. The acute margin of the heart was identified angiographically as the lowest point in the "C" described by the RCA in the left and right anterior oblique views (Fig. 4.12).

   c. "Posterior descending branch" was used to designate the branch that follows the posterior interventricular groove and is angiographically identified by the posterior septal penetrating branches (Fig. 4.12). Compared with the anterior septal penetrating branches, the posterior ones are shorter, frequently being similar in length to the penetrating branches in the free wall of the left ventricle. For this reason, our favored means of identifying the posterior descending branch (and, hence, the dominant artery) was the myocardial blush phase during coronary angiography in the left anterior oblique projection, especially with a caudal tilt, when available. We used the term "codominant circumflex and RCA" for cases in which two branches, one from each of these arteries, coursed into the posterior descending groove, providing septal perforators (Table 4.2).

   d. "Posterolateral" was used to designate branches that provide flow to some portion of the posterolateral wall of the left ventricle, extending as far as the obtuse margin and sometimes including the posteromedial papillary muscle (Fig. 4.8).

TABLE 4.2. *Incidence of coronary anomalies and patterns, as observed in a continuous series of 1950 angiograms*

Variable	Number	Percentage
Coronary anomalies (total)	110	5.64
Split RCA	24	1.23
Ectopic RCA (right cusp)	22	1.13
Ectopic RCA (left cusp)	18	0.92
Fistulas	17	0.87
Absent left main coronary artery	13	0.67
Circumflex arising from right cusp	13	0.67
LCA arising from right cusp	3	0.15
Low origination of RCA	2	0.1
Other anomalies	3	0.27
Coronary dominance patterns		
Dominant RCA	1641	89.1
Dominant LCA (circumflex)	164	8.4
Codominant arteries (RCA, circumflex)	48	2.5

LCA = left coronary artery; RCA = right coronary artery.

Correlations (Table 4.3)

After identifying the variant anatomic patterns, we related them to the following variables: sex, the presence of coronary disease (criterion: >50% obstruction of vessel with a lumen larger than 1.5 mm), the presence of a primary cardiomyopathy (myocardial systolic dysfunction in the absence of coronary disease and/or a clinical history of myocardial infarction able to justify contractile dysfunction). Coronary anomalies were classified according to the scheme

TABLE 4.3. *Correlations*

Variable	Number	Percentage
Men with coronary anomalies	66/1369	4.82
Women with coronary anomalies	44/581	7.6
Patients with CAD and coronary anomalies	63/1290	4.96
Patients without CAD and coronary anomalies	57/1950	8.6
Patients with aortic valve anomalies	75/1950	3.8
Patients with aortic valve anomalies and coronary anomalies	20/75	26.7
Patients with cardiomyopathy	96/1950	4.92[a]
Patients with cardiomyopathy and coronary anomalies	5/96	5.2[a,b]
Patients without cardiomyopathy but with coronary anomalies	105/1854	5.7[b]

[a] P = .90 (NS)
[b] P = .85 (NS).
CAD = coronary artery disease

described in the section entitled Coronary Anomalies, as summarized in Table 4.4 in the Coronary Anomalies section.

Results (Tables 4.1 through 4.3)

Coronary artery obstructive disease was present in 1287 patients (66%) (Table 4.1). The incidence was greater in men (78%) than in women (40%) (*P* < .0001). Coronary variants were identified in 110 individuals (5.6%) (Table 4.2). Such variants were more common in women (7.6%) than in men (4.8%; *P* = .008) (Table 4.3). Primary myocardial impairment (hypokinesia in the absence of obstructive coronary lesions) was not observed more frequently in patients with coronary anomalies (5.2%) than would be expected in the general population. Seventy-five patients (3.8%) had aortic valve disease that was probably of congenital origin, based only on asymmetry of the aortic sinuses. In 20 (27%) of these cases, coronary variants or anomalies were also present. The incidence of coronary variants was significantly higher than that encountered in the patients with coronary artery obstructive disease (4.9%; *P* < .0001) or in the series as a whole (5.6%; *P* < .0001). The incidence of coronary anomalies seemed to be mildly increased in the patients without coronary disease (8.6%; *P* = .001) compared to those with coronary disease. A dominant RCA pattern was present in 89.1% of the general population. The circumflex artery was dominant in only 8.4%, and codominance (RCA, circumflex) was observed in 2.5% (Table 4.2).

Discussion

The most frequent coronary variants (Table 4.2) were split RCA or double posterior descending artery (1.23%) and anomalous origination of the RCA from an ectopic site close to, or at, the right anterior aortic sinus (1.13%) (Table 4.2). These were the only two variants that were present in more than 1% of the cases. According to the "more than 1% incidence" criterion, these morphologies should be considered normal variants.

Because absence of a common left main trunk was observed in only 0.67% of the cases, this pattern should be considered a coronary anomaly, at least as defined by our angiographic criteria. Coronary fistulas were seen in 0.87% of the cases: these were usually small, multiple fistulas that opened into the left ventricle. Admittedly, many of the cineangiograms had too short a running time to identify some of the smaller fistulas. Ad hoc prospective studies may indicate that small coronaro-cameral fistulas (see pages 60–63) are present in more than 1% of normal hearts.

A similar case may be made with regard to muscular bridges. In our series, such bridges were encountered in only five cases (0.003%), but this variant is detected with much increased frequency when more precise, prospective angiographic and anatomic techniques are used (see pages 56–57). Specific angiographic studies intended to rule out myocardial bridges should include multiple views of the LAD (at

least) after intracoronary nitroglycerin administration,[11] which was not routinely done in our series.

In previous angiographic studies reported in the literature, the total incidence of coronary anomalies has ranged from 0.2 to 1.5%, and the frequency of individual anomalies has varied, mainly because of the use of different methods and study criteria.[76,96,206,435] The fact that we detected coronary anomalies on 5.6% of our angiograms was primarily related to the meticulous, prospective quality of our analysis.

Our study had two main intrinsic limitations. First, coronary angiography does not always allow the accurate detection (or exclusion) of some anatomic features that may be relevant for describing normal human coronary arteries. We especially allude to the exclusion of certain associated congenital heart anomalies that may affect the coronary morphology to a greater or lesser extent. Whereas coronary angiography can reliably exclude major congenital defects such as transposition of the great vessels or common truncus arteriosus, this modality may fail to detect minor aortic valve anomalies.[227] We were especially interested in identifying abnormal aortic valves, as there is a notable association between anomalies of the aortic sinuses and those of coronary origination.[227,348] We elected to analyze the coronary patterns in patients who had structurally normal hearts, but minor congenital anomalies of the aortic valve may have been overlooked.

The study's second limitation was that, in our patient population, the usual indication for coronary angiography was clinical evidence of coronary artery obstructive disease or presumption of such disease. It is theoretically possible that congenital anomalies indeed predispose patients to coronary artery disease; if so, our population did not represent the general population. For this reason, we separately analyzed the incidence of coronary artery disease in both the subset with coronary anomalies and the larger population with normal coronary patterns. Despite these limitations, we thought that an angiographic ad hoc analysis was the only practical way to assess the frequency of coronary anomalies in a large clinical series. Autopsy studies of a large series would have been quite difficult and expensive to carry out.

As seen in Table 4.2, less frequent anomalies were also encountered in our series: some of these and other anomalies observed by the authors over the last several years are the object of the angiographic atlas of coronary anomalies that accompanies the following systematic discussion.

CORONARY ANOMALIES

Table 4.4 presents a list of coronary anomalies that aims at being comprehensive and rational but is yet historical and nontheoretical. Additional coronary anomalies could potentially occur, but we have never encountered such anomalies and are unaware of any descriptions of them. Examples could include (1) anomalous origination of the LAD from a posterior septal perforator and (2) anomalous course of a

TABLE 4.4. *Classification of coronary anomalies in (normal) human hearts*

A) Anomalies of origination and course
   1) Absent left main trunk (split origination of LCA)
   2) Anomalous location of coronary ostium within aortic root or near proper aortic sinus of Valsalva (for each artery):
      a) High
      b) Low
      c) Commissural
   3) Anomalous location of coronary ostium outside normal "coronary" aortic sinuses
      a) Right posterior aortic sinus
      b) Ascending aorta
      c) Left ventricle
      d) Right ventricle
      e) Pulmonary artery Variants:
         1) LCA arising from posterior facing sinus
         2) Cx arising from posterior facing sinus
         3) LAD arising from posterior facing sinus
         4) RCA arising from anterior right facing sinus
         5) Ectopic location (outside facing sinuses) of any coronary artery from pulmonary artery
            • From anterior left sinus
            • From pulmonary trunk
            • From pulmonary branch
      f) Aortic arch
      g) Innominate artery
      h) Right carotid artery
      i) Internal mammary artery
      j) Bronchial artery
      k) Subclavian artery
      l) Descending thoracic aorta
   4) Anomalous origination of coronary ostium from opposite, facing "coronary" sinus (which may involve joint origination or adjacent double ostia). Variants:
      a) RCA arising from left anterior sinus, with anomalous course:
         1) Posterior atrioventricular groove* or retrocardiac
         2) Retroaortic[a]
         3) Between aorta and pulmonary artery[a]
         4) Intraseptal[a]
         5) Anterior to pulmonary outflow[a] or precardiac
         6) Posteroanterior interventricular groove[a]
      b) LAD arising from right anterior sinus, with anomalous course:
         1) Between aorta and pulmonary artery
         2) Intraseptal
         3) Anterior to pulmonary outflow or precardiac
         4) Posteroanterior interventricular groove

   c) Cx arising from right anterior sinus, with anomalous course:
      1) Posterior atrioventricular groove
      2) Retroaortic
   d) LCA arising from right anterior sinus, with anomalous course:
      1) Posterior atrioventricular groove[a] or retrocardiac
      2) Retroaortic[a]
      3) Between aorta and pulmonary artery[a]
      4) Intraseptal[a]
      5) Anterior to pulmonary outflow[a] or precardiac
      6) Posteroanterior interventricular groove[a]
   5) Single coronary artery
B) Anomalies of intrinsic coronary arterial anatomy
   1) Congenital ostial stenosis or atresia (LCA, LAD, RCA, Cx)
      a) Coronary ostial dimple
      b) Coronary ectasia or aneurysm
   2) Absent coronary artery
   3) Coronary hypoplasia
   4) Intramural coronary artery (muscular bridge)
   5) Subendocardial coronary course
   6) Coronary crossing
   7) Anomalous origination of posterior descending artery from anterior descending branch or septal penetrating branch
   8) Absent PD (split RCA)
      Variants:
      a) (Proximal + distal) PDs, both arising from RCA
   9) Absent LAD (split LAD). Variants:
      a) LAD + first large septal branch
      b) LAD, double
   10) Ectopic origination of first septal branch
C) Anomalies of coronary termination
   1) Inadequate arteriolar/capillary ramifications?
   2) Fistulas from RCA, LCA, or infundibular artery to:
      a) Right ventricle
      b) Right atrium
      c) Coronary sinus
      d) Superior vena cava
      e) Pulmonary artery
      f) Pulmonary vein
      g) Left atrium
      h) Left ventricle
      i) Multiple, right + left ventricles
D) Anomalous collateral vessels

[a] If a single, common ostium is present, the pattern is considered to represent "single" coronary artery.
Cx = circumflex; LAD = left anterior descending coronary artery; LCA = left coronary artery; PD = posterior descending branch; RCA = right coronary artery.

coronary artery inside the atrial septum. Our proposed classification scheme is based on our own experience as angiographers and a thorough review of the pertinent literature. It stresses a meticulous, orderly approach in which each feature of the normal coronary anatomy is viewed as a criterion for potential anomalies. We prefer to combine the traditional headings ''anomalies of origin'' and ''anomalies of course,''[115,287] because a coronary artery's proximal course can be abnormal only if that artery's origin is abnormal (except in the case of intramural or subendocardial coronary arteries). Rather than favoring alphabetical-numerical listings, we prefer descriptive, clear terminology that identifies each anomaly. Moreover, we prefer to avoid labeling an anomaly with the name of its purported discoverer.

In this section, most of the descriptions of coronary anomalies are followed by case presentations that illustrate the anomalies' typical features. Because our institution has a limited collection of anatomic specimens, the illustrations are primarily angiographic. Additionally, relevant clinical and functional correlations are presented. A general discussion of the clinical and functional consequences of coronary anomalies is included at the end of this chapter.

The clinical features of major coronary anomalies that tend to manifest in the pediatric age group are described in Chapter 5, which also discusses the surgical treatment of those anomalies.

INDIVIDUAL ANOMALIES OF ORIGINATION AND COURSE

Absent Left Main Trunk (Split Origination of the LCA)

Isolated absence of a left main trunk is defined as that condition in which both the LAD and the circumflex artery originate directly from the center section of the left sinus of Valsalva, without having a common trunk.[94,391] In 2000 consecutive autopsies, Vlodaver and associates[413] found this anomaly in 1% of the cases. In a prospective analysis of a continuous series of 1950 angiograms (see pages 38–43), researchers at the Texas Heart Institute concluded that the incidence of absent left main trunk (as thereby defined) was only 0.55%, suggesting that this entity is properly classified as an anomaly. The left main trunk should also be considered to be absent when the LAD or circumflex artery originates ectopically, outside the left coronary sinus (this condition is known as secondary absence of a left main trunk). On the contrary, when both the LAD and the circumflex artery originate ectopically, an ectopic left main trunk may be present if the LAD and circumflex arteries share a proximal, conjoined stem of any length (see pages 50–54). The clinical relevance of isolated absence of a left main trunk appears to be limited,[430] as this anatomic pattern, *per se,* cannot be expected to produce any functional ischemic effect. In cases involving an absent left main trunk, special techniques must be used for selective catheterization and angiography, as mentioned earlier (page 39); moreover, angioplasty of either the LAD or the circumflex artery may necessitate certain technical adaptations. The coronary ostia are usually smaller than would be expected in the presence of a common left main trunk, and the routine preformed guiding catheter may subselectively cannulate the target vessel, resulting in its obstruction. Typically, the Judkins left coronary catheter will selectively cannulate the LAD, and the Amplatz left coronary catheter will tend to cannulate the circumflex artery. In contrast to patients who have a left main trunk, those with an absent left main trunk cannot develop left main stenosis, the most severe form of coronary disease.

(See Case Report 4.1 in the Atlas of Case Reports)

Anomalous Origination of a Coronary Ostium at or Near the Normal Aortic Sinus of Valsalva

As discussed earlier, an exact definition of normal versus abnormal coronary origination from the aortic root would depend on the completion of studies in large populations, which could be done only from an anatomic standpoint. Meanwhile, it seems safe to state that coronary arteries which arise above the sinotubular ridge or junction and/or which are located next to the aortic commissures[234,496] are anomalous, even when located in the vicinity of the expected sites in the proper sinus of Valsalva (Fig. 4.6). A "commissural" coronary ostium should probably be defined as an ostium located less than 5 mm away from an aortic valve commissure (or apex of the intercuspal triangle). In this group of anomalies, "high" origination tends to overlap with ectopic origination from the ascending aorta. We propose that ostia located less than 1 cm "above normal" be included in this group; this classification would be especially valuable for angiographic purposes, since the sinotubular junction often cannot be precisely identified.

A more subtle variation, which usually goes unrecognized, is anomalously low origination within the proper coronary sinus (Fig. 4.7). This condition is recognizable anatomically and angiographically because the involved ostium is located close to the lower rim of implantation of the aortic cusp. Preformed coronary catheters often fail to allow selective cannulation because they are designed to be aimed specifically at the mid portion of the right and left aortic sinuses and, more importantly, because the proximal stems of these ectopic coronary arteries may be tangential[508]—rather than orthogonal—with respect to the aortic wall. Angiographic studies of such anomalies frequently require the use of more than one catheter, multiple injections of a contrast medium (including initial subselective injections to locate the anomalous ostium), and a prolonged catheter manipulation and fluoroscopy time.

In these cases, selective catheterization is especially important, because tangential origination of such ectopic arteries leads to an increased incidence of ostial coronary stenosis (involving atherosclerosis and/or congenital ostial ridges or fibrous thickening), as seen in *Case Report 4.3,* below. Multiple angiographic projections may be necessary for proper visualization of such ostial stenoses. Tangential origination seems to be a definite anatomic risk factor for coronary artery obstructive disease. Otherwise, this anomaly apparently causes no clinical repercussions except for difficult cannulation during coronary angioplasty. However, because aortic valve replacement is usually accomplished via an aortotomy just above the sinotubular junction of the ascending aorta, high origination of the RCA may interfere with this surgical approach. Implantation of the ring of an aortic valve prosthesis should not be hindered if these anomalies are recognized beforehand (especially in cases involving low origination of the RCA).

(See Case Reports 4.2 Through 4.7 in the Atlas of Case Reports)

Anomalous Location of a Coronary Ostium Outside the Normal "Coronary" Aortic Sinuses

Ectopic Coronary Ostium Located at or near the Right Posterior Aortic Sinus (Noncoronary)

The right posterior coronary sinus is commonly termed "noncoronary" because coronary ostia are only rarely, if ever, observed in this sinus.[77,219,285,435,526,527,529] A fundamental condition for including a case in this category is the presence of a normal, trifoliate aortic valve. Some of the patients reported in the literature have had, or could have had, substantial anomalies of the aortic valve, mainly of the bicuspid kind. In most true cases of these anomalies, the ectopic ostium has a commissural location: usually it is the LCA ostium that is located next to the posterior left commissure. In itself, this anomaly is benign unless it involves a tangential origin (as it frequently does), in which case it may carry an increased risk of ostial stenosis and/or enhanced spasticity. During coronary angiography, this anomaly causes difficult cannulation as a result of its unexpected location and its tangential or slitlike nature. When this anomaly is suspected after initial unsuccessful attempts to cannulate, biplane aortography is recommended. The right anterior oblique and straight lateral projections are the most contributory ones for establishing posterior origination of the LCA. The relationship between the ostium and the aortic sinuses should be documented, preferably using the right anterior oblique projection with a cranial tilt and selective injections. For selective catheterization, the operator must be highly skilled and patient.[179,219,300,529] The Amplatz or Multipurpose curved catheters offer the best chance of success. Alternatively, the Sones catheter, advanced from the brachial artery, offers a favorable approach. In addition, intravascular ultrasound has recently been used to identify this anomaly (Fig. 4.13).[527]

This anomaly should be ruled out when selective cannulation cannot be achieved with Judkins left-sided catheters and nonselective angiography shows a longer than usual left main trunk. The anomaly is generally considered benign,[19,186,411] and the literature contains only one case in which origination of the left main artery from the noncoronary sinus led to a clinical event, namely the occurrence of a large, fatal anterior myocardial infarction in a 12-year-old girl.[529] The mechanism of coronary occlusion in this case was probably clot formation in the slitlike ostium of the anomalous vessel.

In the presence of this anomaly, angioplasty of any LCA's branches would also offer unusual difficulties because of precarious selective cannulation and back-up support.

(See Case Reports 4.8 and 4.9 in the Atlas of Case Reports)

Ectopic Coronary Ostium Arising Outside the Aortic Root, in the Ascending Aorta

An ectopic coronary ostium located outside the aortic root, in the ascending aorta, can be present at different levels but

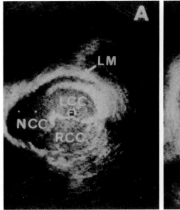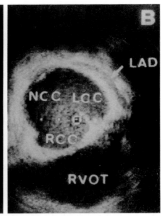

FIGURE 4.13. A. Intraaortic ultrasound image showing the left main coronary artery (LM, white arrow) originating from the square coronary sinus. **B.** The artery courses posteriorly around the left coronary sinus and gives rise to the left anterior descending artery (LAD, white arrow). The ultrasound transducer's position (in the left coronary sinus in view **A** and the right coronary sinus in view **B**) is indicated by the dark central square with the surrounding bright halo of ring-down artifact. The imaging field is scaled by 8-mm divisions. LCC = left coronary cusp; NCC = noncoronary cusp; RCC = right coronary cusp; RVOT = right ventricular outflow tract. (From Lo et al. Anomalous origin of left main coronary artery from the noncoronary sinus: an intravascular ultrasound observation. Cathet Cardiovasc Diagn 1997;42:431. Reprinted with permission.)

usually involves the anterior/left surface of the aorta.[180,201,234,344,390] In the rare cases reported in the literature, the site of coronary origination has ranged from just above the sinotubular junction to the origin of the innominate artery, several centimeters above the aortic valve. This condition differs from the previously discussed milder anomalies (page 45) in that, here, the ostium is clearly located above the sinotubular region of the aortic root; the ectopic coronary arteries frequently have slitlike orifices and a tangential proximal course along the aortic wall, on which they lie, loosely attached to the aortic tissue. Occasionally, the proximal coronary segment is intramural, inside the aortic wall, and is intussuscepted for 0.5 to 5.0 cm.[325] Once the ectopic coronary artery reaches the epicardial surface, it regains a normal location and course. The RCA is the most frequently ectopic artery, but the LCA (or, separately, the LAD and circumflex artery) may also originate ectopically. Although an ectopic proximal artery course is not a pathologic condition in itself, the artery may be predisposed to have a more active atherosclerotic buildup, especially at the ostium, perhaps because of rheologic factors and unusual shear stress.[409]

Angiography of this type of anomaly is frequently challenging and incomplete. The basic initial condition that should alert the angiographer is the absence of a coronary ostium at the expected site. In such cases, the first step is to rule out ostial atresia or occlusion, as suggested by retrograde filling of the distal "missing" artery from the contralateral ostium or a conal branch. The second step is to rule out necrosis of the dependent myocardium, in which case occlusion without collateral filling could be hypothesized. It is frequently necessary to obtain a biplane aortogram to visualize the anomalous vessel, even though nonselectively. On the basis of biplane aortographic data, the ascending aorta, especially the anterolateral segment, should be probed with special catheters to identify and selectively cannulate the ectopic ostium. The most helpful catheters for this purpose are the Sones, Multipurpose, and Amplatz models (especially the left, with its shorter curve) and only occasionally the routine Judkins catheters. Once the anomalous coronary artery has been selectively cannulated, angiography must be carried out in multiple projections, with special emphasis on those that show tangential views of the proximal segment, to rule out ostial stenosis.

Angioplasty of these vessels can be quite difficult, because of the unusual ostial features (intrinsic obstruction, a slitlike orifice, and a tangential proximal course),[259] which render selective catheterization with the larger guiding catheters unfeasible. During cardiac surgery, coronary arteries of this type may create unexpected problems if the anomaly is unsuspected. To avoid damaging the anomalous artery, the aortotomy should be carried out, after careful dissection of the ectopic vessel, at a higher level than usual, especially during aortic valve replacement.

Because congenital aortic valve anomalies are associated with an increased risk of coronary ectopia (see also Chapter 3), adequate preoperative evaluation by means of selective angiography is mandatory for such aortic valve anomalies, even in the absence of clinical evidence of coronary obstructive disease. Routine echocardiography will rarely identify such anomalies.

(See Case Report 4.10 in the Atlas of Case Reports)

Ectopic Coronary Ostium Arising from the Left Ventricle

To our knowledge, there have been only a few reports[81, 289,464] of origination of the RCA from an otherwise normal left ventricle, just below a congenitally insufficient and/or stenotic aortic valve, in adults (Fig. 4.14). This condition should be strictly defined as origination of a nutrient coronary vessel (providing flow to the myocardium) from the left ventricle. This definition excludes unrelated anomalies such as aorto-left ventricular tunnel and sinusoidal-coronary collaterals. Only in the presence of severe congenital stenosis or atresia, within the spectrum of left ventricular hypoplasia,[163,477,496] do the latter anomalies tend to occur, constituting a venting mechanism for the overloaded left ventricle, as occurs in the right ventricle in cases of pulmonary atresia with intact ventricular septum.[280] In such cases, communication between left ventricular intertrabecular spaces and normally originating epicardial coronary arteries (which may be stenotic or atretic) represents congenital collateral or vi-

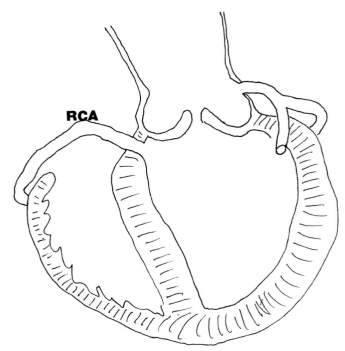

FIGURE 4.14. Schematic diagram showing anomalous origination of the right coronary artery (RCA) from the subvalvular left ventricular outflow tract. This anomaly probably represents the most extreme degree of caudal migration of the right coronary ostium (see Fig. 4.7).

carious circulation[484] and, therefore, should be regarded as a different entity from primary ectopia of the coronary artery.

Especially in the absence of significant aortic insufficiency, the anomalous artery that originates from the left ventricle will be seen to have diastolic flow into the left ventricle, in the presence of collateral flow from the opposite, normally originating coronary artery. In such cases, selective catheterization of the ectopic ostium is expected to be quite problematic. An ischemic effect on the dependent myocardium may be demonstrable, especially by means of nuclear scintigraphy.

Ectopic Coronary Ostium Arising From the Right Ventricle (see Chapter 6)

"Origination of a coronary artery from the right ventricle" is usually a misnomer for a complex congenital heart condition in which pulmonary atresia and an intact ventricular septum coexist with multiple right ventricular sinusoids, which functionally drain during systole into the neighboring coronary vessels;[31,129,163] during diastole, however, these sinusoids drain coronary blood to the right ventricle, in competition with nutrient flow to the myocardium (see Chapter 6). This condition has never been observed in an otherwise normal heart.

Ectopic Coronary Artery Arising from the Pulmonary Artery

As a major coronary anomaly that commonly manifests in the pediatric age group,[43,104] ectopic coronary artery originating from the pulmonary artery is more thoroughly discussed in Chapter 5. The present chapter covers general anatomic and nosologic considerations regarding this condition.

Anomalous origination of a coronary artery from the pulmonary artery is defined as that condition in which a coronary artery carrying nutrient flow anatomically arises from the pulmonary main trunk.[49] Indeed, a coronary artery is also connected to the main pulmonary artery (or its branches) in some cases of coronary fistulas.[26] To further confuse this issue, anomalous origination of a conal branch from the main pulmonary artery may result in a condition that resembles a coronary fistula both angiographically and anatomically. Interestingly, in anomalous origination of a coronary artery from the pulmonary artery, the direction of the fistulous flow is toward the pulmonary artery,[8,113,306,318,339,452] as seen in coronary-to-pulmonary fistulas. Nevertheless, in the present condition, blood flow originates from the contralateral, normally originating, coronary artery; whereas in coronary-to-pulmonary fistulas, flow originates from the coronary aortic ostium of the artery that has the fistulous communication.

The following forms of ectopic origination of one or more coronary arteries from the pulmonary artery have been reported.[73,197,277,278,426]

- Anomalous LCA arising from the posterior facing sinus of the pulmonary artery or from the pulmonary trunk or branches (the most common form, abbreviated as ALCAPA)[467]
- (Isolated) circumflex artery arising from the pulmonary artery (posterior facing sinus) or one of its branches[57,74,169,292]
- (Isolated) LAD arising from the posterior facing sinus of the pulmonary artery[98]
- RCA originating from the anterior facing sinus of the pulmonary artery or from the pulmonary trunk or its branches[102,251,264,378,420]
- Simultaneous RCA and LCA arising from the pulmonary artery[398,451,465,474] (sometimes originating in a single common trunk[503])
- Small (right infundibular or conal) branch arising from the anterior facing sinus of the pulmonary artery

Occasionally, ostial stenosis involving a ridge or fibrous buildup is observed in the pulmonary arterial wall.[252] This condition may significantly decrease fistulous flow.

Anomalous origination of the entire LCA from the pulmonary artery (ALCAPA) has distinct clinical features that are discussed in Chapter 5. In the literature and in clinical practice, several taxonomic classification criteria have been proposed, mainly in response to the clinical need for distinguishing between subtypes of ALCAPA that have different prognostic and therapeutic implications. This anomaly's clinical manifestations and anatomophysiologic forms are not adequately characterized by the terms "infantile" or "adult" or similar fuzzy descriptors (see Chapter 5) but, rather, require a more complex terminology.

ALCAPA varies greatly with respect to clinical presentation, prognostic implications, and the optimal choice and timing of therapy. Its treatment depends on multiple anatomic, functional, and clinical variables, including the following factors:

- The coronary dominance pattern (the larger the RCA, the better the results of simple ligation of the ectopic vessel and the overall prognosis)
- Obstruction of the ectopic ostium (the more severe the obstruction, the better the natural prognosis)
- The extent of acquired coronary artery obstructive disease (the more extensive the disease, the more severe the myocardial ischemia)
- Epicardial versus intramural collateral patterns (the former pattern promotes fistulous flow, and the latter one favors nutrient flow)
- The myocardial oxygen demand (which is related to left ventricular dilation, diastolic volume overload secondary to a left-to-right shunt and mitral regurgitation, and systemic vasoconstriction)
- The pulmonary artery pressure (the higher the pressure, the lower the fistulous flow)[276]
- Body weight and lifestyle factors

Less common, clinically different conditions—anomalous origination of the RCA, LAD, or circumflex artery from the pulmonary artery—are presented here, as they are usually compatible with prolonged, frequently asymptomatic, survival in the adult age group].

Anomalous Origination of the RCA, LAD, or Circumflex Artery From the Pulmonary Artery

Each of these three anomalies has different pathophysiologic consequences and clinical presentations. *Origination of the RCA from the pulmonary artery* has been described in several recent isolated case reports.[117,130,214,226,251,252,264,312,378,387,400,416,420] In most instances, the ectopic ostium was described as being located at the anterior right pulmonary cusp, and the RCA was dominant, with a posterior descending branch. In such cases, collateral circulation between the LCA and the RCA follows the patterns seen in atherosclerotic occlusion of the coronary arteries: the atrial, infundibular, right anterior, and septal branches may contribute to variable degrees in individual cases (Fig. 4.15A). The septal branches are usually the dominant source of collateral flow (from the LAD to the posterior descending artery). These enlarged vessels, with their fistulous flow, are prominently displayed not only during angiography but also during echocardiography with Doppler interrogation (Fig. 4.15). In adults, the condition is typically recognized because of a heart murmur or when angiography is performed for ac-

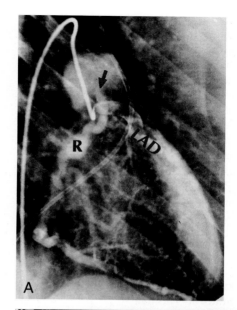

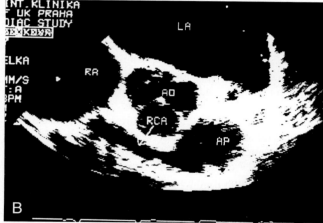

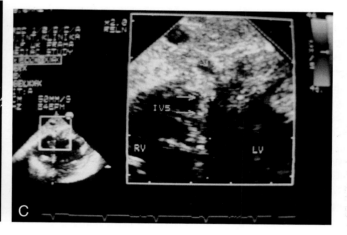

FIGURE 4.15. Anomalous origination of the RCA in a 36-year-old woman. A strictly systolic murmur was present on precordial auscultation. **A.** Angiogram of the LCA in the right anterior oblique projection (late frame). Residual contrast material is seen in the LCA. The mildly enlarged right coronary artery (R) drains into the pulmonary artery (arrow). LAD = left anterior descending artery. **B.** Transesophageal echocardiogram showing the three aortic valve sinuses (AO), next to the pulmonary artery (AP), from which the right coronary artery (RCA) originates from an anterior-right position. LA = left atrium; RA = right atrium. **C.** Color Doppler image of the ventricular septum in a four-chamber view, showing several sites of high-velocity (fistulous) flow (arrows) within the interventricular septum (IVS). LV = left ventricle; RV = right ventricle. (Photos courtesy of Dr. J. Veselka of Prague, Czech Republic.)

quired coronary obstructive disease, but some patients report angina[214] (frequently atypical) or have silent ischemia, as manifested by a positive stress test without angina.[130] Only in occasional cases does myocardial impairment cause congestive heart failure in patients of pediatric age.[400] Most adult patients with anomalous origination of the RCA from the pulmonary artery have normal left and right ventricular function, and there are no reports of sudden death related to this anomaly. Surgical treatment is similar to that for AL-CAPA; in fact, the first surgical reimplantation into the aorta of an ectopic coronary artery originating from the pulmonary artery involved an anomalous RCA (see Chapter 5). Location of the ectopic coronary ostium in the anterior cusp, adjacent to the aorta (Fig. 4.15*B*), greatly expedites surgical correction (see Chapter 5), and extracorporeal circulation is frequently not required.

An isolated *circumflex artery*[57,74,169,292] *or LAD*[98,309] may originate anomalously *from the pulmonary artery*. These anomalies are quite rare but are well recognized in the litera-

ture. Each condition is an instance of absent common left main trunk, and only one of the two left-sided arteries is ectopic. Therefore, with respect to its clinical presentation, this condition is much less severe than ALCAPA: the territory at risk for ischemia is more limited, and the sources of collateral flow are more abundant. Indeed, both the RCA and the normally originating left coronary branch provide collateral and fistulous flow. In most cases, the clinical presentation is benign. With LAD originating from the pulmonary artery, only one case of clinical ischemia resulting in a myocardial infarction has been reported.[98] Clinical findings typically include a heart murmur (usually only systolic, but possibly also continuous), atypical angina, and an unexpectedly abnormal stress test or angiogram. Although there are no reports of sudden death related to these anomalies, such an event is surely a possibility, especially during strenuous exertion. The anomalous LAD ostium is commonly located in the posterior left sinus, next to the aorta (in the facing cusps), and can usually be transferred surgically into the aorta with the aid of extracorporeal circulation and transection of the pulmonary artery (see Chapter 5). The ectopic circumflex artery more typically originates from a pulmonary branch (the proximal right or left), and reimplantation necessitates careful dissection.

Unlike in ALCAPA, the ratio of fistulous to nutrient flow seems to favor nutrient flow, so that myocardial ischemic manifestations tend to be more limited and to occur only with maximal exercise. Frequently, a relatively obstructive ectopic coronary ostium will also limit the fistulous flow. The amount of absolute flow probably perpetuates an intrinsic mechanism of progressive enlargement of the involved vessels.[103]

Although ectopic origination of a coronary artery from the pulmonary artery is routinely subjected to surgical repair, the need for repair has not been well established.[125] In the absence of major clinical manifestations (recurrent angina, myocardial infarction, ventricular arrhythmias, syncope, or aborted sudden death), anomalous origination from the pulmonary artery may not, in itself, be an automatic indication for surgery, especially if the anomalous vessel is a smaller one such as a nondominant RCA or a circumflex artery. In such cases, stress testing is frequently negative for reversible ischemia in adult patients, although mild fixed myocardial uptake defects are frequently found on nuclear images, because of old scar tissue and/or a rich collateral network, which replaces myocardial tissue.[125,264] Progressive enlargement of the dilated coronary vessels, with the risk of intimal changes, mural thrombosis, and/or accelerated atherosclerosis, is a possibility in these cases, just as in primary coronary fistula. This factor tends to encourage early intervention (during childhood or the patient's teen years), because otherwise the extremely dilated vessels with increased flow would be transformed, by surgical correction during adult life, into aneurysmatic vessels with normal flow, yielding a persistently poor prognosis because of the risk of mural thrombosis. After correction of this anomaly, coronary ectasia may undergo reversal in young patients but will not generally do so in older ones. The survival of untreated older patients is an indication, if not proof, of the benign nature of the anomaly in such instances. Moreover, the surgical risks may be substantially greater and the potential benefits fewer in older patients, causing many physicians to prefer continued medical treatment and some surgeons to prefer simple ligation (versus the more complex reimplantation) of the ectopic vessel.

(See Case Report 4.11 in the Atlas of Case Reports)

Ectopic Coronary Ostium Arising from the Aortic Arch, Innominate Artery, Right Carotid Artery, Internal Mammary Artery, Bronchial Artery, Subclavian Artery, or Descending Thoracic Aorta

The literature contains rare reports of extracardiac origination of the coronary arteries from the aortic arch,[63] innominate artery,[86] right carotid artery,[63] internal mammary artery,[329,330] bronchial artery,[63] subclavian artery,[330] or descending thoracic aorta[63] in humans. Most of these reports mention accompanying major congenital heart defects.[63,330] In such cases, the proximal coronary trunk's ectopia reproduces, in humans, the normal coronary pattern seen in various animals (see Chapter 1). Reports of bronchial origination of a coronary artery (see also Coronary-Bronchial Fistula, page 62) should be examined critically: because both the bronchial and the coronary arteries are normally subject to the same systemic pressure, no flow could be expected in the absence of a congenital coronary obstruction or a suprasystemic pulmonary pressure with an inverted patent ductus arteriosus (usually in the presence of a hypoplastic left heart syndrome). In cases of uncomplicated extracardiac origination of the coronary arteries from the systemic circulation, no myocardial ischemic effects are generally expected.

Anomalous Origination of a Coronary Artery from the Opposite, Facing Sinus of Valsalva

As stated earlier, the right, left, LAD, and circumflex coronary arteries are defined by virtue of their territory of distribution, not by their origination.[147] When a coronary artery arises anomalously from the opposite-from-normal sinus of Valsalva, the artery's intrinsic name and nature (or function) remain unchanged, and only its origin and proximal course are anomalous.[208] Of necessity, the artery's proximal course is abnormal in these cases, as the artery connects with the contralateral, in situ vascular network. Because these anomalies are characterized by abnormal origination of an otherwise ''normal'' coronary artery from the opposite sinus of Valsalva, it is important that the *essence* of a coronary artery (in contradistinction to, and independently of, its *origin*) be clearly defined.

Indeed, conceptually the human heart has not two, but three, coronary arteries: the RCA, LAD, and circumflex. The essence of each of these arteries was discussed previously (pages 35–38), and it becomes clear in light of the spectrum of possible variations described in this section.

The RCA is essentially that artery that courses in the right atrioventricular groove and provides nutritive branches to the free wall of the right ventricle. Branches that supply the right ventricular infundibulum, or conus, often originate directly from the right aortic sinus and are not an essential part of the RCA. The same is true of the sinus or atrioventricular nodal arteries and the posterior descending branch: all of these branches may originate anomalously without changing the nature of the RCA.

Similarly, the LAD is essentially that artery that courses along the anterior interventricular groove and provides perforating branches to most of the anterior ventricular septum. It is not essential that the LAD provide a diagonal branch (although it usually does) or reach the apex, but it is essential for the LAD to course mostly in the anterior subepicardial space. Cases in which a large, entirely intramyocardial first septal artery provides most of the anterior perforating branches in the absence of an anterior subepicardial artery are regarded as anomalous.

Finally, the circumflex artery is essentially that artery that follows the left atrioventricular groove and provides branches to the free wall of the left ventricle, supplying the obtuse margin of the heart. The precise extent of the essential territory of the circumflex artery is a matter of conventional agreement, and no authoritative (empirical) decision has yet been made in this regard.

In any case of anomalous origination of a coronary artery from the opposite sinus of Valsalva, specific attention should be devoted to the ostial location and anatomy, crossing pathway(s), and pathophysiologic and clinical consequences.

Ostial Location and Anatomy

The anomalous coronary artery originating from the contralateral sinus of Valsalva may arise directly from the aorta. Alternatively, the anomalous artery may arise jointly, by way of a mixed trunk,[419] with the coronary artery that normally originates from that cusp. In such a case, a single coronary artery is generally present. When the anomalous coronary artery has an independent aortic ostium, usually it is adjacent to the ostium of the coronary artery that normally arises from that sinus; moreover, the independent additional ostium frequently has a slitlike appearance[395] and an increased likelihood of intrinsic pathology (Fig. 4.16).[344,532] Occasionally, intussusception of the anomalous proximal trunk into the aortic wall is also observed.[340,384]

Crossing Pathways

After arising from the contralateral sinus of Valsalva, an anomalous coronary artery can take one of at least five (or six) crossing pathways—not four, as sometimes stated in the literature.[323] Each of these paths has a peculiar, consistent topographic anatomy[422,504] (Fig. 4.17).

Path 1 may be labeled *"retrocardiac"* to differentiate it from the "retroaortic" one (both paths being generically "posterior"). The retrocardiac path is located behind the tricuspid and mitral valves, at the posterior atrioventricular groove. It frequently goes unrecognized[40,323,327] but is an important alternative route. When an anomalous RCA takes this course, it constitutes the terminal branch of a superdominant circumflex artery, which reaches the right ventricular infundibulum. This condition is usually classified as "single LCA," since no RCA originates from the right sinus of Valsalva. We object to this nomenclature, because it erroneously suggests that these patients have no RCA. In reality, however, the RCA is perfectly developed, although it has an anomalous pattern *(see Case Report 4.16 in the Atlas of Case Reports).*

When the circumflex artery[293] originates from the right sinus of Valsalva jointly with the RCA and has a posterior course (behind the atrioventricular valves), the anomalous trunk that extends to the crux of the heart is indeed a mixed

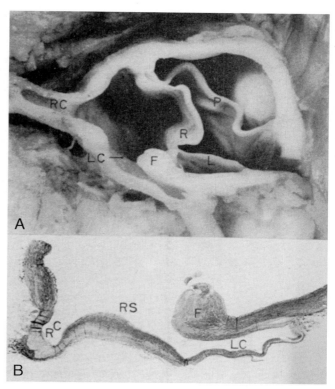

FIGURE 4.16. A. Gross view of a cross-section of the ascending aorta at upper levels of aortic valvular insertions. The right (RC) and left (LC) coronary arteries each arise from the right aortic sinus (RS). As the left coronary artery proceeds toward the patient's left, it makes an oblique angle with the aorta and creates a flap (F) in relation to its ostium. **B.** Section through the same plane as that shown in view **A,** showing the wall of the right aortic sinus from which arise the right and left coronary arteries. The oblique course of the ectopically arising left coronary artery creates, along with the aortic wall, a flap (elastic tissue stain, original magnification x5). L, P, and R = left, posterior, and right aortic cusps, respectively. (From Mahowald et al. Ectopic origin of a coronary artery from the aorta: sudden death in 3 of 23 patients. Chest 1986;89: 669. Reprinted with permission.)

trunk, not a simple RCA.[341] Similarly, the coronary artery that arises from the left cusp is indeed the LAD, not a true LCA, and the left main trunk is absent. Therefore, in such an instance, the diagnosis is absent left main trunk with anomalous origination of the circumflex artery from the distal RCA.

Similarly, the whole LCA may arise from the right anterior sinus jointly with the RCA and have a posterior course behind the atrioventricular valves. In such a case, the proximal trunk is a mixed one, not a "single RCA." The trunk distal to the crux of the heart is indeed an LCA that gives rise first to the circumflex-obtuse marginal and then to the LAD systems. Again, this condition is usually referred to as single RCA, and the above-mentioned objections to this terminology apply (see Single Coronary Artery).

Path 2, the *retroaortic* anomalous path (Fig. 4.17), is the

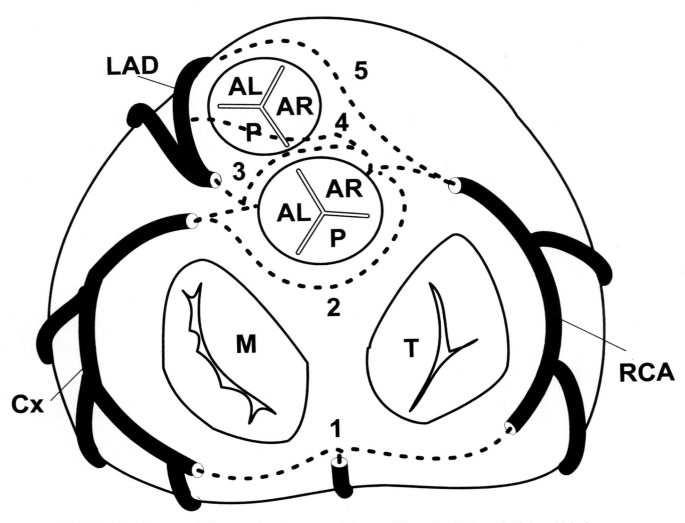

FIGURE 4.17. Conceptual diagram showing most of the possible paths (1 through 5) by which the RCA, LAD, and circumflex artery (Cx) can potentially connect with the opposite coronary cusps. Paths: 1, retrocardiac; 2, retroaortic; 3, preaortic, or between the aorta and pulmonary artery; 4, intraseptal (supracristal); 5, prepulmonary (precardiac). The aortic and pulmonary cusps are labeled according to their position in space: AL = antero-left; AR = antero-right; P = posterior; M = mitral valve; T = tricuspid valve.

path most commonly associated with this type of anomaly, specifically involving origination of the circumflex artery from the right sinus of Valsalva.[41,334,365] This anomaly's incidence in the general population ranges from 0.1 to 0.9%,[21a,41] including cases in which the circumflex artery has a separate origin, adjacent to the RCA ostium, and those in which the circumflex artery arises jointly with the RCA from a common short, mixed trunk. The anomalous retroaortic circumflex path courses just next to the posterior wall of the aorta, in the sulcus between the atria and the aorta (the transverse sinus), and finally reaches a normal location in the left atrioventricular groove, providing pathognomonic angiographic features.[41] Cardiac surgeons should be especially aware of this anomalous coronary path, because placement of sutures at the aortic or mitral annulus during valve

replacement might compromise the aberrant vessel. Otherwise, the anomaly, in itself, is not expected to have any clinical consequences.[336]

The same retroaortic path can also be observed, although less frequently,[324] when the RCA originates from the left sinus (either directly or, more often, from a common mixed trunk), and when the entire LCA originates from the right sinus. The retroaortic path is not seen, however, when the LAD has an isolated ectopic origin.

Path 3, the *preaortic* anomalous path, (Fig. 4.17) courses *"between the aorta and pulmonary artery."* This terminology alludes to the fact that an anomalous RCA or LAD or left main trunk (but never the isolated circumflex artery) subepicardially crosses the aortopulmonary septum or space. Embryologically, the aortopulmonary septum is initially intact, formed by the truncal swellings or ridges that subdivide the primitive common truncus. The fact that a coronary artery can be observed to cross the area of the embryologic aortopulmonary septum testifies to the lateness of definition of the proximal coronary anatomy, which occurs well after the completion of truncal septation (see Chapter 1). This path usually entails ostial abnormalities,[213,324,346] but it rarely, if ever, involves systolic compression (unlike path 4, which is intramyocardial).[44]

Recently, crossing of the aortopulmonary septum by the RCA, LAD, or left main artery has been presumed to be the culprit for clinical ischemic manifestations and/or sudden death.[25,32,47,140,159,272,324,335,338,384,494] This subject is addressed in the final section of the present chapter, which discusses the pathophysiologic mechanisms and clinical relevance of coronary anomalies.

Path 4, known as the *intraseptal* path (Fig. 4.17), is mainly located inside the upper, anterior interventricular septum (which embryologically is derived from the conal septum). This path joins the left-sided subepicardial coronary system at the upper anterior interventricular groove, where the LAD meets the aberrant trunk (which never directly joins the left main or circumflex artery). This anomalous path is mostly intramural (intramyocardial) and is frequently recognized angiographically because of its systolic phasic narrowing, as in a muscular bridge.[352,491] Also, the intramural anomalous trunk almost always produces one or two septal perforators that indicate the intraseptal portion of the arterial trunk.[57] In the differential diagnosis based on angiographic data, these two features (intramyocardial course and origin of septal vessels) should be considered characteristic of path 4 (not paths 3 or 5). Whether the anomalous vessel is an RCA,[324] LAD, or left main trunk, it immediately surfaces epicardially on the right side of the heart, beyond the level of the ventricular septum. The anomalous artery then continues until it joins a normal distal RCA (in the case of an anomalous RCA) or an aortic orifice located next to the RCA (in the case of an anomalous LAD or left main trunk). This anomalous path is sometimes called supracristal, but this nomenclature is erroneous, as the anomalous vessel runs behind the crista supraventricularis of the right ventricle and does not directly cross it (Fig. 4.4).

Path 5, also known as the *precardiac* or *prepulmonic* path, is characterized by its subepicardial location, on the anterior wall of the right ventricular outflow tract, or infundibulum. Again, this path may be taken by an ectopic RCA,[263,324,488] LAD, or left main trunk, but never by an isolated ectopic circumflex artery. It is particularly common in patients with tetralogy of Fallot (see Chapter 6), in which the LAD originates ectopically from the right coronary sinus and courses anterior to the hypoplastic, stenotic pulmonary infundibulum. The right-sided point of connection for an ectopic LAD or left main artery is usually the proximal RCA; alternatively, the anomalous artery may connect directly to a supplementary aortic ostium adjacent to the RCA's ostium. If the ectopic vessel with an anterior (prepulmonary) course is

the RCA, it arises from the proximal LAD (not the left main artery), crosses the pulmonary infundibulum, and quickly joins the right atrioventricular groove, regaining a normal course from that point on. The anomalous precardiac vessel frequently gives rise to infundibular but never septal branches.

The presence of a *sixth anomalous path* could be postulated if one considers that the apical route could constitute an alternative origination pathway, as exemplified by cases in which the posterior descending artery originates from the LAD or vice versa (see pages 54–59).

In many cases, the patient will have multiple simultaneous ectopic pathways.[419,498]

Pathophysiologic and Clinical Consequences

This subject is discussed extensively in the last section of this chapter (see Pathophysiologic Mechanisms and Clinical Implications of Coronary Anomalies).

(See Case Reports 4.12 Through 4.34 in the Atlas of Case Reports)

Single Coronary Artery

When a single aortic ostium or origination provides for all of the coronary blood flow, the condition is frequently called single coronary artery.[7,143,167,198,242,283,356,357,360,423,479] It comprises a mixed group of anomalies of coronary origination, already described under other headings, whose only common element is the presence of a single aortic ostium.[40] In the general population, the incidence of single coronary artery is approximately 0.024%,[242,360] so this condition is clearly an anomaly.

In the majority of cases diagnosed as "single left" coronary artery, a thorough anatomic study will reveal that another, small ostium exists in the right coronary cusp and leads to a conal or infundibular branch. In such cases, the diagnosis of single coronary artery is still correct, because the RCA originates (with respect to its essence) from the left ostium. In cases of "single right" coronary artery, no coronary artery, however small, is seen to arise from the left coronary cusp.

The primary classification (and terminology) for single coronary arteries should be based on the location of the single ostium[242,360] (in the right anterior cusp, left anterior cusp, or an ectopic position[180,198]), not on the nature of the single artery itself.[44] Indeed, the anomalous vessel's single proximal trunk should not be designated the RCA or LCA according to the cusp of origination; rather, it should be considered a common mixed trunk, since it gives rise to both the right and left coronary branches, which are labeled (as in a normal coronary tree) according to their respective areas of distribution.[419]

All of the combinations listed in Table 4.5 can occur, and most of them have been reported in the literature. These combinations should be described according to their ostial

TABLE 4.5. *Single Coronary Arteries: Classification Criteria*

Sinus of Origination
1) Right anterior sinus
2) Left anterior sinus
3) Posterior sinus
4) Ectopic sinus, at:
   A) Ascending aorta
   B) Systemic artery
   C) Pulmonary artery
Pathways Followed by Each Ectopic Branch Arising From the Proximal Trunk[a]
1) Retrocardiac (circumflex, LCA or RCA)
2) Retroaortic (circumflex, LCA, or RCA)
3) Preaortic (LCA or RCA)
4) Intraseptal (LCA, LAD, or RCA)
5) Precardiac (LCA, LAD, or RCA)

   [a] Any individual case may involve more than one anomalous path.

location, their sequence of origination, and the proximal course of their anomalous coronary branches.[362] Excluded from this list are several conditions that resemble single coronary artery but involve ectopic origination of a coronary artery from the opposite cusp, from an additional ostium adjacent to the normal coronary ostium for that cusp. To conclusively establish the diagnosis of single coronary artery, angiographers and anatomists should verify (1) the presence of a single ostium in one sinus, jointly with the absence of an ostium in the opposite sinus, and (2) the lack of origination of any other coronary artery from an ectopic site. This process is usually quite simple for anatomists but may be harder for angiographers, who may encounter difficulties in ascertaining that the artery in question indeed supplies all of the heart and that no additional ectopic coronary artery exists.

Functionally, single coronary artery has essentially the same clinical implications as ectopic coronary origination from the opposite sinus but with separate ostia; nevertheless, a single coronary artery is not as susceptible to tangential origin or ostial ridge pathology as are ectopic coronary arteries with independent ostia. Coronary blood flow is not affected by the simple presence of a single proximal trunk that supplies coronary flow to the entire heart, unless congenital or acquired obstructive disease is present in the proximal mixed trunk.[22,457] In such a case, the hemodynamic repercussions would be quite severe,[244,423] as the whole heart could become ischemic without having any possible source of collateral circulation. Although definitive studies are not available, the incidence of atherosclerotic disease does not appear to be increased in the mixed trunk. An ectopic single coronary ostium[180,198] could, indeed, be more susceptible to congenital (ostial) or acquired obstructive disease, but the rarity of this anomaly precludes adequate analysis.

During coronary angioplasty, a few minor adjustments are necessary in patients with a single coronary artery.[21,149,375,427] In the presence of a single ostium, even the temporary

creation of an ostial obstruction (by means of a large guiding catheter or any other instrument, such as the bulky directional atherectomy device) would be poorly tolerated and could cause symptoms (angina, dyspnea, light-headedness) and important changes in physiologic variables, including blood pressure. In general, angioplasty of the common trunk is absolutely contraindicated, even with the use of stents, not only because of the increased perioperative risk but, more importantly, because of the risk of postoperative restenosis resulting in sudden death (a risk that is expected to be even higher than after angioplasty of the left main trunk).

During coronary artery bypass surgery, the presence of a single coronary artery should not affect any technical decisions, except for suggesting the absolute need for as many arterial conduits as possible. Proximal mixed trunk obstruction is particularly relevant in this regard, because it tends to progress to total occlusion soon after successful bypass surgery. In contrast to venous grafts, arterial grafts are expected to provide longer-lasting conduits. If graft occlusion does eventually occur, it will likely be fatal because of the presence of total occlusion of the native circulation.

ANOMALIES OF INTRINSIC CORONARY ARTERIAL ANATOMY

Congenital Ostial Stenosis or Atresia

The literature contains occasional reports[30,51,139,337,423] of coronary arteries that are atretic[160,455,475,492] or stenosed because of a membrane or fibrotic ridge[195] located at, or near, the aortic orifice in an otherwise normal heart. In cases of atresia, only a dimple is seen from the aortic side.[13] Histologically, when the obstructive element is congenital, it invariably consists of fibrous tissue. A stenosis observed during angiography, surgery, or autopsy may be subject to debate regarding its nature (congenital versus acquired).[139,337] The condition may be associated with a coronary anomaly, sometimes involving tangential origination of a coronary artery.[326,346] Indeed, atherosclerotic growth may occur early in life at the site of a congenital ostial fibrotic plaque.[259] Coronary ostial or proximal occlusion frequently occurs in the context of pulmonary valve atresia with intact ventricular septum (see Chapter 6); in extreme cases, both the RCA and the LAD may be affected by ostial atresia.[396] Isolated coronary ostial atresia (total occlusion) probably represents the extreme degree of improper formation of the aortic ostium, and its presence often raises two questions: first, is the condition congenital or acquired, and second and more importantly, is it truly a case of ostial atresia or is it anomalous origination? The congenital cases could be regarded as instances of neonatally or fetally acquired ostial occlusion, which occurs after a normal distal coronary tree has already developed (however, such occlusion would most likely occur after embryologic development). Ostial atresia in the left coronary system can potentially occur, not only at the aortic connection site but also at the left main bifurcation, the site of embryologic fusion of the circumflex and LAD arteries with the left main trunk. Collateral circulation to the occluded artery is established prenatally and is provided by neighboring coronary arteries. Unlike anomalous origination of a coronary vessel, this anomaly includes one or more of the following features: (1) more than one (collateral) connection is present; (2) the proximal occluded artery (close to the occlusion) has a larger diameter than the intermediate segment(s) or collateral(s); (3) the proximal anatomy of the occluded vessel is characterized by a cul-de-sac, or blind pouch, that adjoins an aortic sinus; (4) during stress testing, the dependent myocardial territory may show ischemic damage or reversible ischemia, indicating that the obstruction had a relatively late onset and that the collateral circulation is inadequate for maximal myocardial demand; and 5) the site of ostial atresia is sometimes recognizable as a dimple in the related aortic sinus (see the next section).

The fact that myocardial fibrosis and segmental hypokinesia are frequently seen in these cases suggests that early myocardial development may have been normal and that the coronary stenosis or atresia developed or progressed during a later stage of fetal life or during the neonatal period. In cases that involve a primitively atretic proximal coronary artery formation (during the embryologic period), one would expect to find ectopic origination of the affected artery and normal development of the dependent myocardium. Coronary artery ''isolation'' is a variant of ostial atresia, caused by juxtaposition of an abnormal aortic cusp with the aortic sinus wall, which leads to obliteration of the underlying coronary ostium.[253,500]

(See Case Report 4.34 in the Atlas of Case Reports)

Coronary Ostial Dimple

In the recent literature,[14,361] the term ''coronary ostial dimple'' has been used for an anomalous finding (a depression in the wall of the aorta at an aortic sinus deprived of functional coronary origination) that may have some embryogenetic implications.[14,361] We refer to cases in which either (1) the sinus opposite the one with the single coronary ostium or (2) the noncoronary (right posterior) sinus in a normal two-coronary heart has a depression in its mid portion that does not lead to a coronary artery.[361] Although this dimple may be the remnant of an embryologic coronary bud,[458] its developmental implications are unclear, especially in light of recent evidence that the primitive coronary network seems to induce penetration into the aortic wall without the independent, active participation of the wall itself (see Chapter 2).

Coronary Ectasia or Aneurysm

In the foregoing discussion of normal coronary artery diameter, ectasia and aneurysm were defined as localized dilations in an otherwise normal-sized coronary artery. Studies in which a Doppler coronary flow wire is used to measure blood flow velocity in coronary aneurysms have helped to characterize ectasia by revealing a significant reduction in peak flow velocity. The possibility should be considered that an eventual decrease in coronary reserve could be related not only to development of acquired stenosis but also (and probably mainly) to the presence of mural thrombosis with distal embolization.[61] Aneurysmal rupture is also a possible complication, especially with larger lesions that have a degenerated arterial wall.[61,109]

Anatomically, ectasia may be divided into two types: primary and secondary. In *primary ectasia*,[46,354] a localized coronary segment has a disproportionately large diameter in comparison to neighboring segments[69,84,162,239,253,255,354,431,485,487,493,501] and a localized decrease in flow velocity, as indicated angiographically by streamlining and slow runoff of contrast media. Morphologically, ectasia is defined as an increase in the diameter of a coronary segment by >50% with respect to normal.[371] Differentiating primary, congenital ectasia from acquired (atherosclerotic) ectasia may be quite difficult in individual cases.[31,379,380]

In contrast, *secondary ectasia* is characterized by diffuse (global) coronary dilation (with respect to the dependent myocardial territory) secondary to increased or fistulous flow.[103] Here, we are referring not to minor forms of coronary ectasia related to myocardial hypertrophy (such as aortic stenosis or athlete's heart) but especially to the form related to coronary fistulas with greatly increased blood flow. In such cases, the coronary diameter is actually appropriate for the increased flow and is excessive only with respect to nutrient myocardial flow. *The coronary flow velocity is actually increased, not decreased as in primary ectasia.* Additional, disproportionate, localized coronary aneurysmal dilation is typically seen in ALCAPA and in older patients with larger coronaro-cameral fistulas.[85]

Patients with primary or secondary ectasia usually have a highly abnormal intrinsic coronary wall anatomy, with medial degeneration, intimal thickening, and eventually ulceration and mural thrombi.[61,138,209,371,471] Even in patients of pediatric age, congenital primary coronary aneurysms are frequently hard to distinguish from acquired aneurysms resulting from medial degeneration, as in Kawasaki's arteritis.[128,290,522] In adults, the distinction is even more conjectural.[229] Histologic findings are typical only in the acute stages of the disease. A clearly documented history of arteritis and gradual resolution of the coronary aneurysm with time can be considered strong evidence of an acquired etiology.

(See Case Reports 4.8 and 4.11 in the Atlas of Case Reports)

Absent Coronary Artery

This nomenclature is generally a misnomer, used to identify *apparently ''missing'' coronary arteries or branches*[24,34,95,178,224] in the absence of adequate documentation. True congenital (embryologic) absence of a coronary artery is expected to lead to hypoplasia of the dependent myocardium as a result of a lack of essential nutrients during embryonic development.[499]

As suggested by R. D. Leachman (oral communication, 1989), some cases of syndrome X (angina and myocardial ischemia in the absence of coronary obstruction) may be caused by a defective number of capillaries per myocardial fiber. This syndrome has never been definitely documented and is not identical with what has been called "absent coronary artery" in the literature.

On angiographic grounds, the most frequent reasons[95] for an apparently missing coronary artery are coronary ectopia (misdiagnosed), coronary occlusion with lack of demonstrable collateral retrograde filling,[225,433] or an alternative coronary artery tree pattern that may not be recognized on angiography. Although the literature includes sporadic cases in which an absent coronary artery was reported to cause chest pain,[178] cardiomyopathy,[34] or a myocardial infarction,[224] absence of a coronary artery has never been established as a specific congenital entity.

(See Case Report 4.6 in the Atlas of Case Reports)

Coronary Hypoplasia

Several reports have appeared in the literature alluding to a poorly defined entity called coronary hypoplasia.[87,137,261, 322,425] Earlier in this chapter, we discussed the difficulty of demonstrating congenital inadequacy of coronary vessel size. Normal coronary arterial size should be defined in terms of both resting metabolic needs and coronary reserve. Epicardial coronary branches normally maintain an ideal luminal diameter ratio with respect to the dependent myocardial bed or territory or capillary network.[205,230,233,281,301] Gould[145] theorized that flow velocity is the most practical parameter for measuring the adequacy of vessel diameter: a higher than normal flow velocity would imply a vessel size that is restricted in comparison to the distal arteriolar-capillary network. However, this type of measurement was previously quite impractical; it became clinically possible only recently, with the introduction of flow velocity wires, and has not yet been used to substantiate the claim of coronary hypoplasia. A more practical diagnostic method may be based on the simultaneous (1) angiographic appearance of a "hypoplastic" coronary branch (that has a small diameter with respect to the apparent area of dependent myocardium) and (2) demonstration of local reversible ischemia (reduced coronary reserve) during stress testing with myocardial nuclear scintigraphy. We are not aware of any cases in the literature in which the diagnosis of hypoplasia could be soundly based on such combined evidence, and any report that portrays a small coronary artery as a pathologic congenital entity[472] should be viewed with skepticism. In most cases, the terminology is used incorrectly, and the dependent myocardial bed is actually served by alternative sources (unusual coronary patterns),[322] or coronary spasm or diffuse disease is present. Roberts and coworkers[322] observed "hypoplastic" right or circumflex arteries in 8 of 3400 consecutive autopsies (0.0024%), according to the dubious criterion of an "absent dominant vessel" (see Absent Posterior Descending Branch).

(See Case Report 4.35 in the Atlas of Case Reports)

Intramural Coronary Artery (Muscular Bridge)

On anatomic grounds, the general rule in human hearts is that large coronary arteries and their branches are situated in the loose connective tissue of the subepicardial space. Nevertheless, the septal penetrating branches are normally intramyocardial, and other usually subepicardial branches are found to be intramural in more than 1% of instances.[68,157,316]

In several mammals and in birds, most of the coronary arteries are intramyocardial (see Chapter 1), apparently without having adverse functional consequences. Three considerations are relevant in defining and discussing muscular bridges in humans: (1) nosologic considerations (what constitutes a muscular bridge? is it an anomaly?); (2) functional considerations (are muscular bridges able to cause disease?); and (3) prognostic considerations (do muscular bridges lead to unexpected pathologic events such as spasm, thrombosis, or atherosclerotic changes?).

An intramural coronary artery[136] is defined as a coronary artery that has a segment of variable length covered by myocardial fibers but that otherwise lies subepicardially.[266] These fibers constitute the "bridge," whereas the underlying coronary segment is not the bridge but, rather, is the "bridged artery." Fine anatomic dissection, with the use of microscopy, has indicated a high incidence of myocardial fibers overriding otherwise subepicardial coronary arteries or branches, as reported in detail by Polacek.[306]

In clinical angiographic studies, detection of the intramyocardial course of a coronary artery depends on systolic compression,[9,307] a narrowing of the lumen ("milking effect") seen during systolic myocardial contraction. Phasic narrowing of a coronary artery may also occur in other conditions, such as in the presence of ventricular aneurysms or pericardial fibrous bands.[10] This angiographic marker is highly predictive of an intramyocardial coronary course, but it is actually seen in only a minority of anatomically detectable cases. Administration of a vasodilator (typically, intracoronary nitroglycerin in a 100- to 300-μg bolus[12,187]) greatly facilitates the angiographic recognition of systolic narrowing. Also, multiple angiographic views of the involved vessel may add relevant information. Systolic narrowing is generally considered to be caused by coronary compression by myocardial fibers that are oriented circumferentially with respect to the heart (and tangentially with respect to the involved vessel). It is usually best seen in projections that are tangential to the cardiac wall over which the involved artery is located *(see Case Report 4.36 in the Atlas of Case Reports)*. A less reliable, indirect indicator of an intramural coronary segment is the "U sign,"[12] caused by the artery's subclinically accentuated descent from its epicardial location into the myocardium. In more severe muscular bridges, the myocardial bundle over the involved coronary segment is thicker, and the involved artery may be surrounded by circumferentially oriented myofibers.[79,124,265]

With intravascular ultrasonography[12,51,116,134,191] or coronary flow velocity measurements,[116,127,204,352,353,388] it is possible to examine intramyocardial coronary arteries more precisely, because these imaging methods can recognize phasic changes in the coronary cross-section and flow velocity (see Case Report 50, Fig. CR4.50). Unfortunately, the relatively stiff intravascular diagnostic device may cause artifacts both by straightening the artery's U-shaped course and by causing spasm or abnormal compression. According to some recent intravascular ultrasound studies,[12,51,116,191] the systolic milking effect may involve circumferential as well as asymmetric flattening of the vessel, probably depending on the depth of the myocardial bridge.

The question of whether this entity is a coronary anomaly, or an exceptional finding versus a less frequent but normal variant, seems to be answerable on the basis of anatomic and angiographic studies: muscular bridges are present in more than 1% of normal human hearts[11,38,182] and are observed especially often in the presence of ventricular hypertrophy,[11,316] whether it is secondary (aortic stenosis, hypertension), primary (hypertrophic cardiomyopathy)[203] and/or associated with adrenergic stimulation.[133] The proximal LAD is the most common site of muscular bridges,[20,195] and other coronary arteries only rarely have such bridges.[266,362,432]

With respect to the hemodynamic repercussions of an intramyocardial coronary course,[92,93,101,120,158,164,181,210,246,256,305,352,401,417] the discussion is still open. Because an intramyocardial course is normal for large arteries (e.g., septal perforators in humans, and most coronary arteries in many other animals) and because the LAD often has an intramyocardial course without causing ischemic manifestations, this condition should be regarded as only rarely capable of causing pathologic consequences.[50,64,79,196,207,210,491] Unfortunately, the literature contains a large series of poorly documented claims to the contrary.[35,36,59,91,101,119,189,228,257,265,304,405] Of the many patients who undergo angiography because of suspected ischemic heart disease but who do not have fixed obstructive coronary disease, some indeed have a muscular bridge associated with abnormal (usually electrocardiographic) stress test results. This association is especially common in the presence of ventricular hypertrophy, which frequently accompanies muscular bridges and causes nonspecific ST changes in the resting and/or exercise electrocardiogram.

A few authors claim to have demonstrated dependent myocardial ischemia by means of a more specific method, nuclear myocardial scintigraphic stress testing,[33,148,268,274,308,321,319] and some authors have observed relief after coronary stenting or surgical resection of muscular bridges.[5,39,152,166,204,248,257,420,482] Local lactate production during elec-

tronic pacing was also attributed to systolic narrowing, especially during severe tachycardia.[417,482]

Systolic stenosis (which is rarely critical in the absence of maximal, induced vasodilation) is quite unlikely to result in an absolute flow reduction, since 75 to 85% of human coronary flow occurs during diastole, which is not affected by muscular bridges. Indeed, intramural pressure at the capillary level is much more effective at reducing flow than is external, partial compression of a short coronary segment, and it is the intramural pressure that normally modulates phasic flow to the myocardium, even in the absence of a muscular bridge.[168] In a normal heart, during systole, the intramural pressure is higher than the intracoronary pressure[459] (and, hence, the aortic pressure), especially in the subendocardial layers of the left ventricular myocardium, where the capillary bed becomes totally compressed[376]; during systole, coronary flow from the epicardium to the intramural space is abruptly reduced, while flow in the coronary veins is enhanced.[168] In this sense, the left ventricular myocardium normally behaves like a sponge that becomes phasically compressed. Superimposed systolic narrowing of an epicardial vessel cannot greatly change this basic hemodynamic behavior,[210] although such narrowing may cause a minor local disturbance in the phasic dynamics.[135,204] The recent introduction of flow-meter wires has permitted investigators to describe typical phasic changes in instantaneous flow velocity but has not provided reliable data about global blood flow rates.[12,116,127,204,352,353,388]

Still, intramyocardial coronary arteries can have prognostic and clinical relevance with respect to the occurrence of certain rare, potentially important events,[181,183,207] especially coronary spasm (which is only occasionally mentioned in the literature[54,132,153,211,271,358]), thrombosis (which is quite rarely reported[3,121]), and coronary atherosclerotic changes.[112,124,293] Numerous anatomic,[293] angiographic,[182,236,297] and intravascular ultrasound[135] reports document the relatively frequent presence of a coronary atherosclerotic plaque at the proximal bend of an intramural LAD and a consistent absence of intimal changes in the intramural segment.[112,184,223,293,294] In these cases, it is the proximal atheroma (accompanying an intramyocardial LAD) that is the most likely cause of an occasionally positive stress test during myocardial scintigraphy.[271]

(See Case Reports 4.36 and 4.50 in the Atlas of Case Reports)

Subendocardial Coronary Course

In rare cases, the RCA, LAD, or circumflex pursues a subendocardial course after penetrating the myocardial layers.[172,282] In this manner, the LAD may reach the anterior portion of the right ventricular cavity. More frequently, it is the RCA that becomes subendocardial where its posterior, distal segment (just proximal to the crux, in the lower part of the right atrium) adjoins the tricuspid valve annulus.[439] This unusual location of a sizable coronary artery may be more than a curiosity, especially during surgery for debridging of a coronary artery, or tricuspid valve replacement or valvuloplasty. The literature includes reports of cases in which a simple, nonextracorporeal approach to correcting a muscular bridge of the LAD became a surgical nightmare because of perforation of the right ventricle during unroofing of a segment of the intramyocardial LAD in an unexpected subendocardial location.[90] Unfortunately, no angiographic clues allow this anomaly to be diagnosed before surgery. A subendocardial coronary artery might be viewed as an intermediate stage in a spectrum of "coronary malpositions" ranging from the normal subepicardial location to intramyocardial coronary artery and to coronaro-cameral fistula.

Coronary Crossing

As a rule, epicardial coronary arteries do not cross one another. The literature contains only a few angiographic (but not anatomic) reports[273] that describe crossing of adjacent branches, apparently at the subepicardial level. This phenomenon should not be confused with superimposition of coronary branches during angiography when the vessels lie in different planes. In almost all reported cases and in the few cases seen by these authors, the crossed arteries were obtuse marginal branches. By examining this feature in several angiographic views, the observer can occasionally verify that both arteries are indeed subepicardial (instead of papillary muscles, penetrating coronary branches, or subendocardial collateral vessels). Coronary crossing affects secondary vessels and only rarely causes clinical problems, such as difficulty in identifying a branch to be grafted during coronary artery bypass.

(See Case Report 4.37 in the Atlas of Case Reports)

Anomalous Origination of the Posterior Descending Artery from the Anterior Descending Branch or a Septal Penetrating Branch

According to a consistent rule of coronary morphology, anterior septal penetrating branches do not reemerge on the opposite side of the ventricular septum. In cases of posterior descending artery occlusion, however, they are frequently a source of collateral connection with the facing, posterior septal vessels. Only rarely have cases been reported of an unusually large anterior septal branch that not only penetrates the whole extent of the septum but also reappears, in a subepicardial position, in the posterior interventricular groove, and produces the terminal portion of the posterior descending branch.[55,367] One might doubt the congenital nature of such an anomaly (versus an acquired occlusion of the posterior descending artery with collateral circulation from an anterior septal branch), especially in the context of coronary atherosclerosis. In a more common and clinically relevant pattern, the posterior descending branch originates congenitally from the distal LAD after encircling the cardiac apex (see the next section).

Absent Posterior Descending Branch (Split RCA)

As a rule, the posterior descending branch is a single, continuous vessel that originates from the RCA or circumflex artery, at the crux of the heart, and courses in the posterior interventricular groove. Occasionally, the posterior descending branch comprises two segments: one that originates normally from the distal RCA at the cardiac crux and courses only in the upper posterior portion of the interventricular groove; and another segment that originates from the mid RCA, close to the acute margin of the heart, and reaches the distal posterior portion of the interventricular groove.[147,470] Alternatively, the LAD or circumflex artery may supply part or all of the posterior descending branch, causing it to appear interrupted or split (Fig. 4.18). This phenomenon is a nosologic curiosity, but it may become clinically relevant in surgical grafting of the "posterior descending branch" or while attempting myocardial scintigraphic/coronary angiographic correlations.

(See Case Reports 4.38 and 4.39 in the Atlas of Case Reports)

"Absent LAD"

In the human heart, the anterior subdivision of the LCA (the LAD) generally features anteroseptal and anterolateral (diagonal) branches as it courses along the anterior interventricular groove and tapers toward the cardiac apex. In some instances, a large subepicardial anterior artery is not encountered in the interventricular groove because one of the following alternative patterns is present:

1. The proximal anterior descending artery[100,345] or a supernumerary aortic ostium[296] gives rise to a single large first septal branch that supplies most of the secondary anteroseptal branches, leaving a small or absent mid-distal subepicardial LAD (which is improperly called atretic).
2. The proximal LAD splits into two smaller, parallel branches ("split LAD"),[372] which run along the anterior interventricular groove.
3. A large diagonal artery originates quite proximally from the LAD and runs parallel to it, giving rise to all the anterolateral branches. Beyond the origin of the first septal branch, the residual distal LAD is left with limited dependent territory and appears as a very small vessel, where a bypass graft could not typically be implanted.
4. A highly dominant RCA gives rise to most of the anterior septal penetrating branches by producing an anomalous LAD[177] (via the direct intraseptal[56] or the anterior prepulmonic[40,418] route, unusually prominent posterior septal branches, or a wrap-around-the-apex posterior descending branch).

In similar cases, the small size of the LAD might lead to the erroneous conclusion that the LAD territory is ischemic because of the unusual coronary pattern. In the absence of

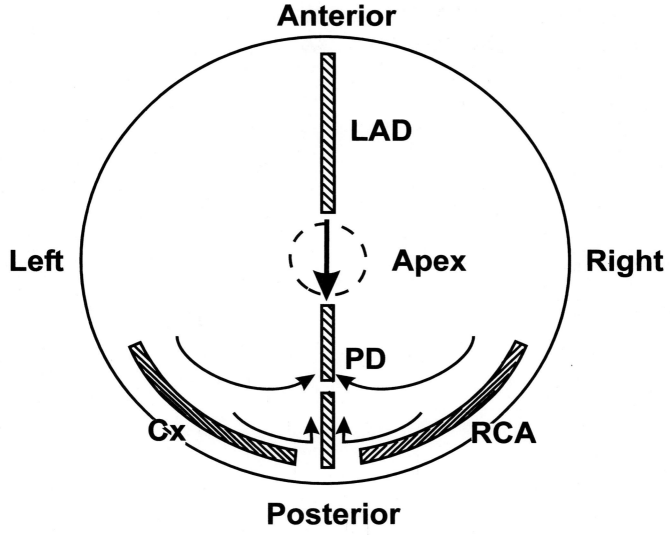

FIGURE 4.18. Schematic representation of the cardiac surface from an apical viewpoint, showing the possible alternative sources of the posterior descending artery (PD). This vessel may be a single trunk that originates from the circumflex artery (Cx), the RCA, or the LAD. The posterior descending artery may also be split into two segments with separate originations from the mid or distal RCA, the mid or distal circumflex artery, or the LAD.

acquired obstructive disease, however, functional testing (especially myocardial scintigraphic stress testing) will consistently rule out a diminished coronary reserve.[433] These coronary patterns become clinically relevant during surgical revascularization of the LAD territory, when the surgeon should be aware of the unusual anatomy.

(See Case Reports 4.35, 4.40, and 4.41 in the Atlas of Case Reports)

Ectopic Origination of the First Septal Branch

The first septal branch is commonly the largest (longest) septal vessel,[100] both because it provides for the uppermost portion of the ventricular septum (which has the largest di-

ameter in comparison to the other segments closer to the apex) and because it frequently has richer ramifications, which could reach even the atrioventricular node. This large vessel is occasionally seen to originate ectopically[296,311,403] from the following:

- The right anterior cusp
- The RCA
- The left coronary cusp[295]
- The left main trunk
- The first diagonal branch
- The proximal circumflex artery
- An anomalous RCA, LAD, LCA, or mixed trunk with an intraseptal course

ANOMALIES OF TERMINATION: CORONARY FISTULAS

As the coronary artery tree branches and propagates peripherally, it undergoes continuous tapering until it reaches the arteriolar level (the last segment of the coronary circulation to have a tunica media). The arterioles eventually drain into the capillary network, and only occasionally do they maintain small communications with sinusoidal intratrabecular spaces. *A sizable communication between a coronary artery and (1) a cardiac cavity or (2) any segment of the systemic or pulmonary circulation is generally called a coronary fistula.*[377] Any structure with a pressure lower than that of the systemic aorta (i.e., equal to the proximal coronary pressure) can drain blood flow from a coronary artery if an abnormal communication occurs, allowing fistulous flow. In reviewing the anatomic literature, starting with the historic early reports of Vieussens (1706) and Thebesius (1708), Baroldi and Scomazzoni[508] analyzed recurrent, lively discussions[525] that have occurred over the centuries about coronaro-cameral communications in the normal heart. These authors concluded that two types of communications normally exist in the human heart, as alternatives to normal drainage into the coronary veins/coronary sinus system:

1. Communications originating at the arteriolar level are established indirectly by means of *arterio-sinusoidal vessels* (which are irregularly shaped, measure 50 to 250 μm in diameter, lack a tunica media, and drain into any cardiac cavity), or directly by means of *arterioluminal vessels* (which are 40 to 200 μm in diameter, have a thin media, and drain into any cardiac cavity).
2. Venous communications or thebesian veins (first described by Thebesius [1686–1732], who injected various substances into the coronary sinus) are direct communications between a coronary vein and a cardiac cavity. They are especially common in the right atrium (where they measure up to 2 mm in size) and in the right ventricle.

The exact nature of these small coronaro-cameral connections remains unclear. However, they should probably not be called fistulas, because they do not involve substantial fistulous flow.

Angiographically, it is usually impossible to visualize the smaller coronary artery to cardiac cavity communications without the use of wedge injections.[128] Baroldi and Scomazzoni found such communications in almost all specimens by injecting the coronary arteries with latex or neoprene, which is fluid at room temperature but solidifies at 40 to 50 °C. The injections were made at 200 mm Hg of continuous pressure and were followed by further manual compression to enhance fluid progression during the 5- to 10-minute preparation period. To visualize veno-cameral communications, these investigators injected the coronary sinus with the same plastic material (of a different color), at 70 mm Hg of pressure, a few minutes after the beginning of the arterial injec-

tions. Appearance of the plastic gel in a cardiac cavity was considered evidence of an arterio- or veno-cameral communication. An important but unproved condition for accurately establishing this diagnosis was that the plastic gel not get past the capillary level. Using these techniques, Baroldi and Scomazzoni[508] demonstrated 200-μ arterioluminal communications in 86% of the left ventricles and 50% of the right ventricles but not in the atria; they also demonstrated $\leq$2-mm veno-cameral communications in the left ventricle, right ventricle, and right atrium but almost never in the left atrium.

The relationship between these findings and angiographic observations or functional status is not immediately clear. During angiography, only arterial injections are made, and any communication with a cardiac cavity is visualized at the end of contrast runoff. Clinically, however, it is impossible to know whether the capillary bed is or is not perfused by "fistulous" blood, which would differentiate potentially damaging (arterio-cameral) communications from benign (veno-cameral) ones.

Only during RCA injections (especially when performed subselectively and under high pressure) is contrast material frequently observed to drain into the anterior right ventricle and the right atrium.[128] This finding is not to be confused with the presence of thebesian veins. It merely shows that coronary veins of the right atrium and ventricle often drain directly into these cavities, without communicating with the coronary sinus.

Most likely, what appear as coronaro-cameral communications on angiography correspond to the >200-μ anatomic channels seen by Baroldi and Scomazzoni in normal hearts. Nevertheless, these channels should be subjected to specific studies, using proper techniques. The definition of coronaro-cameral fistulas is clear when larger vessels are involved, but it is not totally clear when smaller, multiple vessels are involved.[56,170,343] Small angiographic fistulas tend to occur only occasionally in patchy aggregates, affecting the smaller ramifications of several adjoining coronary branches or arteries, and typically involving the apical portions of both the left and right ventricles but never the outflow tracts. In such instances, the flow pattern indicates the presence of multiple small communications with limited flow, which is generally only diastolic into the left ventricle but systolo-diastolic into the right ventricle.[56,170] These communications do not cause ectasia of the proximal feeding arteries, nor do they tend to enlarge with time.[291]

This subject is being discussed extensively herein because of widespread persistent ignorance about the exact nature of the smaller communications between coronary vessels and cardiac cavities.[332] The overwhelming current tendency in the literature and in practice is to group these entities under the general heading of coronary fistulas and to imply that nutrient blood is shunted away from the myocardium.[111] Numerous reports have been published regarding patients with angina, ischemia, myocardial infarction, or arrhythmias in the presence of multiple small, patchy coronaro-cameral communications. However, overwhelming evidence (based mainly on nuclear myocardial imaging data[342]) strongly suggests that these small communications are benign abnormalities that have no functional or prognostic consequences. Drainage of a coronary vein into the right ventricle or atrium is not only clinically irrelevant but normal. Both of these conditions are indeed coronaro-cameral communications, but they should not be confused with large coronaro-cameral fistulas, which are discussed later in this chapter.

Because of the widespread use of right ventricular biopsy techniques, cut arterial vessels are sometimes observed on angiograms, especially in patients subjected to repeated biopsies, as after heart transplantation.[220,343] This angiographic finding correlates with the inclusion of a sizable arterial segment in the biopsy specimen. Most such small communications eventually disappear with time, and we know of no reports of clinical consequences such as progressive enlargement of a fistula.

Another common entity that may be confused with a coronary fistula is a coronaro-cameral communication at the site of a large myocardial infarction, which is typically complicated by an organized mural clot.[448] The communication involves a ruptured artery or (more likely) vein, affecting either the native circulation in the necrotic area or neovessels grown into the myocardial scar or mural clot. Like small coronaro-cameral connections, these communications should be differentiated from congenital coronary fistulas.[343]

In conclusion, we propose that the term coronary fistula be used to identify only some of the many[313] normal or abnormal communications that can exist between a coronary vessel and a cardiac cavity or some other vessel; *the smaller, anatomic but not functional, communications should be called ''coronaro-cameral micro-communications.''* In contrast, a *functional coronary fistula* is characterized by at least one of the following features: (1) definite signs of fistulous flow (for instance, the affected feeding vessel will have a luminal diameter at least 50% greater than the ''expected'' diameter); (2) angiographically clear and prompt visualization of the receiving cardiovascular structure, where a step-up in the concentration of oxygen (or any other injected substance) should be apparent; (3) evidence of volume overload in the affected cardiac chambers;[118] and (4) evidence of steal (or ischemia) involving the myocardial nutrient blood flow,[269,369,524] ideally during segmental (nuclear) testing of the coronary reserve.[154,270]

The physiologic mechanisms that may lead to coronary steal in fistulas are essentially related to a diastolic pressure drop caused by fistulous runoff into a low-pressure cavity (*see Case Report 4.42 in the Atlas of Case Reports*). Whereas normally the aortic pressure is only mildly decreased (as in mild aortic insufficiency), the intracoronary pressure in the fistulous artery may undergo progressive diminution, especially during diastole, if the fistulous flow is large. Essentially, it is the balance between the inflow (coronary, ostial size) and the outflow (fistulous versus nutrient) that determines whether the absolute nutrient coronary flow is adequate or deficient. Multiple factors may af-

fect this balance, depending on the physiologic state and morphologic variant involved. For example, physical exercise tends to lower intramyocardial arteriolar resistance and increase the pressure in the systemic venous cavities (the usual recipients of coronary fistulous flow), inducing a favorable shift in the balance between nutrient and fistulous flow. Whereas distal coronary obstructive changes at the fistulous runoff site favorably affect coronary nutrient flow, proximal obstructive changes in the involved coronary artery or in the purely nutrient distal branches unfavorably affect such flow. Systemic hypertension is usually well tolerated, but hypotension of any etiology can be expected to have a critical adverse effect on the balance between nutrient and fistulous flow.

Traditionally, steal has been considered to be heralded by angina, electrocardiographic ischemic ST-T changes (at rest or during exercise), myocardial infarction, or arrhythmia. In trying to quantify the amount of stolen flow, some authors have directed their attention to the ratio between the fistulous flow and proximal flow in the affected nutrient artery.[264] This ratio can indeed establish the relative amount of steal (the percentage of proximal coronary flow that drains into the fistula) or the absolute amount of fistulous flow. Nevertheless, it does not prove the existence of a metabolically relevant steal phenomenon, based on the needs of the dependent myocardium at rest and under maximal functional demand conditions. The diagnosis of a steal phenomenon can be firmly established only by myocardial scintigraphy, which measures relative or absolute markers of myocardial ischemia in the affected area, both at rest and during evaluation of the coronary functional reserve.

The possibility that fistulous communications can indeed steal essential blood flow intended for the competing dependent myocardial vascular bed may be related to decreased driving pressure at the entry into the nutrient coronary branches. Acquired obstruction of the ostia of nutrient branches arising from the aneursymatic main artery is probably common in older patients (*see Case Report 4.42 in the Atlas of Case Reports*). It is not yet clear whether exercise or pharmacologic vasodilating agents can transiently change the pressure-flow-resistance values in cases of coronary fistulas; the expectation is that coronary arteriolar resistance will drop but that the fistulous opening cannot change.

Because functional coronaro-cameral fistulas,[88] as defined above, can carry large volumes of blood[523] (typically 1200 to 1500 mL/min or 20 to 25 mL/sec), use of a large-lumened angiographic catheter and a mechanical injector is necessary for adequate visualization of the involved vessels. Indeed, the angiographer should not be limited to the qualitative diagnosis of a coronary fistula and its receiving chamber or vessel[15,78,190,284,320,381,415] but should also aim for complete visualization of the nutrient myocardial branches. These vessels need special protection during interventional therapeutic procedures, whether surgical or catheter-mediated. In fact, the primary objective of any intervention in such cases should be to preserve, and possibly enhance, nutrient myocardial flow, rather than simply to eliminate the fistulous tract. The absence of nutrient coronary branches arising from a fistulous tract should suggest an alternative diagnosis, namely ruptured aneurysm of an aortic sinus.[447] With the larger fistulas, a large quantity of contrast medium should be injected (about 20 mL/sec for at least 2 seconds), and the fistula should be examined in different projections, depending on its specific anatomy. It is prudent to avoid small-lumened catheters with only end holes (coronary pre-formed catheters) with high injection pressure and to use large-lumened catheters with side holes (like an NIH® or a Gensini® angiographic catheter). Alternatively, one may use a coronary angioplasty guiding catheter (large-lumened), kept in position by a 0.014-inch guidewire.

The proximal tract of a fistulous coronary artery should be regarded as an atypical example of a "mixed trunk" rather than as a simple coronary artery (which is defined as a vessel that provides exclusively nutrient flow).

Over the years, torrential flow will induce clinically important morphologic changes in the walls of a fistulous coronary artery. The fistulous tract—but not the distal, exclusively nutrient branches—will undergo progressive changes that range from simple dilation (as would be expected because of the increased blood flow) to frank aneurysm formation[18,126,262,288,382,522] (recognizable only because dilation is greater than in the adjacent vessel), intimal ulceration, medial degeneration, intimal rupture, atherosclerotic deposition, calcification,[288] side branch (nutrient) obstruction,[434] and mural thrombosis.[45,434,442] The ultimate, dreaded but rare, complication of the increased wall stress is coronary rupture into adjacent cardiac structures[61] or the pericardium.[156] Because the vessel wall's reaction to the prolonged increased flow is so variable, the observer should be cautious in estimating the amount of fistulous flow on the basis of luminal diameter alone. Vessel size, in itself, may be a fallacious parameter: in the most extreme case, a very large, aneurysmatic fistula could eventually become thrombosed, totally obliterating fistulous runoff to the distal vessel.[118,150,249,364]

In indicating whether intervention is necessary,[399] the amount of dilation of a fistulous vessel has recently become more relevant[52,118,333] than the amount of fistulous flow or symptoms and/or signs of myocardial ischemia.[114,389] Catheter-based[269] or surgical[63] intervention at an early age is generally recommended for patients with large fistulas, because of the risk of rupture and mural clotting[434,442]; moreover, aortic sinus disruption caused by an extremely enlarged coronary ostium can result in aortic insufficiency. Late atherosclerotic and thrombotic changes[218] will evolve even after total obliteration of the fistula. With respect to the optimal timing of surgery, another major consideration should be that reversibility of the ectasia is consistently reported only after surgical correction of fistulas in pediatric cases[118] and is never observed in older patients.[52] Because of these factors, many authorities have concluded that, once a large coronary fistula has been diagnosed, the optimal time for correction

is during the patient's fifth to fifteenth year of life; the timing of surgery in such cases should not be based on the time of onset of symptoms, the absolute amount of fistulous flow,[389] or signs of congestive failure or myocardial ischemia during stress testing. If the diagnosis is missed in the 5- to 15-year age range (as it frequently is), the indications for, and timing of, intervention may change because of variance of the risk-benefit ratio.[406] Older patients[445,495] may still do very well at surgery but may have more frequent complications (especially peri- and postoperative myocardial ischemic events[303,311,533] and extracardiac complications); moreover, after normalization of blood flow, their remaining risk of coronary thromboembolic disease in the excessively ectatic coronary segments will at least equal that of patients treated medically.[533] The recent introduction of catheter devices for the obliteration of coronary fistulas[87,161,217,303,314,315,368,402,441] will be further discussed in Chapter 5.

Concomitant obstructive coronary disease, in either the affected vessel or an unaffected one, may be the most common reason for clinical recognition of a coronary fistula and for surgical intervention in older patients.

Fistulous coronary connections usually involve structures that adjoin the coronary arteries, such as the coronary veins and the four cardiac cavities.[118,237,338,381,406,435,443,444] Less frequently, in otherwise normal hearts, a coronary fistula will drain into an extracardiac structure such as the pulmonary artery or its main branches or the superior vena cava.[18,466] Coronary-to-main pulmonary artery fistulas are usually small, multiple,[16] and of no clinical significance. Congenital coronary-pulmonary connections are sometimes seen in the context of other congenital heart defects, especially critical pulmonary valve stenosis or atresia or (even more frequently) pulmonary branch stenosis or atresia, or coarctation of the aorta.

Although the literature contains frequent references to "coronary-to-bronchial artery fistulas,"[17,41,144,171,347,366,373] we doubt the existence of such an entity. Both of these arteries are, in fact, systemic in patients with a normal cardiovascular anatomy, and fistulous flow cannot be expected to occur between two vascular sites that have identical pressure regimens. Communications have indeed been observed with special frequency between a coronary artery and a lung segment with a chronic infection[1] (bronchiectasia, sequestration, or pseudosequestration); in these cases, the involved vessels behaved more like neovascularizations or collaterals[220,349] than like fistulas.[17,173] Only occasional reporters have suggested that a "coronary to bronchial anastomosis" exists and can cause a myocardial infarction.[17,279] In congenitally sequestered pulmonary lobes, the systemic arterial supply is usually derived from the descending or abdominal aorta; in pseudosequestered lobes, however, it may originate from intercostal, mediastinal, subclavian, and pericardial arteries,[17,173,243,279] which probably connect with pulmonary arterial branches,[20] not bronchial ones.

Coronary-to-pulmonary communications may also appear after cardiac surgery, even heart transplantation (see Case

Report 4.44 in the Atlas of Case Reports). In these cases, the communication is not congenital, and the so-called fistulous artery consistently drains into a left lower pulmonary branch. Most of these connections develop after some degree of postoperative pleuropericarditis (and/or pulmonary atelectasis) has occurred; the inflammatory process must cause the formation of neovessels, which may connect with the lower-pressure pulmonary circulation via the subpleural plexus. Again, these neocommunications have no fistulous flow and are not connected with bronchial arteries or veins but only with pulmonary arteries (curiously, but probably because of a specific tropism, they are never connected with pulmonary veins).

For a more clinical discussion of coronary fistulas in pediatric patients, see Chapter 5.

(See Case Reports 4.43 through 4.49 in the Atlas of Case Reports)

COLLATERAL CORONARY ARTERIES: NORMAL VERSUS ANOMALOUS

"Anastomotic[508] or collateral coronary arteries" is a term that should be used to identify arterial sources other than normal, primary coronary vessels. Generally, collateral arteries are believed to develop after a coronary occlusion,[221] but detailed anatomic studies have shown that collaterals measuring less than 1 mm in luminal diameter (mostly about 0.3 mm[508] and provided with a thin media and endothelium), are extremely common in the normal human heart. Anatomically, these vessels connect either different, contiguous branches of the same artery or contiguous branches of opposite (right and left) coronary arteries. Because the number of collateral vessels in human hearts is quite high, coronary branches should not generally be considered "terminal" in anatomic terms. Functionally, however, most anastomotic circles are inactive and not visualized on coronary angiograms. In the acute stage of coronary occlusion with clinical myocardial infarction, collateral circulation is usually absent both physiologically and angiographically. Only in the subacute and chronic stages of coronary occlusion do collateral vessels become consistently apparent on angiographic studies. The origins of such collaterals are both homolateral and contralateral.

Typically, congenital "anomalous collaterals"[55] are >1-mm anastomotic communications between adjacent, unobstructed coronary arteries or branches. It is conceivable that these collaterals represent an unusual congenital pattern, but it is frequently impossible to rule out a previous transient coronary occlusion. In healthy individuals, normal (angiographically invisible) collaterals probably tend to be closed as a result of an absence of flow between arteries with the same pressure regimens; after a coronary occlusion, however, these collaterals may slowly open and enlarge as a result of the onset of a pressure gradient (this process is known as collateral recruitment). Flow-mediated vasodilation may be the mechanism of progressive enlargement of

anastomotic circles, as in coronary fistulas or ALCAPA (see Fig. CR4.11). When a coronary occlusion (usually involving thrombosis) resolves either spontaneously or because of intervention late after the development of large collaterals, these vessels can frequently still be visualized on coronary angiograms, where they may appear as "anomalous or inappropriate" collaterals. "Anomalous collateralization," a rare condition, tends to occur between the distal branches of the circumflex artery and RCA at the posterior atrioventricular groove.[55]

With respect to functional and prognostic implications, the only effect of anomalous collaterals (measuring >1 mm in luminal diameter, in the absence of coronary occlusion) would be protective, in the event that one of the connected coronary vessels became occluded.[55] Indeed, one postulated mechanism of preconditioning of the ischemic myocardium involves the development of intercoronary anastomotic circles during episodes of reversible ischemia; such collaterization would precede the final occlusive event and diminish its ischemic consequences.

In the absence of coronary occlusions, the largest collaterals are seen in cases of anomalous origination of a coronary artery from the pulmonary artery. In such cases, the collaterals are normal and appropriate, as they are governed by hemodynamic gradients established between the ectopic vessel and a normally originating coronary artery (see page 48).

PATHOPHYSIOLOGIC MECHANISMS AND CLINICAL IMPLICATIONS OF CORONARY ANOMALIES

This section summarizes the possible mechanisms by which coronary anomalies may produce clinical consequences. It also proposes a scheme for classifying coronary anomalies according to the involved pathophysiologic mechanism(s). First, however, it presents a brief summary of basic coronary physiology, based on Gould's excellent recent review,[145] to which interested readers are directed for a more in-depth discussion of this subject.

Overview of Normal Coronary Physiology

The primary source of energy for the resting, working heart is the oxidative metabolism of free fatty acids, which normally supplies 70 to 90% of the myocardial oxygen demand. At rest, the oxygen requirement of the myocardium is much greater (8 to 10 mL/min/100 g) than that of skeletal muscle (0.115 mL/min/100 g). Grossly, 20% of the myocardial oxygen requirement is dedicated to the basal metabolism (in the unloaded heart), and 1% is devoted to electrical activity. Volume work (15%) demands less energy than pressure work (64%). With exercise or an increased pressure workload, the oxygen demand is increased: a 50% increase in myocardial contractility, pressure work, or the heart rate causes almost a 50% increase in the oxygen demand. During exercise, the maximal workload is 3 to 4.5 times greater than at rest; normally, this increased workload results in coronary flow that is 3 to 4.5 times greater than baseline flow.

The oxygen content of systemic arteries is about 80 vol%, whereas that of systemic and coronary veins is 60 vol% and 5 vol%, respectively. This finding reflects the unusually high amount of oxygen extracted by the myocardium under basal conditions (extraction being submaximal at rest).

The myocardial capillary density is about 3500/mm^2 (compared with 400/mm^2 in the skeletal muscles); 50 to 70% of the left ventricular myocardial capillaries are patent at rest, and essentially 100% are recruited during maximal workload conditions.

The capillaries have a diameter of about 3 μ during systole and 4 μ during diastole, evidencing the normal phasic increase in intramural pressure. The intercapillary distance is about 17 μ at rest, versus 11 to 14 μ during maximal capillary recruitment. A normal adult myocardial cell has a transverse diameter of about 18 μ (versus 50 μ for adult skeletal muscle cells), but hypertrophic myocytes can increase that diameter to 30 μ. Therefore, the surface for metabolic exchanges is about 15 times larger in normal myocardial cells than in skeletal fibers.

Compared with the subepicardium, the subendocardium normally has a similar basal flow rate but an increased wall stress, intramural systolic pressure, and oxygen demand; it also has a decreased maximal flow rate (coronary reserve), tissue oxygen concentration at rest, and venous oxygen saturation.

The major regulators of coronary blood flow are (1) the intramural pressure, (2) the aortic (coronary) pressure, which has an elective dependence on the diastolic mean pressure and time (as about 85% of the coronary blood flow occurs during diastole under basal conditions), (3) the myocardial metabolic rate, (4) the parasympathetic and sympathetic nerves, (5) endothelial function (autocrine), and (6) blood viscosity, which is greatly increased in polycythemia.

Coronary stenosis does not affect the resting blood flow until more than 90% of the luminal diameter becomes compromised. The coronary reserve (maximal vasodilatory capacity) is normal in the presence of 0 to 60% luminal narrowing, but it progressively decreases to 0% when the degree of stenosis approaches 90%. In the coronary circulation, vascular resistance is the sum of the proximal (subepicardial) and distal (arteriolar) resistance. Proximal resistance is negligible for proximal stenoses of up to 80 to 90%, but it becomes severe for stenoses of more than 90%. Endogenous vasodilators (especially nitrous oxide) and pharmacologic vasodilators will electively affect distal arteriolar resistance in the absence of significant ($\geq$90%) proximal stenosis. With stenoses greater than 90%, the peripheral vasodilating reserve is lost.

Under baseline conditions, the coronary system is subject to a "low-flow/high-resistance" state. In contrast, exercise or coronary vasodilator (adenosine or dipyridamole) stress/testing results in a "high-flow/low-resistance" state, in which a proximal coronary stenosis becomes more evident. Recent investigations[509–512] have suggested that the coronary tree has a dual mechanism of vasodilation: endothelium-dependent vasodilation of coronary vessels measuring >200 μm in diameter and nonendothelium-dependent vasodilation of arteriolae measuring <150–200 μm in diameter. Nitroglycerin acts by means of the first type of mechanism,[122] which essentially affects only the proximal, epicardial coronary arterial tone (capacitance vessels), where it is converted into its active form (nitric oxide) by the endothelium.[199] In contrast, adenosine directly stimulates smooth-muscle-cell A$_2$ receptors in arterioles (resistance vessels), without affecting capacitance vessels. Papaverine seems to affect both capacitance and resistance vessels. Myocardial perfusion imaging for determining coronary functional reserve is essentially based on these physiologic parameters.

A coronary anomaly may produce physiologic dysfunction or clinical consequences under the circumstances listed in Table 4.6, as discussed in the literature[70,72,238,327] and summarized in the following sections.

TYPES OF PATHOPHYSIOLOGIC MECHANISMS AND/OR CLINICAL IMPLICATIONS

This section discusses mechanisms reported to be involved in causing clinical manifestations or changes in the clinical outlook for patients with congenital coronary anomalies. The clinical relevance of coronary anomalies has recently been recognized by the American Heart Association, the American College of Cardiology, and the American Academy of Pediatrics.[534] The fact that 24% of sudden deaths in athletes can be related to coronary anomalies[534] underscores the importance of this subject.

Misdiagnosis of the Coronary Anatomy

Unusual coronary anatomic patterns may be confusing and easily misdiagnosed.[95,185] Misdiagnosis may adversely affect the treatment strategy and outcome, as well as the patient's psychosocial status and insurability. The following conditions may be particularly hard to recognize and/or interpret.

(Pseudo) Absence of a Coronary Artery

Labeling a coronary artery that is not visualized directly or by means of collateral, retrograde circulation as "absent," "occluded," or "missing" is usually erroneous in the absence of an acute myocardial infarction. Further studies, including ascending (and descending) aortography and selective subclavian or carotid angiography, with follow-through to the mediastinum (possibly using digital subtraction technology), should be performed in these cases.

TABLE 4.6. *Pathophysiologic mechanisms and coronary anomalies (functional classification)*

Pathophysiologic Mechanism	Coronary Anomaly	Proof of Action		
		Certain	Possible	Unlikely
Misdiagnosis	Missing coronary artery	+		
	Hypoplastic coronary artery		+	
Myocardial ischemia, primary (fixed)	Absent coronary artery			+
	Hypoplastic coronary artery			+
	Ostial atresia	+		
	Ostial stenosis	+		
	Coronary fistula		+	
	ALCAPA	+		
	Muscular bridge			+
Myocardial ischemia, secondary (episodic)	Tangential origin		+	
	Ectopic origin (opposite sinus)		+	
	Myocardial bridge		+	
	Coronary ectasia		+	
	Coronary fistula		+	
	ALCAPA, neonatal	+		
	ALCAPA, adult		+	
Increased risk of fixed coronary atherosclerotic disease	Coronary fistula		+	
	ALCAPA	+		
	Coronary ectasia		+	
	Ectopic origin		+	
	Muscular bridge (proximal)		+	
Secondary aortic valve disease	Coronary aneurysm		+	
	Coronary fistula		+	
	ALCAPA		+	
Increased risk of bacterial endocarditis	Coronary fistula		+	
Ischemic cardiomyopathy (hibernation)	ALCAPA	+		
	Coronary fistula		+	
	Ectopic ostia		+	
Volume overload	Coronary fistula	+		
	ALCAPA	+		
Unusual technical difficulties during coronary angioplasty	Ectopic ostia	+		
	Split left coronary artery		+	
	Coronary fistula		+	
Complications during cardiac surgery	Ectopic ostia	+		
	Muscular bridge	+		

ALCAPA = anomalous origination of the left coronary artery from the pulmonary artery.

(Pseudo) Hypoplasia of a Coronary Artery

Most cases of so-called hypoplasia of a coronary artery actually involve alternative coronary branch patterns. True congenital coronary hypoplasia is probably a misdiagnosis, and the term should generally be avoided. Nevertheless, detailed angiographic studies should be performed to clarify the specific coronary distribution pattern for each myocardial segment. Only rarely during nuclear scintigraphic stress testing will the examiner find an association between a small coronary artery and reversible myocardial ischemia of the dependent myocardium that could strictly be classified as coronary hypoplasia (a doubtful congenital entity).

Myocardial Ischemia

Myocardial ischemia may result directly from coronary anomalies themselves (primary myocardial ischemic anomalies). Alternatively, it may be related to the fact that some coronary anomalies increase the probability of developing fixed obstructive disease (secondary myocardial ischemic anomalies) or transient ischemic events (secondary episodic myocardial ischemic anomalies).

The primary function of the coronary arteries is to provide metabolic myocardial perfusion. In dealing with coronary anomalies, clinicians are often frustrated by an unclear relationship between anatomy and function. This relationship is much more variable and subtle than in atherosclerotic obstructive coronary disease.[71,155,235,238,438,481,506]

Primary Myocardial Ischemia

Primary, or obligatory, myocardial ischemia is typically caused by obvious obstructive conditions such as congenital ostial stenosis or atresia, even in the presence of a rich collateral circulation. In these cases, myocardial perfusion testing is consistently positive for ischemia (fixed or reversible). By means of a different mechanism, primary myocardial ischemia can also occur in anomalies like fistulas, which cause nutrient myocardial flow to compete with fistulous flow (in a lower-resistance circuit, organized in parallel) under conditions of limited supply, as in the case of a single, restrictive proximal coronary trunk. This phenomenon rarely occurs in the usual coronary fistula; it is more often associated with anomalous origination of a coronary artery from the pulmonary artery, in which the collateral circulation originating from the normal coronary arteries preferentially tends to drain blood into the ectopic coronary ostium in the pulmonary artery, while bypassing the myocardial bed.[80,206] The dramatic improvement in left ventricular function that is frequently seen after effective repair of this anomaly is clear evidence that a chronic hibernation state may exist well beyond infancy.[53,73,174,193,216,232,317,363] Despite earlier statements to the contrary in the literature, primary myocardial ischemia cannot be assumed to occur routinely because of an anomalous course alone,[83,300] specifically when a coronary artery courses between the pulmonary artery and the aorta.[335,476] The simplistic notion that such an anomalous course could be subject to an external scissors-like compression mechanism[44,58,151,200,383,410] is not generally sustainable in the light of current information. Indeed, these patients usually do not have reproducible angina or ischemia during stress testing, and they tend to live out their entire lives without any ischemic manifestation. Nevertheless, a few of them have ischemic events—usually sudden death,[65,108,188, 236,250,261,383,385] a myocardial infarction,[261] or syncope—in the absence of coronary thrombosis or obvious stenosis.[58, 110,208] Such patients may have a tangential slitlike ostium[272, 322] or ostial ridges[472] or membranes,[66,319,409] but they rarely have a critical fixed stenosis.[213] At the present time, routine surgical correction (generally by means of bypass grafting) cannot be recommended on the basis of such anomalies alone; it would, however, be appropriate for survivors of sudden cardiac death or transient ischemia who have a positive provocation test. Despite exceptions widely reported in the literature, myocardial ischemia cannot usually be documented by stress testing, whether the patient has an isolated coronary intramyocardial course,[388] multiple coronaro-cameral micro-communications,[71,258,291] or coronary aneurysms or ectasia. If these conditions indeed lead to myocardial ischemia,[26] it is generally because of additional acquired features, as described in the following section.

Secondary, Episodic Myocardial Ischemia

Paradoxically, many coronary anomalies that, in fact, arise during the fetal period never produce clinical manifestations until many years later, if at all. One would expect that a congenital disease, especially a potentially lethal one, would not allow for normal life (as it frequently does, in the presence of negative stress tests), although it could suddenly cause a catastrophic event. In most cases, the congenital lesion by itself is not capable of causing the final event; rather, the congenital lesion increases the risk potential for

episodes of superimposed spasm,[265,266,338] intravascular clotting,[3,207,260,434,442,470] or accentuation of systolic narrowing in myocardial bridges, as brought about paradoxically by vasodilators.[74,246]

In recent years, the literature has included many case reports[25,26,208,272,298,384,395,411,502] that testify to the ischemic nature (in the dependent myocardial region) of adverse clinical events (myocardial infarction,[32,79,143,486] chest pain,[44] syncope,[461] ischemic cardiomyopathy,[461] or sudden death[58, 79,240,241,453,461,469]) in patients with various coronary anomalies. Angiographic and autopsy studies[25,32,208,393] (carried out some variable time after the ischemic insult was substantially resolved, even if by death) have consistently failed to reveal the critical coronary obstructions or occlusions that would be expected in such cases. The implication is that a transient obstruction occurred, but this phenomenon could not be well documented. If such an obstruction can resolve that quickly, it must be caused by a coronary spasm in most cases. Platelet clot formation or full thrombosis is unlikely to be missed in angiographic or anatomic studies performed shortly after the event occurs.[3,384] Provocative testing designed to document coronary spastic potential must be more widely performed in clinical practice, to elucidate the pathophysiologic mechanism and prognosis, thereby facilitating rational therapeutic decision-making.[132,153,211] Spasm is probably involved in (1) most cases of ectopic coronary origination from the aorta, with tangential orientation of the proximal trunk and a slitlike orifice or ostial ridge[25,259,489] and (2) some muscular bridges (intramyocardial coronary arteries), especially the more extensive ones, in which long, thick myocardial bands cover a proximal main coronary trunk. It is likely, but not fully certain, that phasic bending of the intramyocardial coronary segment is a stimulus to spasm—even more than is systolic narrowing itself.[211,359] Provocative testing of endothelial dysfunction or excessive spasticity occasionally yield positive results.[132,153,211]

Conceivably, a coronary artery that originates from the opposite coronary sinus and courses between the aorta and the pulmonary artery could behave in a peculiar manner (previously unreported), especially during or after exercise or prolonged athletic training, leading to relevant clinical repercussions. We allude to stretching of the abnormal vessel against the aortic wall while that vessel is being subjected to the opposing forces of right and left ventricular dilation brought about by exercise. Indeed, during strenuous exercise, the cardiac output of young, trained athletes may increase to 25 to 30 L/min: under these circumstances, the dramatic increase in diastolic return flow to the ventricles is only partially compensated by an increased heart rate; a major increase in diastolic volume also results, which must be accompanied by important increases in aortic pressure and wall tension (both of which greatly exceed the respective pulmonary values) and also in right and left ventricular wall tension. By their nature and position, the coronary arteries (especially the LAD) are intrinsically anchored to the ventricular masses and may be subjected to unusual stretching

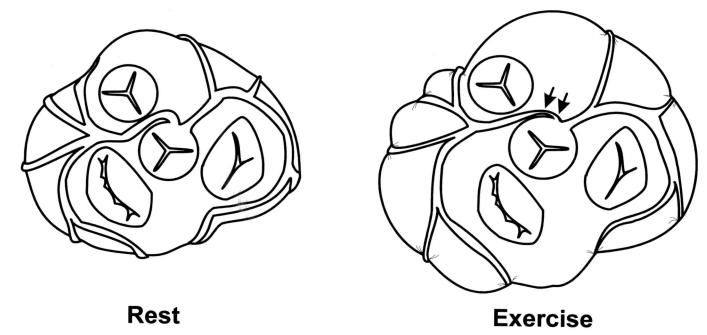

Rest

Exercise

FIGURE 4.19. Schematic representation of a possible mechanism of transient ischemia in patients with anomalous origin of the coronary artery from the opposite sinus. During exercise (right panel), physiologic cardiac enlargement may lead to stretching of the epicardial coronary arteries that are anchored to the myocardium, and compression of the proximal trunk against the aortic wall (arrows) may occur.

during exercise. If, on top of this physiologic condition, one superimposes an anomaly in which a coronary artery arises from the opposite side of the aorta and transverses the aortopulmonary septum adjacent to the aortic perimeter, compression of the anomalous coronary vessel by the aortic wall becomes likely (Fig. 4.19). Coronary compression might have two types of consequences: (1) direct diminution of coronary blood flow at a time of maximal demand and (2) coronary ''mechanical stimulation'' with a potential for secondary spasm (as when a coronary artery is mechanically stimulated by a catheter) or endothelial activation resulting in local platelet activation and/or autocrine vasomotor dysfunction. This abnormal physiologic state could persist during the immediate recovery period after strenuous exercise, when diastolic filling remains increased. Apparently, many of the sudden deaths reported to have been caused by such coronary anomalies occurred during the recovery phase after strenuous exercise.

Increased Risk of Fixed Coronary Atherosclerotic Disease

Some authors have suggested that fixed coronary atherosclerotic disease[77,113,215,294,430,473] could be a general consequence of the anomalous course of a coronary artery. However, recent studies,[435] including the angiographic analysis reported on pages 38–43, seem to indicate that most anomalous coronary vessels are not predisposed to early atheroscle-

rosis. The only certainty is that patients with congenital coronary anomalies have a much greater chance of being identified if they also have atherosclerotic coronary disease,[22] since coronary angiography is a most common diagnostic modality for ischemic heart disease.

In a recent study[528] designed to determine whether anomalies of coronary origin and course influence the location of atherosclerotic coronary disease, we documented no such influence. Indeed, in reviewing the Texas Heart Institute's database of 36,883 consecutive coronary angiograms, we encountered only 69 cases (0.2%) involving coronary anomalies of origination. Of this population, which was studied because of suspected coronary artery disease, 35 patients (51%) actually had such disease. Of the 105 proximal coronary arteries (LAD, RCA, and circumflex) studied in this subgroup of patients, 66 (63%) had a normal origin, and the other 39 (37%) were ectopic; obstructive disease was observed in 53% (35/66) of the normal segments and 30% (12/39) of the ectopic ones ($P = 0.027$).

The specific entity consisting of an ectopic, tangential ostium, maybe with a congenital fibrous ridge, may indeed increase the risk of additional ostial fixed, progressive obstructions,[75,260] probably because of unfavorable local rheologic factors. More studies are needed in this regard, including detailed anatomic analyses or adequate angiographic views of the anomalous ostia, accompanied by functional correlations. Highly atypical diffuse severe obstructive coronary disease has recently been documented in most cases involving extreme overload of the right ventricle (pulmonary atresia with intact ventricular septum[129,142]) or the left ventricle (aortic valve atresia).[63] The obstructive lesions have been attributed to shrinkage and, even more, to fibrous intimal proliferation.[88,129] These lesions occur in the presence of high-velocity collateral flow, which vents the overloaded ventricular cavities. Surgical palliation of hemodynamic right ventricular overload may delay the progression of coronary pathology but also may eliminate critically important coronary collateral sources in the presence of severe proximal obstructions (see Chapter 6). Single coronary artery is not generically associated with an increased incidence of atherosclerosis; should atherosclerosis occur in the common trunk, however, the clinical consequences would be unusually severe, because the dependent myocardial territory includes the whole heart and no collateral circulation can develop.[262]

Secondary Aortic Valve Disease

In patients with coronary anomalies, clinically important aortic valve disease may result from (1) an independent congenital defect associated with coronary anomalies or (2) an acquired defect secondary to longstanding coronary anomalies, especially those involving greatly increased fistulous flow and enlarged coronary ostia—primarily coronary fistula and ectopic origination of the LCA from the pulmonary artery. As previously noted, when a coronary ostium attains a greatly enlarged diameter, the structure of the aortic cusp and the adjoining leaflet may be critically altered, resulting in aortic regurgitation. When a coronary artery originates ectopically from the pulmonary artery, it is the normal contralateral coronary artery (the source of collateral and fistulous flow) that may cause such impairment of the aortic valve.

Increased Risk of Bacterial Endocarditis

The earlier literature contains a few scattered reports concerning an increased risk of bacterial endocarditis or endoarteritis in patients with coronary anomalies, especially coronary fistulas. This risk is probably related more to coexisting aortic valve anomalies (even if their repercussions are initially minor) than to the coronary anomaly itself. The current extreme rarity of endocarditis[450] under such conditions may be caused by extensive use of antibiotics in the general population and routine prophylaxis for endocarditis in the presence of ''heart murmurs,'' even in the absence of a definite diagnosis.

Cardiomyopathy

A cardiomyopathy is more likely to accompany ALCAPA or left coronary atresia than anomalous origination of the RCA, LAD, or circumflex artery (individually) from the pulmonary artery. As previously discussed, myocardial ischemic damage occurs prenatally in coronary atresia but neonatally in anomalous origination of a coronary artery from the pulmonary artery.

Some amazing observations have been widely confirmed in regard to the nature and behavior of chronic ischemia in pediatric patients with ALCAPA. Anatomically and histologically, this cardiomyopathy may involve cardiomegaly, left ventricular dilation, myocardial hypertrophy, secondary mitral insufficiency, changes associated with an acute myocardial infarction, and various degrees of interstitial, patchy, or diffuse fibrosis. After surgical correction of these anomalies, myocardial function may be recovered, often to an amazing extent. Not only are the results of nuclear myocardial perfusion studies dramatically improved or completely normalized but cardiomegaly, mitral regurgitation, and left ventricular systolic dysfunction may totally disappear.[454] In these cases, recovery is similar to that observed after revascularization of critical left main lesions but is consistently more extensive. This phenomenon clearly reflects the presence of a hibernating myocardium. Additionally, it is interesting to note that myocardial hypertrophy is a probable result of ischemia in young persons, and myocardial reabsorption (possibly by means of apoptosis) may occur after the chronic ischemia has been resolved.

Diffuse cardiomyopathy is also observed in some cases of anomalous origination of the LCA from the right anterior cusp. In such cases, ischemia is probably the original cause of the cardiomyopathy, but, as previously discussed, this event must be caused by clinical or subclinical episodic obstruction (spasm and/or clotting), followed by spontaneous revascularization.[461] In these cases, revascularization can prevent further worsening but may not produce a total recovery of myocardial function.

Volume Overload

A coronary fistula may cause cardiac enlargement and volume (diastolic) overload by creating significant shunting of blood through the fistula. Depending on the degree of fistulous flow and the size of the recipient cavity or vessel, different cardiac cavities will be affected to varying degrees. Coronary fistulas that drain into a systemic vein, coronary sinus, right-sided cardiac cavity, or pulmonary artery (including anomalous origination of a coronary artery from the pulmonary artery) will cause left-to-right shunting at systemic or near systemic pressures, resulting in volume overload (with cavitary dilation and an increased diastolic workload). Pulmonary hypertension is only rarely observed in cases involving coronary fistulas draining to the right ventricle or pulmonary artery, because the degree of shunting is never excessive[52] (i.e., greater than the systemic cardiac output or entailing a pulmonary-to-systemic flow ratio of >2:1). Volume overload may be poorly tolerated by patients who also have ischemia and/or a primary cardiomyopathy, as in ALCAPA.

Unusual Technical Difficulties During Coronary Angioplasty

Coronary anomalies of origin and course may increase the technical difficulty of coronary angioplasty for acquired or congenital obstructive disease.[27,62,67,392] Selective catheterization and guiding catheter support may be impaired, especially when a coronary artery originates tangentially and ectopically, outside the center of the aortic cusp.[60,436] In the absence of a left main coronary trunk, each individual left trunk (the LAD and circumflex artery) is smaller than normal, and the guiding catheter may easily become wedged.[391] A discussion of the adaptations needed during catheter interventions in these cases is beyond the scope of this book but is included elsewhere in the literature on interventional cardiology.[60,393,436]

(see Case Report 4.16 in the Atlas of Case Reports)

Complications During Cardiac Surgery

Ectopic coronary arteries may complicate the surgical treatment of associated cardiac conditions.[468] For instance, when an ectopic artery encircles or courses near the aortic or mitral valve annulus,[267] the artery may be injured during creation of the aortotomy or suture line at the time of aortic or mitral valve replacement.[267,328] During otherwise routine coronary artery bypass surgery, the surgeon may discover that the target coronary artery has an intramyocardial course. In such cases, the anomalous artery may not be found, or its unroofing may result in transmural perforation of the cardiac wall. Moreover, anomalous coronary branching patterns such as split RCA or LAD may confuse surgeons who are unfamiliar with them and may result in incomplete or erroneous bypass grafting.

REFERENCES *(in alphabetical order until #438)*

1. Abergel E, Aouate JM, Geslin J, et al. Dilatation des bronchs localisee. Etiologie meconnue de fistule coronaro bronchique. Arch Mal Coeur 1990;83:271.
2. Abrams HL, Barnhard HJ, Gruntzig AR, et al. Coronary arteriography. A practical approach. 1st ed. Boston: Little, Brown, 1983:10–72.
3. Agirbasli M, Martin GS, Stout JB, et al. Myocardial bridge as a cause of thrombus formation and myocardial infarction in a young athlete. Clin Cardiol 1997;20:1032.
4. Ahmad M, Merry SL, Haibach H. Evidence of impaired myocardial perfusion and abnormal left ventricular function during exercise in patients with isolated systolic narrowing of the left anterior descending coronary artery. Am J Cardiol 1981;48:832.
5. Akilli A, Kultursay H, Akin M, et al. Stenting of myocardial bridging. J Invasive Cardiol 1997;9:529.
6. Alam M, Brymer J, Smith S. Transesophageal echocardiographic diagnosis of anomalous left coronary artery from the right aortic sinus. Chest 1993;103:1617.
7. Allen GL, Snider TH. Myocardial infarction with a single coronary artery. Arch Intern Med 1966;117:261.
8. Alstrup P, Madsen T, Jagt T. Left coronary artery originating from the pulmonary artery: correction and total myocardial blood flow measurements. J Cardiovasc Surg (Torino) 1978;19:169.
9. Amplatz K, Anderson R. Angiographic appearance of myocardial bridging of the coronary artery. Invest Radiol 1968;3:213.
10. Angelini P, Leachman RD, Autrey A. Atypical phasic coronary narrowing. Cathet Cardiovasc Diagn 1986;12:39.
11. Angelini P, Trivellato M, Donis J, et al. Myocardial bridges: a review. Prog Cardiovasc Dis 1983;26:75.
12. Angelini P. Myocardial bridges revisited. Cathet Cardiovasc Diagn 1994;32:40.
13. Angelini P. The case of a fascinating dimple. Am J Cardiol 1993;72:102.
14. Anversa P, Sonnenblick EH. Ischemic cardiomyopathy: pathophysiologic mechanisms. Prog Cardiovasc Dis 1990;32:1.
15. Arani D, Greene D, Krocke F. Coronary artery fistulas emptying into the left heart chambers. Am Heart J 1978;96:438.
16. Ashraf SS, Shaukat N, Fisher M, et al. Bicoronary-pulmonary fistulae with coexistent mitral valve prolapse: a case report and literature review of coronary-pulmonary fistula. Eur Heart J 1994;15:571.
17. Aupetit JF, Gallet M, Boutarin J. Coronary-to-bronchial artery anastomosis complicated with myocardial infarction. Int J Cardiol 1988;18:93.
18. Aydogan U, Onursal E, Cantez T, et al. Giant congenital coronary artery fistula to left superior vena cava and right atrium with compression of left pulmonary vein simulating cor triatriatum—diagnostic value of magnetic resonance imaging. Eur J Cardiothorac Surg 1994;8:97.
19. Bahrati S, Lev M. The pathology of congenital heart disease. Armonk, NY: Futura Publishing, 1996.
20. Baim DS, Klinen H, Silverman JF. Bilateral coronary artery-pulmonary artery fistulas. Report of five cases and review of the literature. Circulation 1982; 65:810.
21. Baljepally RM, Pollock SH, Magram MY. Transluminal angioplasty of a single coronary artery anomaly during acute myocardial infarction—a case report. Angiology 1993;44:981.
21a. Baltaxe HA, Wixson D. The incidence of congenital anomalies of the coronary arteries in the adult population. Radiology 1977;122:47.
22. Barendra C, Chan CN, Tan A. Single coronary artery: a case report and review of current literature. Singapore Med J 1995;36:335.
23. Edwards WD. Applied anatomy of the heart. In Giuliani ER, Gersh BJ, McGoon MD, et al., eds: Mayo Clinic practice of cardiology. St. Louis: Mosby, 1996:474–481.
24. Barresi V, Susmano A, Colandrea MA, et al. Congenital absence of the circumflex coronary artery. Clinical and cineangiographic observations. Am Heart J 1973;86:811.
25. Barth CW, Roberts WC. Left main coronary artery originating from the right sinus of Valsalva and coursing between the aorta and pulmonary trunk. J Am Coll Cardiol 1986;7:366.
26. Bartorelli AL, Pepi M, Sganzerla P, et al. Syncope with cardiac arrest as the first manifestation of two congenital left coronary artery-to-main pulmonary artery fistulae. Am Heart J 1994;127:207.
27. Bass TA, Miller AB, Rubin MR, et al. Transluminal angioplasty of anomalous coronary arteries. Am Heart J 1986;112:610.
28. Becker AE, Anderson RH. Cardiac embryology: a help or a hindrance in understanding congenital heart disease? In: Nora JJ, Takao A, eds. Congenital heart disease: causes and processes. Mount Kisco, NY: Futura Publishing, 1984:339–351.
29. Becker AE. Congenital coronary arterial anomalies of clinical relevance. Cor Art Dis 1995;6:187.
30. Bedogni F, Castellani A, La Vecchia L, et al. Atresia of the left main coronary artery: clinical recognition and surgical treatment. Cathet Cardiovasc Diagn 1992;25:35.
31. Befeler B, Aranda JM, Embi A, et al. Coronary artery aneurysms: study of their etiology, clinical course and effect on the left ventricular function and prognosis. Am J Med 1977;62:597.
32. Benge W, Martins JB, Funk DC. Morbidity associated with anomalous origin of the right coronary artery from the left sinus of Valsalva. Am Heart J 1980;99:46.
33. Bennett JM, Blomerus P. Thallium-201 scintigraphy perfusion defect with dipyridamole in a patient with a myocardial bridge. Clin Cardiol 1988;11:268.
34. Bestetti RB, Costa RB, Oliveira JSM, et al. Congenital absence of the circumflex coronary artery associated with dilated cardiomyopathy. Int J Cardiol 1985;8:331.
35. Bestetti RB, Costa RS, Kazava DK, et al. Can isolated myocardial bridging of the left anterior descending coronary artery be associated with sudden death during exercise? Acta Cardiol 1991;46:27.
36. Bestetti RB, Costa RS, Zucolotto S, et al. Fatal outcome associated

with autopsy proven myocardial bridging of the left anterior descending coronary artery. Eur Heart J 1989;10:573.

37. Betriu A, Pare JC, Sanz GA, et al. Myocardial infarction with normal coronary arteries: a prospective clinical-angiographic study. Am J Cardiol 1981;48:28.

38. Bezerra AJC, Prates JC, DiDio LJA. Incidence and clinical significance of bridges of myocardium over the coronary arteries and their branches. Surg Radiol Anat 1987;9:273.

39. Binet JP, Guiraudon G, Langlois J, et al. Angine de poitrine et ponts musculaires sur l'arterie interventriculaire anterieure: a propos de trois cas operes. Arch Mal Coeur 1978;71:251.

40. Bittner V, Nath HP, Cohen M, et al. Dual connection of the left anterior descending coronary artery to the left and right coronary arteries. Cathet Cardiovasc Diagn 1989;16:168.

41. Bjork L. Angiographic demonstration of extracardial anastomoses to the coronary arteries. Radiology 1966;87:274.

42. Blake HA, Manion WC, Mattingly TW, et al. Coronary artery anomalies. Circulation 1964;30:927.

43. Bland EF, White PD, Garland J. Congenital anomalies of the coronary arteries. Am Heart J 1933;8:787.

44. Bloomfield P, Ehrlich C, Folland ED, et al. Anomalous right coronary artery: a surgically correctable cause of angina pectoris. Am J Cardiol 1983;51:1235.

45. Bolognesi R, Tsialtas D, Barbaresi F, et al. Single coronary artery-right ventricular fistula with a partially thrombosed large aneurysm of its proximal tract in a 66-year-old man. Eur Heart J 1994;15:1720.

46. Bove AA, Vlietstra RE. Spasm in ectatic coronary arteries. Mayo Clin Proc 1985;60:822.

47. Brandt B III, Martins JB, Marcus ML. Anomalous origin of the right coronary artery from the left sinus of Valsalva. N Engl J Med 1983; 309:596.

48. Brandt PWT, Partridge JB, Wattie WJ. Coronary arteriography; method of presentation of the arteriogram report and a scoring system. Clin Radiol 1977;28:361.

49. Brooks H. Two cases of abnormal coronary artery of the heart arising from the pulmonary artery. With some remarks upon the effect of this anomaly in producing cirsoid dilatation of the vessels. J Anat Physiol 1884;20:26.

50. Burke AP, Farb A, Virmani R, et al. Sports-related and non–sports-related sudden cardiac death in young adults. Am Heart J 1991;121: 568.

51. Byrum CJ, Blackman MS, Schneider B, et al. Congenital atresia of the left coronary ostium and hypoplasia of the left main coronary artery. Am Heart J 1980;99:354.

52. Carrel T, Tkebuchava T, Jenni R, et al. Congenital coronary fistulas in children and adults: diagnosis, surgical technique and results. Cardiology 1996;87:325.

53. Carvalho JS, Redington AN, Oldershaw PJ, et al. Analysis of left ventricular wall movement before and after reimplantation of anomalous left coronary artery in infancy. Br Heart J 1991;65:218.

54. Carvalho VB, Macruz R, Decourt LV, et al. Hemodynamic determination of coronary constriction in human myocardial bridges. Am Heart J 1984;108:73.

55. Celano C, Peters RW, Fisher ML. Coronary collateral blood flow in a patient with angiographically normal coronary arteries. Cathet Cardiovasc Diagn 1987;13:325.

56. Cha SD, Singer E, Maranhao V, et al. Silent coronary artery-left ventricular fistula: a disorder of the thebesian system. Angiology 1978; 29:169.

57. Chaitman BR, Bourassa MG, Lesperance J, et al. Aberrant course of the left anterior descending coronary artery associated with anomalous left circumflex origin from the pulmonary artery. Circulation 1975; 52:955.

58. Chaitman BR, Lesperance J, Saltiel J, et al. Clinical, angiographic, and hemodynamic findings in patients with anomalous origin of the coronary arteries. Circulation 1976;53:122.

59. Chambers JD Jr, Johns JP, Davees TS. Myocardial stunning resulting from systolic coronary artery compression by myocardial bridging. Am Heart J 1994;128:1036.

60. Chan CNS, Berland J, Cribier A, et al. Angioplasty of the right coronary artery with origin of all three coronary arteries from a single ostium in the right sinus of Valsalva. Am Heart J 1993;126:985.

61. Chapman RW, Watkins J. Rupture of right coronary artery aneurysm into the right atrium. Br Heart J 1978;40:938.

62. Charney R, Spindola-Franco H, Grose R. Coronary angioplasty of anomalous right coronary arteries. Cathet Cardiovasc Diagn 1993;29: 233.

63. Cheatham JP, Ruyle NA, NcManus BM, et al. Origin of the right coronary artery from the descending thoracic aorta: angiographic diagnosis and unique coronary artery anatomy at autopsy. Cathet Cardiovasc Diagn 1987;13:321.

64. Chee TP, Jensen DP, Padnick MB, et al. Myocardial bridging of the left anterior descending coronary artery resulting in subendocardial infarction. Arch Intern Med 1981;141:1703.

65. Cheitlin MD, De Castro CM, McAllister HA. Sudden death as a complication of anomalous left coronary origin from the anterior sinus of Valsalva: a not-so-minor congenital anomaly. Circulation 1974;50: 780.

66. Cheitlin MD. Congenital coronary artery anomalies: pathologic aspects. In: Virmani R, Forman MB, eds. Non-atherosclerotic ischemic heart disease. New York: Raven, 1989:81–98.

67. Chen H, Lo P, Wu C, et al. Coronary angioplasty of a single coronary artery with an anomalous origin in the ascending aorta. J Invas Cardiol 1997;9:188.

68. Chen JN, Liao R. A study of the myocardial bridges on the coronary arteries in the Chinese. Acta Anat Sinica 1965;8:106.

69. Chen YT, Hwang CL, Kan MN. Large, isolated, congenital aneurysm of the anterior descending coronary artery. Br Heart J 1993;70:274.

70. Cheng TO. Anomalous coronary arteries. Int J Cardiol 1993;40:183.

71. Cheng TO. Left coronary artery-to-left ventricular fistula: demonstration of coronary steal phenomenon. Am Heart J 1982;104:870.

72. Cheng TO. Prevalence and relevance of coronary artery anomalies. Cathet Cardiovasc Diagn 1997;42:276.

73. Cherian KM, Bharati S, Rao SG. Surgical correction of anomalous origin of the left coronary artery from the pulmonary artery. J Card Surg 1994;9:386.

74. Chopra PS, Reed WH, Wilson AD, et al. Delayed presentation of anomalous circumflex coronary artery arising from pulmonary artery following repair of aortopulmonary window in infancy. Chest 1994; 106:1920.

75. Ciampricotti R, El Gamal M. Vasospastic coronary occlusion associated with a myocardial bridge. Cathet Cardiovasc Diagn 1988;14:118.

76. Cieslinski G, Rapprich B, Kober G. Coronary anomalies: incidence and importance. Clin Cardiol 1993;16:711.

77. Click RL, Holmes DR Jr, Vlietstra RE, et al. Anomalous coronary arteries: location, degree of atherosclerosis and effect on survival: a report from the Coronary Artery Surgery Study. J Am Coll Cardiol 1989;13:531.

78. Teno LA, Santos JL, Bestetti RB, et al. Congenital circumflex coronary artery fistula with drainage into the left ventricle. Tex Heart Inst J 1993;20:304.

79. Corrado D, Thiene G, Cocco P, et al. Non-atherosclerotic coronary artery disease and sudden death in the young. Br Heart J 1992;68: 601.

80. Cowie MR, Mahmood S, Ell PJ. The diagnosis and assessment of an adult with anomalous origin of the left coronary artery from the pulmonary artery. Eur J Nucl Med 1994;21:1017.

81. Culbertson C, De Campli W, Williams R, et al. Congenital valvular aortic stenosis and abnormal origin of the right coronary artery: rare combination with important clinical implications. Pediatr Cardiol 1995;16:73.

82. Culham JAG. Abnormalities of the coronary arteries. In: Freedom RM, Mawson JB, Yoo SJ, Benson LN, eds. Congenital heart disease: textbook of angiocardiography. Armonk NY: Futura Publishing, 1997:849–867.

83. Dalal JJ, West RO, Parker JO. Isolated anomaly of the left anterior descending coronary artery. Cathet Cardiovasc Diagn 1984;10:189.

84. Daoud AS, Pankin D, Tulgan H, et al. Aneurysms of the coronary artery: report of ten cases and review of the literature. Am J Cardiol 1963;11:228.

85. Davidson PH, McCrackan BH, McIlveen JJS. Congenital coronary arteriovenous aneurysm. Br Heart J 1955;17:569.

86. Davis JS, Lie JT. Anomalous origin of a single coronary artery from the innominate artery. Angiology 1977;28:775.

87. De Feyter PJ, Wardeh R, Majid PA. Exercise-induced and variant form of angina pectoris in a patient with hypoplasia of the left coronary artery: clinical, metabolic and angiographic observations. Eur J Cardiol 1981;12:147.

88. De Nef JJ, Varghese PJ, Losekoot G. Congenital coronary artery fistula: report of 17 cases with a note on natural history of lesion. Br Heart J 1971;33:150.

89. De Wolf D, Terriere M, De Wilde P, Reidy JF. Embolization of a coronary fistula with a controlled delivery platinum coil in a 2-year-old. Pediatr Cardiol 1994;15:308.

90. de Zwaan C, Wellens HJ. Left ventricular aneurysm subsequent to cleavage of myocardial bridging of a coronary artery. J Am Coll Cardiol 1984;3:1345.

91. Dean JW, Mills PG. Abnormal ventricular repolarization in association with myocardial bridging. Br Heart J 1994;71:366.

92. Den Dulk K, Brugada P, Braat S, et al. Myocardial bridging as a cause of paroxysmal atrioventricular block. J Am Coll Cardiol 1983; 1:965.

93. Desseigne P, Tabib A, Loire R. Myocardial bridging on the left anterior descending coronary artery and sudden death: an autopsy study of 19 cases. Arch Mal Coeur 1991;84:511.

94. Dicicco BS, McManus BM, Waller BF, et al. Separate aortic ostium of the left anterior descending and left circumflex coronary arteries from the left aortic sinus of Valsalva (absent left main coronary artery). Am Heart J 1982;104:153.

95. Donaldson RM, Raphael MJ. Missing coronary artery: review of technical problems in coronary arteriography resulting from anatomical variants. Br Heart J 1982;47:62.

96. Donaldson RM, Raphael M, Radley-Smith R, et al. Angiographic identification of primary coronary anomalies causing impaired myocardial perfusion. Cathet Cardiovasc Diagn 1983;9:237.

97. Donaldson RM, Raphael MJ, Yacoub MH, et al. Hemodynamically significant anomalies of the coronary arteries. Thorac Cardiovasc Surg 1982;30:7.

98. Donaldson RM, Thornton A, Raphael MJ, et al. Anomalous origin of the left anterior descending coronary artery from the pulmonary trunk. Eur J Cardiol 1979;10:295.

99. Doorey AJ, Wills JS, Blasetto J, et al. Usefulness of magnetic resonance imaging for diagnosing an anomalous coronary artery coursing between aorta and pulmonary trunk. Am J Cardiol 1994;74:198.

100. Dorald BE, Essex HW. The coronary septal artery. An anatomic and electrocardiographic study. Am J Physiol 1954;176:143.

101. Dottori V, Torre F, Spagnolo S, et al. The intramyocardial coronary artery and the muscular bridge. The physiopathological and surgical considerations in a clinical case. G Ital Cardiol 1993;23:787.

102. Doty DB, Chandramouli B, Schieken RE, et al. Anomalous origin of the left coronary artery from the right pulmonary artery. J Thorac Cardiovasc Surg 1976;71:787.

103. Drexler H, Zeiher AM, Wollschlager, et al. Flow-dependent coronary artery dilation in humans. Circulation 1989;80:466.

104. Driscoll DJ, Nihill MR, Mullins CT, et al. Management of symptomatic infants with anomalous origin of the left coronary artery from the pulmonary artery. Am J Cardiol 1981;47:642.

105. Driscoll DJ. Congenital coronary artery anomalies. In: Garson A, Bricker TJ, McNamara DG, eds. The science and practice of pediatric cardiology. Philadelphia: Lea & Febiger, 1990:1453–1461.

106. Drory Y, Turetz Y, Hiss Y, et al. Sudden unexpected death in persons less than 40 years of age. Am J Cardiol 1991;68:1388.

107. Duerinckx AJ, Bogaert J, Jiang H, et al. Anomalous origin of the left coronary artery: diagnosis by coronary MR angiography. AJR 1995; 164:1095.

108. Duran AC, Angelini A, Frescura C, et al. Anomalous origin of the right coronary artery from the left aortic sinus and sudden infant death. Int J Cardiol 1994;45:147.

109. Ebert PA, Peter RH, Gunnells JC, et al. Resecting and grafting of coronary artery aneurysm. Circulation 1971;43:593.

110. Edelstein J, Juhasz RS. Myocardial infarction in the distribution of a patent anomalous left circumflex coronary artery. Cathet Cardiovasc Diagn 1984;10:171.

111. Edward JE. Anomalous coronary arteries with special reference to arteriovenous-like communications. Circulation 1958;17:1001.

112. Edwards JE, Burnsides C, Swarm RL, et al. Arteriosclerosis in the intramural and extramural portion of coronary arteries in the human heart. Circulation 1956;13:235.

113. Edwards JE. The direction of blood flow in coronary arteries arising from the pulmonary trunk (editorial). Circulation 1964;29:163.

114. Effler DB, Sheldon WC, Turner JJ, et al. Coronary arteriovenous fistulas: diagnosis and surgical management: report of 15 cases. Surgery 1967;61:41.

115. Engel HJ, Torres C, Page HL. Major variations in anatomical origin of the coronary arteries: angiographic observations in 4250 patients without associated congenital heart disease. Cathet Cardiovasc Diagn 1975;1:157.

116. Erbel R, Ge J, Rupprecht HJ, et al. Comparison of intravascular ultrasound and angiography in the assessment of myocardial bridging. Circulation 1994;89:1725.

117. Eugster GS, Oliva PB. Anomalous origin of the right coronary artery from the pulmonary artery. Chest 1973;63:294.

118. Farooki ZQ, Nowlen T, Hakimi M, et al. Congenital coronary artery fistulae: a review of 18 cases with special emphasis on spontaneous closure. Pediatr Cardiol 1993;14:208.

119. Faruqui AMA, Maloy WC, Felner JM, et al. Symptomatic myocardial bridging of coronary artery. Am J Cardiol 1978;41:1305.

120. Feld H, Guadanino V, Hololander G, et al. Exercise-induced ventricular tachycardia associated with a myocardial bridge. Chest 1991;99: 1295.

121. Feldman AM, Baughman KL. Myocardial infarction associated with a myocardial bridge. Am Heart J 1986;111:784.

122. Feldman RL, Pepine CJ, Conti CR. Magnitude of dilatation of large and small coronary arteries by nitroglycerin. Circulation 1981;64:324.

123. Fernandes F, Alam M, Smith S, et al. The role of transesophageal echocardiography in identifying anomalous coronary arteries. Circulation 1993;88:2532.

124. Ferreira AG Jr, Trotter SE, Konig B Jr, et al. Myocardial bridges: morphological and functional aspects. Br Heart J 1991;66:364.

125. Finley JP, Howman-Giles K, Gilday DL, et al. Thallium-201 myocardial imaging in anomalous left coronary artery arising from the pulmonary artery. Am J Cardiol 1978;42:675.

126. Floyd WL, Young WG, Johnsrude IS. Coronary arterial-left atrial fistula. Case with obstruction of the inferior vena cava by a giant left atrium. Am J Cardiol 1970;25:716.

127. Flynn MS, Kern MJ, Aguirre FV, et al. Intramyocardial muscle bridging of the coronary artery: An examination of a diastolic "spike and dome" pattern of coronary flow velocity. Cathet Cardiovasc Diagn 1994;32:36.

128. Freedom RM, Culham JAG, Moes CAF. Anomalies of the coronary arteries. In: Freedom RM, Culham JAG, Moes CAF, eds. Angiocardiography of congenital heart disease. New York: Macmillan, 1974: 405–421.

129. Freedom RM, Benson LN. The etiology of myocardial ischemia: surgical considerations. In: Freedom RM, ed. Pulmonary atresia with intact ventricular septum. New York: Futura, 1989:233.

130. Fu M, Hung JS, Yeh SJ, et al. Reversal of silent myocardial ischemia by surgery for isolated anomalous origin of the left anterior descending coronary artery from the pulmonary artery. Am Heart J 1992;124: 1369.

131. Gaither NS, Rogan KM, Stajduhar K, et al. Anomalous origin and course of coronary arteries in adults: identification and improved imaging utilizing transesophageal echocardiography. Am Heart J 1991; 122:69.

132. Gallet B, Adams C, Hlitgen M, et al. Myocardial bridge of the left anterior descending coronary artery and myocardial infarction: does coronary spasm play a part? Arch Mal Coeur Vaiss 1991;84:517.

133. Galli M, Politi A, Zerboni S. "Functional myocardial bridging" and "hyperkinetic state": a rare association as a cause of acute myocardial infarction. G Ital Cardiol 1997;27:1286.

134. Ge J, Erbel R, Meyer J, et al. Comparison of intravascular ultrasound and angiography in the assessment of myocardial bridging. Circulation 1994;89:1725.

135. Ge J, Jeremias A, Simon HU, et al. A new and characteristic coronary flow pattern in patients with myocardial bridging demonstrated by intracoronary FloWire. Circulation 1997;96:704.

136. Geiringer E. The mural coronary artery. Am Heart J 1951;41:359.

137. Gentzler RD, Gault JH, Liedtke AJ, et al. Congenital absence of the left circumflex artery in the systolic click syndrome. Circulation 1975; 52:490.

138. Ghahrani A, Iyengar R, Cunha D, et al. Myocardial infarction due to congenital coronary arterial aneurysm (with successful saphenous vein bypass graft). Am J Cardiol 1972;29:863.

139. Ghosh PK, Friedman M, Vidne BA. Isolated congenital atresia of the left main coronary artery and atherosclerosis. Ann Thorac Surg 1993; 55:1564.

140. Gibbs HH, Spokojny AM, Molloy TJ, et al. Percutaneous transluminal

coronary angioplasty of a right coronary artery arising from the left main coronary artery. Cathet Cardiovasc Diagn 1993;30:37.

141. Gibson R, Nihill MR, Mullins CE, et al. Congenital coronary artery obstruction associated with aortic valve anomalies in children: report of two cases. Circulation 1981;64:857.

142. Gittenberger-de Groot AC, Sauer U, Bindl L, et al. Competition of coronary arteries and ventriculo-coronary arterial communications in pulmonary atresia with intact ventricular septum. Int J Cardiol 1988; 18:243.

143. Glover MV, Kuber MT, Warren SE, et al. Myocardial infarction before age 36: risk factor and arteriographic analysis. Am J Cardiol 1982;49:1600.

144. Gobel FL, Anderson CF, Baltaxe HA, et al. Shunts between the coronary and pulmonary arteries with normal origin of the coronary arteries. Am J Cardiol 1970;25:655.

145. Gould KL: Coronary artery stenosis. New York: Elsevier Science Publishers, 1991:7–71.

146. Grant RT, Regnier M. The comparative anatomy of the cardiac coronary vessels. Heart 1926;13:285.

147. Green CE. Unusual coronary anatomy and variations. In: Green CE. Coronary cinematography. Philadelphia: Lippincott-Raven, 1996: 19–38.

148. Greenspan M, Iskandrian AS, Catherwood E, et al. Myocardial bridging of the left anterior descending artery: evaluation using exercise thallium-201 myocardial scintigraphy. Cathet Cardiovasc Diagn 1980; 6:173.

149. Grenadier E, Beyar R, Amikam S, et al. Two-vessel PTCA of single anomalous coronary artery. Am Heart J 1992;123:220.

150. Griffiths SP, Ellis K, Hardof AJ, et al. Spontaneous complete closure of a congenital coronary fistula. J Am Coll Cardiol 1983;2:1169.

151. Grollman JH Jr, Mao SS, Weinstein SR. Arteriographic demonstration of both kinking at the origin and compression between the great vessels of an anomalous right coronary artery arising in common with a left coronary artery from above the left sinus of Valsalva. Cathet Cardiovasc Diagn 1992;25:46.

152. Grondin P, Bourassa MB, Noble J, et al. Successful course after supraarterial myotomy for myocardial bridging and milking effect of the left anterior descending artery. Ann Thorac Surg 1977;24:422.

153. Grover M, Mancini GB. Myocardial bridge associated with pacing-induced coronary spasm. Am Heart J 1984;108:1540.

154. Gupta NC, Beauvais J. Physiologic assessment of coronary artery fistula. Clin Nucl Med 1991;16:40.

155. Gutgesell HP, Pinsky WW, DePuey EG. Thallium-201 myocardial perfusion imaging in infants and children. Value in distinguishing anomalous left coronary artery from congestive cardiomyopathy. Circulation 1980;61:596.

156. Haberman JH, Howard ML, Johnson ES. Rupture of the coronary sinus with hemopericardium. A rare complication of coronary arteriovenous fistula. Circulation 1963;28:1143.

157. Hackett D, Hallidie-Smith KA. Spontaneous closure of coronary artery fistula. Br Heart J 1984;52:477.

158. Hansen BF. Myocardial covering on epicardial coronary arteries. Prevalence, localization, and significance. Scand J Thorac Cardiovasc Surg 1982;16:151.

159. Hanzlick R, Stivers RR. Sudden death in a marathon runner with origin of the right coronary artery from the left sinus of Valsalva (letter to editor). Am J Cardiol 1983;51:1467.

160. Harada K, Ito T, Suzuki Y, et al. Congenital atresia of left coronary ostium. Eur J Pediatr 1993;152:539.

161. Hartnell GG, Jordan SC. Balloon embolization of a coronary arterial fistula. Int J Cardiol 1990;29:381.

162. Hartnell GG, Parnell BM, Pridie RB. Coronary artery ectasia: its prevalence and clinical significance in 4,993 patients. Br Heart J 1985; 54:392.

163. Hausdorf G, Gravinghoff L, Keck EW. Effects of persisting myocardial sinusoids on left ventricular performance in pulmonary atresia with intact ventricular septum. Eur Heart J 1987;8:291.

164. Herreira AG Jr, Trotter SE, Koning B Jr, et al. Myocardial bridges: morphological and functional aspects. Br Heart J 1991;66:364.

165. Higgins CB, Wexler L. Reversal of dominance of the coronary arterial system in isolated aortic stenosis and bicuspid aortic valve. Circulation 1975;52:292.

166. Hill RC, Chitwood WR Jr, Bashore TM, et al. Coronary flow and regional function before and after supra-arterial myotomy for myocardial bridging. Ann Thorac Surg 1981;31:176.

167. Hillestad L, Eie H. Single coronary artery. Acta Med Scand 1971; 189:409.

168. Hoffman J. The effect of intramyocardial forces on the distribution of intramyocardial blood flow. J Biomed Eng 1979;1:33.

169. Honey M, Lincoln JCR, Osborne MP, et al. Coarctation of the aorta with right aortic arch. Report of surgical correction in two cases: one with associated anomalous origin of left circumflex coronary artery from the right pulmonary artery. Br Heart J 1975;37:937.

170. Housman LB, Morse J, Litchford B, et al. Left ventricular fistula as a cause of intractable angina pectoris. Successful surgical repair. JAMA 1978;240:372.

171. Hughes M. Anomalous origin of the right coronary artery from the left anterior descending coronary artery. Cathet Cardiovasc Diagn 1997;42:308.

172. Huhta JC, Edwards WD, Danielson GK. Supravalvular mitral ridge containing the dominant left circumflex coronary artery. J Thorac Cardiovasc Surg 1981;81:577.

173. Hung K, Hsieh I, Chern M, et al. Pulmonary pseudosequestration receiving arterial supply from a coronary artery fistula. Angiology 1996;47:925.

174. Hurwitz RA, Caldwell RL, Girod DA, et al. Clinical and hemodynamic course of infants and children with anomalous left coronary artery. Am Heart J 1989;118:1176.

175. Hutchins GM, Bulkley BH, Miner MM, et al. Correlation of age and heart weight with tortuosity and caliber of normal human coronary arteries. Am Heart J 1977;94:196.

176. Hutchins GM, Nazarian IH, Bulkley BH. Association of left dominant coronary arterial system with congenital bicuspid aortic valve. Am J Cardiol 1978;42:57.

177. Ilia R, Gilutz H, Gueron M. Mid left anterior descending coronary artery originating from the right coronary artery. Int J Cardiol 1991; 33:162.

178. Ilia R, Jafari J, Weinstein JM, et al. Absent left circumflex coronary artery. Cathet Cardiovasc Diagn 1994;32:349.

179. Ilia R. Anomalous origin of the right coronary artery high above the noncoronary sinus of Valsalva. Cathet Cardiovasc Diagn 1994;35: 184.

180. Ilia R, Weinstein JM, Battler A. Single coronary artery originating above the left sinus of Valsalva. Int J Cardiol 1995;48:97.

181. Shotar A, Busittil A. Myocardial bars and bridges and sudden death. Forensic Sci Int 1994;68:143.

182. Irving GI. The angiographic prevalence of myocardial bridging in man. Chest 1982;81:198.

183. Virmani R, Farb A, Burke AP. Ischemia from myocardial coronary bridging: fact or fancy? Hum Pathol 1993;24:687.

184. Ishii T, Hosoda Y, Osaka T, et al. The significance of myocardial bridge upon atherosclerosis in the left anterior descending coronary artery. J Pathol 1986;148:279.

185. Ishikawa T, Brandt PWT. Anomalous origin of the left main coronary artery from the right anterior aortic sinus: angiographic definition of anomalous course. Am J Cardiol 1985;55:770.

186. Ishikawa T, Otsuka T, Suzuki T. Anomalous origin of the left main coronary artery from the noncoronary sinus of Valsalva. Pediatr Cardiol 1990;11:173.

187. Ishimori T, Raizner AF, Chahine RA, et al. Myocardial bridges in man: clinical correlations and angiographic accentuation with nitroglycerin. Cathet Cardiovasc Diagn 1977;3:59.

188. Isner JM, Shen EM, Martin ET, et al. Sudden unexpected death as a result of anomalous origin of the right coronary artery from the left sinus of Valsalva. Am J Med 1984;76:55.

189. Iversen S, Hake U, Mayer E, et al. Surgical treatment of myocardial bridging causing coronary artery obstruction. Scand J Thorac Cardiovasc Surg 1992;26:107.

190. Jaffe RB, Clancy DL, Epstein SE, et al. Coronary arterial-right heart fistulae. Long-term observations in seven patients. Circulation 1973; 47:133.

191. Jain SP, White CJ, Ventura HO. De novo appearance of a myocardial bridge in heart transplant: assessment by intravascular ultrasonography, Doppler, and angioscopy. Am Heart J 1993;126:453.

192. James TN. Anatomy of the coronary arteries. New York: Paul B. Hoeber, 1961:1–60.

193. Jin Z, Berger F, Uhlemann F, et al. Improvement in left ventricular dysfunction after aortic reimplantation in 11 consecutive pediatric patients with anomalous origin of the left coronary artery from the

pulmonary artery: early results of a serial echocardiographic follow-up. Eur Heart J 1994;15:1044.

194. Johnson AD, Detwiler JH, Higgins CB. Left coronary artery anatomy in patients with bicuspid aortic valves. Br Heart J 1978;40:489.

195. Josa M, Danielson GK, Weidman WH, et al. Congenital ostial membrane of left main coronary artery. J Thorac Cardiovasc Surg 1981; 81:338.

196. Juilliere Y, Berder V, Suty-Selton C, et al. Isolated myocardial bridges with angiographic milking of the left anterior descending coronary artery: a long-term follow-up study. Am Heart J 1995;129:663.

197. Kardos A, Babai L, Rudas L, et al. Epidemiology of congenital coronary artery anomalies: a coronary arteriography study on a Central European population. Cathet Cardiovasc Diagn 1992;42:270.

198. Kelley MJ, Wolfson S, Marshall R. Single coronary artery from the right sinus of Valsalva: angiography, anatomy, and clinical significance. Am J Roentgenol 1977;128:257.

199. Kelm M, Schrader J. Control of coronary vascular tone by nitric oxide. Circ Res 1990;66:1561.

200. Keren A, Tzivoni D, Stern S. Functional consequences of right coronary artery originating from left sinus of Valsalva (letter to editor). Am J Cardiol 1983;51:1241.

201. Kimbiris D, Iskandrian A, Segal BL, et al. Anomalous aortic origin of coronary arteries. Circulation 1978;58:606.

202. King BD, Ambrose JA, Stein JH, et al. Anomalous origin of the right coronary artery from the ascending aorta above the left coronary sinus. Cath Cardiovasc Diag 1982;8:277.

203. Kitazume H, Kramer Jr, Krauthamer D, et al. Myocardial bridges in obstructive hypertrophic cardiomyopathy. Am Heart J 1983;106:131.

204. Klues HG, Schwarz ER, vom Dahl J, et al. Intracoronary stent implantation—a new therapeutical approach in highly symptomatic patients with myocardial bridging. J Am Coll Cardiol 1997;29:220A.

205. Koiwa Y, Bahn RC, Ritman EL. Regional myocardial volume perfused by the coronary artery branch: estimation in vivo. Circulation 1986;74:157.

206. Koops B, Kerber RE, Wexler L, et al. Congenital coronary artery anomalies, experience at Stanford University hospital (1963–1971). JAMA 1973;226:1425.

207. Kracoff OH, Ovsyshcher I, Gueron M. Malignant course of a benign anomaly: myocardial bridging. Chest 1987;92:1113.

208. Kragel AH, Roberts WC. Anomalous origin of either the right or left main coronary artery from the aorta with subsequent coursing between aorta and pulmonary trunk: analysis of 32 necropsy cases. Am J Cardiol 1988;62:771.

209. Krajcer Z, Leachman RD, Lufschanowski R, et al. Anomalous left coronary artery from pulmonary artery. Unusual case complicated by coronary arterial disease and fistula from coronary artery to left ventricle. Chest 1978;74:102.

210. Kramer JR, Kitazume H, Proudfit WI, et al. Clinical significance of isolated coronary bridges: benign and frequent condition involving the left anterior descending artery. Am Heart J 1982;103:283.

211. Kuhn FE, Reagan K, Mohler ER, et al. Evidence for endothelial dysfunction and enhanced vasoconstriction in myocardial bridges. Am Heart J 1991;122:1764.

212. Kurosawa H, Wagenaar SS, Becker AE. Sudden death in a youth. A case of quadricuspid aortic valve with isolation of origin of left coronary artery. Br Heart J 1981;46:211.

213. Kwan T, Feit A, Garcia A, et al. Cardiac catheterization and selective coronary angiography with tortuous aorta and anomalous coronary artery. Angiology 1996;47:705.

214. Ladowski JS, Belvedere DA, Wuest LF. Anomalous origin of the right coronary artery from the pulmonary artery: an unusual cause of angina. Cardiovasc Surg 1995;3:81.

215. Laifer LI, Weiner BH. Percutaneous transluminal coronary angioplasty of a coronary stenosis at the site of myocardial bridging. Cardiology 1991;79:245.

216. Lambert V, Touchot A, Losay J, et al. Midterm results after surgical repair of the anomalous origin of the coronary artery. Circulation 1996;94(Suppl II):38.

217. Latson LA, Forbes TJ, Cheatham JP. Transcatheter coil embolization of a fistula from the posterior descending coronary artery to the right ventricle in a two-year-old child. Am Heart J 1992;124:1624.

218. Lau G. Sudden death arising from a congenital coronary artery fistula. Forens Sci Int 1995;73:125.

219. Lawson A, Dailey M, Soto B. Selective injection of a left coronary artery arising anomalously from the posterior aortic sinus. Cathet Cardiovasc Diagn 1993;30:300.

220. Lazar JM, Uretsky BF. Coronary artery fistula after heart transplantation: a disappearing entity? Cathet Cardiovasc Diagn 1996;37:10.

221. Lazarous DF, Scheinowitz M, Shou M, et al. Effects of chronic systemic administration of basic fibroblast growth factor on collateral development in the canine heart. Circulation 1995;91:145.

222. Le TQ, Laskey WK, McLaughin J, et al. Utility of magnetic resonance imaging in a patient with anomalous origin of the right coronary artery, acute myocardial infarction and near-sudden cardiac death. Cathet Cardiovasc Diagn 1997;42:205.

223. Lee SS, Wu TL. The role of mural coronary artery in prevention of coronary atherosclerosis. Arch Path 1972;93:32.

224. Leitch A, Caves PK. A case of Marfan's syndrome with absent right coronary artery complicated by aortic dissection and right ventricular infarction. Thorax 1975;30:352.

225. Lenox CC, Briner J. Absent proximal coronary arteries associated with pulmonary atresia. Am J Cardiol 1972;30:666.

226. Lerberg DB, Ogden JA, Zuberbuhler JR, et al. Anomalous origin of the right coronary artery from the pulmonary artery. Ann Thorac Surg 1979;27:87.

227. Lerer PF, Edwards WD. Coronary arterial anatomy in bicuspid aortic valve: necropsy study of 100 hearts. Br Heart J 1981;45:142.

228. Lesauskaite VV. A sudden death case with myocardial bridge in the left anterior descending artery. Arkh Patol 1988;50:67.

229. Letac B, Cazor JL, Cribier A, et al. Large multiple coronary artery aneurysm in adult patients: a report on three patients and a review of the literature. Am Heart J 1980;99:694.

230. Leung WHL, Stadius ML, Alderman EL. Determinants of normal coronary artery dimensions in humans. Circulation 1991;84:2294.

231. Levin DC, Fellow KE, Abrams HL. Hemodynamically significant primary anomalies of the coronary arteries: angiographic aspects. Circulation 1978;58:25.

232. Levitsky S, van der Horst RL, Hastreiter AR, et al. Anomalous left coronary artery in the infant: recovery of ventricular function following early direct aortic implantation. J Thorac Cardiovasc Surg 1980; 79:598.

233. Lewis BS, Gotsman MS. Relation between coronary artery size and left ventricular wall mass. Br Heart J 1973;35:1150.

234. Liberthson RR, Dinsmore R, Bharati S, et al. Aberrant coronary artery origin from the aorta: diagnosis and clinical significance. Circulation 1974;50:774.

235. Liberthson RR, Dinsmore RE, Fallon JT. Aberrant coronary artery origin from the aorta. Report of 18 patients, review of literature and delineation of natural history and management. Circulation 1979;59: 748.

236. Liberthson RR, Gang DL, Custer J. Sudden death in an infant with aberrant origin of the right coronary artery from the left sinus of Valsalva of the aorta: case report and review of the literature. Pediatr Cardiol 1983;4:45.

237. Liberthson RR, Sagar K, Berkoben JP, et al. Congenital coronary arteriovenous fistula. Report of 13 patients, review of the literature, and delineation of management. Circulation 1979;59:849.

238. Liberthson RR. Sudden death from cardiac causes in children and young adults. N Engl J Med 1996;334:1039.

239. Lim CH, Tan NC, Tan L, et al. Giant congenital aneurysm of the right coronary artery. Am J Cardiol 1977;39:751.

240. Lipsett J, Bryard RW, Carpenter BF, et al. Anomalous coronary arteries arising from the aorta associated with sudden death in infancy and early childhood. Arch Pathol Lab Med 1991;115:770.

241. Lipsett J, Cohle SD, Berry PJ, et al. Anomalous coronary arteries: a multicenter pediatric autopsy study. Pediatr Pathol 1994;14:287.

242. Lipton MJ, Barry WH, Obrez I, et al. Isolated single coronary artery: diagnosis, angiographic classification, and clinical significance. Radiology 1979;130:39.

243. Livingston DR, Mehta AC, O'Donovan PB, et al. Angiographic dilemma: bronchopulmonary sequestration versus pseudosequestration: case report. Angiology 1986;37:896.

244. Longenecker CG, Reemtsma K, Creech O Jr. Surgical implications of single coronary artery: a review and two case reports. Am Heart J 1961;61:382.

245. Lynch P. Soldiers, sport and sudden death. Lancet 1980;1:1235.

246. MacAlpin RN. Clinical significance of myocardial bridges. Am Heart J 1982;104:648.

247. MacAlpin RN, Abbasi AS, Grollman JH, et al. Human coronary artery size during life. Diagn Radiol 1973;108:567.

248. Mahon NG, Sugrue DD. Treatment of a long segment of symptomatic myocardial bridging with multiple coronary stents. J Invas Cardiol 1997;9:484.

249. Mahoney LT, Schieken RM, Lauer RM. Spontaneous closure of a coronary artery fistula in childhood. Pediatr Cardiol 1982;2:311.

250. Mahowald JM, Blieden LC, Coe JI, et al. Ectopic origin of a coronary artery from the aorta. Sudden death in 3 of 23 patients. Chest 1986; 89:668.

251. Maluf MA, Smith M, Abellan DM, et al. Anomalous origin of the right coronary artery from the pulmonary artery in association with a ventricular septal defect. Tex Heart Inst J 1997;24:226.

252. Marik D, Gately HL, Strauss R, Starr A. Anomalous origin of right coronary artery from pulmonary artery. J Cardiac Surg 1995;10:55.

253. Markis JE, Joffe CD, Cohn PF, et al. Clinical significance of coronary arterial ectasia. Am J Cardiol 1976;37:217.

254. Maron BJ, Roberts WC, McAllister HA, et al. Sudden death in young athletes. Circulation 1980;62:218.

255. Mattern AL, Baker WP, McHale JJ, et al. Congenital coronary aneurysms with angina pectoris and myocardial infarction treated with saphenous vein bypass graft. Am J Cardiol 1972;30:906.

256. Mays AE Jr, McHale PA, Greenfield JR Jr. Transmural myocardial blood flow in a canine model of coronary artery bridging. Circ Res 1981;49:726.

257. Marzu A, Ditano G, Cogade K, et al. Myocardial bridging involving more than one site of the left anterior descending coronary artery: an uncommon cause of acute ischemic syndrome. Cathet Cardiovasc Diagn 1995;34:329.

258. McLellan BA, Pelikan PCD. Myocardial infarction due to multiple coronary-ventricular fistulas. Cathet Cardiovasc Diagn 1989;16:247.

259. Menke DM, Jordan MD, Aust CH, et al. Isolated and severe left main coronary atherosclerosis and thrombosis: a complication of acute angle takeoff of the left main coronary artery. Am Heart J 1986;112:1319.

260. Menke DM, Waller BF, Pless JE. Hypoplastic coronary arteries and high takeoff position of the right coronary ostium. A fatal combination of congenital coronary artery anomalies in an amateur athlete. Chest 1985;88:299.

261. Meyer MH, Stephenson HE, Ketas TE, et al. Coronary artery resection for giant aneurysmal enlargement and arteriovenous fistulae. Am Heart J 1967;74:603.

262. Meyers DG, McManus BM, McCall D, et al. Single coronary artery with the right coronary artery arising from the first septal perforator. Cathet Cardiovasc Diagn 1984;10:479.

263. Mintz GS, Abdulmassih S, Bemis LE, et al. Myocardial ischemia in anomalous origin of the right coronary artery from the pulmonary trunk. Am J Cardiol 1983;51:610.

264. Morales AR, Romanelli R, Boucke RJ. The mural left anterior descending coronary artery, strenuous exercise and sudden death. Circulation 1980;62:230.

265. Morales AR, Romanelli R, Tate LG, et al. Intramural left anterior descending coronary artery: significance of the depth of the muscular tunnels. Hum Pathol 1993;24:693.

266. Morin D, Fischer AP, Sohl BE, et al. Iatrogenic myocardial infarction. A possible complication of mitral valve surgery related to anatomical variation of the circumflex coronary artery. Thorac Cardiovasc Surg 1982;30:176.

267. Moskowitz WB, Newkumet KM, Albrecht GT, et al. Case of steel versus steal: coil embolization of congenital coronary arteriovenous fistula. Am Heart J 1991;121:909.

268. Mouratidis B, Lomas FE, McGill D. Thallium-201 myocardial SPECT in myocardial bridging. J Nucl Med 1995;36:1031.

269. Mukai H, Minemawari Y, Hanawa N, et al. Coronary stenosis and steal phenomenon in coronary-pulmonary fistula—assessment with stress thallium tomography after coronary angioplasty and fistulectomy. Jpn Circ J 1993;57:1021.

270. Munkata K, Sata N, Sasake Y. Two cases of variant from angina pectoris associated with myocardial bridge: a possible relationship among coronary vasospasm, atherosclerosis and myocardial bridge. Jpn Circ J 1992;56:1248.

271. Murphy DA, Roy DL, Sohal M, et al. Anomalous origin of left main coronary artery from anterior sinus of Valsalva with myocardial infarction. J Thorac Cardiovasc Surg 1978;75:282.

272. Muus CJ, McManus BM. Common origin of right and left coronary arteries from the region of left sinus of Valsalva: association with unexpected intrauterine death. Am Heart J 1984;107:1285.

273. Muyldermans LL, Van den Heuvel PA, Ernst SM. Epicardial crossing of coronary arteries: a variation of coronary arterial anatomy. Int J Cardiol 1985;7:416.

274. Nakajima K, Taki J, Bunko H, et al. Demonstration of therapeutic effect in a patient with myocardial bridge by exercise-myocardial SPECT imaging. Clin Nucl Med 1985;10:116.

275. Neches WH, Mathews RA, Park SC, et al. Anomalous origin of the left coronary artery from the pulmonary artery. Circulation 1974;50:582.

276. Nehgme RA, Dewar ML, Lutin WA, et al. Anomalous left coronary artery from the main pulmonary trunk: physiologic and clinical importance of its association with persistent ductus arteriosus. Pediatr Cardiol 1992;13:97.

277. Neufeld HN, Schneeweiss A. Anomalous origin of the coronary arteries from the pulmonary artery. In: Neufeld NH, Schneeweiss A, eds. Coronary artery disease in infants and children. Vol 1. Philadelphia: Lea & Febiger, 1983:30–40.

278. Nohara R, Kambara H, Murakami T, et al. Giant coronary-to-bronchial artery anastomosis complicated by myocardial infarction. Chest 1983; 84:772.

279. O'Connor WN, Stahr BJ, Cottrill CM, et al. Ventriculocoronary connections in hypoplastic right heart syndrome: autopsy serial section study of six cases. J Am Coll Cardiol 1988;11:1061.

280. O'Keefe JH, Owen RM, Bove AA. Influence of left ventricular mass on coronary artery cross-sectional area. Am J Cardiol 1987;59:1395.

281. Ochsner JL, Mills NL. Surgical management of diseased intracavitary coronary arteries. Ann Thorac Surg 1984;38:356.

282. Ogden JA, Goodyear AVN. Patterns of distribution of the single coronary artery. Yale J Biol Med 1970;43:11.

283. Ogden JA, Stansel HC. The anatomic variability of coronary artery fistulae termination in the right and left atria. Chest 1974;65:76.

284. Ogden JA. Congenital anomalies of the coronary arteries. Am J Cardiol 1970;25:474.

285. Ogden JA. Congenital variations of the coronary arteries. A clinicopathologic survey. A thesis presented to the Faculty of the School of Medicine, Yale University, 1968.

286. Ogden JA. Anomalous aortic origin: circumflex, anterior descending or main left coronary arteries. Arch Pathol 1969;88:323.

287. Okita Y, Miki S, Kusuhara K, et al. Aneurysm of coronary arteriovenous fistula presenting as a calcified mediastinal mass. Ann Thoracic Surg 1992;54:771.

288. Okuyama M, Kubota I, Miura T, et al. Anomalous origin of the right coronary artery from the left ventricle in an adult. Jpn Heart J 1995; 36:115.

289. Onouchi Z, Shimazu S, Kiyosawa N, et al. Aneurysms of the coronary arteries in Kawasaki disease. Circulation 1982;66:6.

290. Oshiro H, Shimabukuro M, Nakada Y, et al. Multiple coronary LV fistulas: demonstration of coronary steal phenomenon by stress thallium scintigraphy and exercise hemodynamics. Am Heart J 1990;120:217.

291. Ott DA, Cooley DA, Pinsky WW, et al. Anomalous origin of circumflex coronary artery from right pulmonary artery: report of a rare anomaly. J Thorac Cardiovasc Surg 1978;76:190.

292. Page HL, Engel HJ, Campbell WB, et al. Anomalous origin of the left circumflex coronary artery: recognition, angiographic demonstration and clinical significance. Circulation 1974;50:768.

293. Polacek P. Relation of myocardial bridges and loops on the coronary arteries to coronary occlusions. Am Heart J 1961;61:44.

294. Palomo AR, Schrager BR, Chahine RA. Anomalous origin of the right coronary artery from the ascending aorta high above the left posterior sinus of Valsalva of a bicuspid aortic valve. Am Heart J 1985;109:902.

295. Palomo AR, Schrager BR, Chahine RA. Anomalous separate origin of the septal perforator coronary artery from the left sinus of Valsalva. Cathet Cardiovasc Diagn 1984;10:385.

296. Parashara DK, Ledley GS, Kotler MN, et al. The combined presence of myocardial bridging and fixed coronary artery stenosis. Am Heart J 1993;125:1170.

297. Parsonnet V. Intracavitary coronary arteries. Ann Thorac Surg 1985; 40:206.

298. Patterson FK. Sudden death in a young adult with anomalous origin of the posterior circumflex artery. South Med J 1982;75:748.

299. Paulin SJ. Ectopic origin of the right coronary artery: anterior or posterior—that is the question. Cathet Cardiovasc Diagn 1995;36:379.

300. Paulsen S, Vetner M, Hagerup CM. Relationship between heart weight and the cross-sectional area of the coronary ostia. Acta Pathol Microbiol Scand 1975;83:529.

301. Perloff JK. Congenital anomalies of the coronary circulation. In: The clinical recognition of congenital heart disease. 4th ed. Philadelphia: WB Saunders, 1994:738.

302. Perry SB, Rome J, Keane JF, et al. Transcatheter closure of coronary artery fistulas. J Am Coll Cardiol 1992;124:1624.

303. Phillips DA, Berman J. A variation in the origin of the posterior descending coronary artery. Cardiovasc Intervent Radiol 1984;7:75.

304. Pichard AD, Casanegra P, Marchant E, et al. Abnormal regional myocardial flow in myocardial bridging of the left anterior descending coronary artery. Am J Cardiol 1981;47:978.

305. Piechaud JF, Shalaby L, Kachaner J, et al. Pulmonary artery "stop-flow" angiography to visualize the anomalous origin of the left coronary artery from the pulmonary artery in infants. Pediatr Cardiol 1987;8:11.

306. Polacek P, Zechmeister A. The occurrence and significance of myocardial bridges and loops on coronary arteries. Opuscola Cardiologica. Acta Facultatis Medicae Universitatis Brunensis, Brno, Czech Republic, 1968.

307. Portsmann W, Iwig J. Die intramurale Koronaroarterie im Angiogramm. Fortschr Roentenstr 1960;92:129.

308. Rivitz SM, Yasuda T. Predictive value of dipyridamole thallium imaging in a patient with myocardial bridging but without fixed obstructive coronary artery disease. J Nucl Med 1992;33:1905.

309. Probst P, Pachinger O, Koller H, et al. Origin of anterior descending branch of left coronary artery from pulmonary trunk. Br Heart J 1976;38:523.

310. Raffer SF, Oetgen WJ, Weeks KD Jr, et al. Thallium-201 scintigraphy after surgical repair of hemodynamically significant primary coronary artery anomalies. Chest 1982;81:687.

311. Raht S, Har-Zahav Y, Battler A, et al. Frequency and clinical significance of anomalous origin of septal perforator coronary artery. Am J Cardiol 1986;58:657.

312. Ranniger K, Thilenius OG, Cassels DE. Angiographic diagnosis of an anomalous right coronary artery arising from the pulmonary artery. Radiology 1967;88:29.

313. Reddy K, Mohinder G, Hamby RI. Multiple coronary arteriosystemic fistulas. Am J Cardiol 1974;33:304.

314. Reidy JF, Anjos RT, Qureshi SA, et al. Transcatheter embolization in the treatment of coronary artery fistula. J Am Coll Cardiol 1991;18:187.

315. Reidy JF, Tynan MJ, Qureshi S. Embolization of a complex coronary arteriovenous fistula in a 6 year old child: the need for specialized embolization techniques. Br Heart J 1990;63:246.

316. Reig J, Ruiz de Miguel C, Moragas A. Morphometric analysis of myocardial bridges in children with ventricular hypertrophy. Pediatr Cardiol 1990;11:186.

317. Rein AJJT, Colan SD, Parness IA, et al. Regional and global left ventricular function in infants with anomalous origin of the left coronary artery from the pulmonary trunk: preoperative and postoperative assessment. Circulation 1987;75:115.

318. Reis RL, Cohen LS, Mason DT. Direct measurement of instantaneous coronary blood flow after total correction of anomalous left coronary artery. Circulation 1969;39:229.

319. Rinaldi RG, Carballido J, Giles R, et al. Right coronary artery with anomalous origin and slit ostium. Ann Thorac Surg 1994;58:829.

320. Rittenhouse EA, Doty DB, Ehrenhaft JL. Congenital coronary artery-cardiac chamber fistula. Ann Thorac Surg 1975;20:468.

321. Rivitz SM, Yasuda T. Predictive value of dipyridamole thallium imaging in a patient with myocardial bridging but without fixed obstructive coronary artery disease. J Nucl Med 1992;33:1905.

322. Roberts WC, Glick BN. Congenital hypoplasia of both right and left circumflex coronary arteries. Am J Cardiol 1992;70:121.

323. Roberts WC, Shirani J. The four subtypes of anomalous origin of the left main coronary artery from the right aortic sinus (or from the right coronary artery). Am J Cardiol 1992;70:119.

324. Roberts WC, Siegel RJ, Zipes DP. Origin of the right coronary artery from the left sinus of Valsalva and its functional consequences: analysis of 10 necropsy patients. Am J Cardiol 1982;49:863.

325. Roberts WC, Silver MA, Sapala JC. Intussusception of a coronary artery associated with sudden death in a college football player. Am J Cardiol 1986;57:179.

326. Roberts WC, Waller BF, Roberts CS. Fatal atherosclerotic narrowing of the right main coronary artery: origin of the left anterior descending or left circumflex coronary artery from the right (the true "left-main equivalent"). Am Heart J 1982;104:638.

327. Roberts WC. Major anomalies of coronary arterial origin seen in adulthood. Am Heart J 1986;111:941.

328. Roberts WJ, Morrow AG. Compression of anomalous left circumflex coronary arteries by prosthetic valve fixation rings. J Thorac Cardiovasc Surg 1969;57:834.

329. Robicsek F. Origin of the left anterior descending coronary artery from the left mammary artery. Am Heart J 1984;108:1377.

330. Robicsek R, Sanger P, Daugherty HK, et al. Origin of the anterior interventricular (descending) artery and vein from the left mammary vessels. A previously unknown anomaly of the coronary system. J Thorac Cardiovasc Surg 1967;53:602.

331. Rodgers DM, Wolf NM, Barrett MJ, et al. Two-dimensional echocardiographic features of coronary arteriovenous fistulae. Am Heart J 1982;104:872.

332. Rose AG. Multiple coronary arterioventricular fistulae. Circulation 1978;58:178.

333. Roughneen PT, Bhattacharjee M, Morris PT, et al. Spontaneous thrombosis in a coronary artery fistula with aneurysmal dilatation of the sinus of Valsalva. Ann Thorac Surg 1994;57:232.

334. Rowe L, Carmody TJ, Askenazi J. Anomalous origin of the left circumflex coronary artery from the right aortic sinus: a familial clustering. Cathet Cardiovasc Diagn 1993;29:277.

335. Roynard JL, Cattan S, Artigou JY, et al. Anomalous course of the left anterior descending coronary artery between the aorta and pulmonary trunk: a rare cause of myocardial ischemia at rest. Br Heart J 1994;72:397.

336. Rozenman Y, Schechter D, Gilon D, et al. Anomalous origin of the circumflex coronary artery from the right sinus of Valsalva as a cause of ischemia at old age. Clin Cardiol 1993;16:900.

337. Ruiz CE, Lau FYK. Congenital atresia of left main coronary artery: proposed mechanism for severe disabling angina in a patient with non-atherosclerotic single right coronary artery. A case report. Cathet Cardiovasc Diagn 1991;23:190.

338. Ruszkiewicz A, Opeskin K. Sudden death in pregnancy from congenital malformation of the coronary arteries. Pathology 1993;25:236.

339. Sabiston DC Jr, Neill CA, Taussig HB. Direction of blood flow in anomalous left coronary artery arising from the pulmonary artery. Circulation 1960;22:591.

340. Sacks JH, Londe SP, Rosenbluth A, et al. Left main coronary bypass for aberrant (aortic) intramural left coronary artery. J Thorac Cardiovasc Surg 1977;73:733.

341. Sagkan O, Ornek E, Yesildag O. Left circumflex coronary artery arising as a terminal extension of right coronary artery. A case report. Angiology 1994;45:405.

342. Said SA, Bucx JJ, van de Weel FA. Stress MIBI scintigraphy in multiple coronary-pulmonary fistula: failure to demonstrate "steal" phenomenon. Int J Cardiol 1992;35:270.

343. Said SAM, El Gamal MIH, van der Werf T. Coronary arteriovenous fistulas: collective review and management of six new cases—changing etiology, presentation and treatment strategy. Clin Cardiol 1997;20:748.

344. Saji T, Yamamoto K, Hashiguchi R, et al. Hypoplastic left coronary artery in association with occlusive thickening of a coronary artery with ectopic ostium and with atresia of the left coronary ostium. Jpn Heart J 1985;26:603.

345. Saner HE, Saner BD, Dykoski RK, et al. Origin of anterior descending coronary artery from the first septal perforator. Cathet Cardiovasc Diagn 1984;10:479.

346. Sasson Z, Grande P, Lorett I, et al. Proximal narrowing of anomalous right coronary artery from the left coronary sinus: delineation by Omniplane transesophageal echocardiogram. Can J Cardiol 1996;12:529.

347. Savic B, Birtel FJ, Tholen W, et al. Lung sequestration: report of seven cases and review of 540 published cases. Thorax 1979;34:96.

348. Schang SJ, Pepine CJ, Bemiller CR. Anomalous coronary origin and bicuspid aortic valve. Vasc Surg 1975;9:67.

349. Schaper W, Schaper J. Collateral circulation. Norwell, MA: Kluwer Academic Publishers, 1993.

350. Schlesinger MJ, Zoll PM, Wessler S. The conus artery: a third coronary artery. Am Heart J 1949;38:823.

351. Schlesinger MJ. An injection plus dissection study of coronary artery occlusions and anastomosis. Am Heart J 1938;15:528.

352. Schulte MA, Waller BF, Hull MT, et al. Origin of the left anterior descending coronary artery from the right aortic sinus with intramyocardial tunneling to the left side of the heart via the ventricular septum: a case against clinical and morphologic significance of myocardial bridging. Am Heart J 1985;110:499.

353. Schwarz ER, Klues HG, Dahl J, et al. Functional, angiographic and intracoronary Doppler flow characteristics in symptomatic patients with myocardial bridging: effect of short-term intravenous beta-blocker medication. J Am Coll Cardiol 1996;27:1637.

354. Seabra-Gomes R, Somerville J, Ross DN, et al. Congenital coronary artery aneurysms. Br Heart J 1974;36:329.

355. Serota H, Barth CW, Seus CA, et al. Rapid identification of the course of anomalous coronary arteries in adults: the ''dot'' and ''eye'' method. Am J Cardiol 1990;65:891.

356. Sharbaugh AH, White RS. Single coronary artery. Analysis of the anatomic variation, clinical importance, and report of five cases. JAMA 1974;230:243.

357. Shigenobu M, Ohta T, Senoo Y, et al. Congenital coronary aneurysm associated with a single coronary artery. Cardiovasc Surg 1993;1:79.

358. Shiode N, Kato M, Teragawa H, et al. Vasomotility and nitric oxide bioactivity of the bridging segments of the left anterior descending coronary artery. Am J Cardiol 1998;81:341.

359. Shirai K, Ogawa M, Kawaguchi H, et al. Acute myocardial infarction due to thrombus formation in congenital coronary artery fistula. Eur Heart J 1994;15:577.

360. Shirani J, Roberts WC. Solitary coronary ostium in the aorta in the absence of other major congenital cardiovascular anomalies. J Am Coll Cardiol 1993;21:137.

361. Shirani J, Roberts WD. Coronary ostial dimple (in the posterior aortic sinus) in the absence of other coronary arterial abnormalities. Am J Cardiol 1993;72:118.

362. Shirani J, Zafari AM, Roberts WC. Sudden death, right ventricular infarction, and abnormal right ventricular intramural coronary arteries in isolated congenital valvular pulmonic stenosis. Am J Cardiol 1993;72:368.

363. Shivalkar B, Borgers M, Daenen W, et al. ALCAPA syndrome: an example of chronic myocardial hypoperfusion? J Am Coll Cardiol 1994;23:772.

364. Shubrooks SJ Jr, Naggar CZ. Spontaneous near closure of coronary artery fistula. Circulation 1978;57:197.

365. Silverman KJ, Bulkley BH, Hutchins GM. Anomalous left circumflex coronary artery: ''normal'' variant of uncertain clinical and pathologic significance. Am J Cardiol 1978;41:1311.

366. Silverman ME, White CS, Ziskind AA. Pulmonary sequestration receiving arterial supply from the left circumflex coronary artery. Chest 1994;106:948.

367. Sing SP, Soto B, Nath H. Anomalous origin of posterior descending artery with unusual intraseptal course. J Thorac Imaging 1994;9:255.

368. Skimming JW, Gessner IH, Victorica BE, et al. Percutaneous transcatheter occlusion of coronary artery fistula using detachable balloons. Pediatr Cardiol 1995;16:38.

369. Skimming JW, Walls JT. Congenital coronary artery fistula suggesting a ''steal phenomenon'' in a neonate. Pediatr Cardiol 1993;14:174.

370. Sones FM, Shirey EK. Cine coronary arteriography. Mod Conc Cardiovasc Dis 1962;31:735.

371. Sorrell VL, Davis MJ, Bove AA. Current knowledge and significance of coronary artery ectasia: a chronologic review of the literature, recommendations for treatment, possible etiologies, and future considerations. Clin Cardiol 1998;21:157.

372. Spindola FH, Grose R, Solomon N. Dual left anterior descending coronary artery: angiographic description of important variants and surgical implications. Am Heart J 1983;105:445.

373. St. John Sutton MG, Miller GA, Kerr IH, et al. Coronary steal via large coronary artery to bronchial artery anastomosis successfully treated by operation. Br Heart J 1980;44:460.

374. Stables RH, Knight CJ, Neill JG, et al. Coronary stenting in the management of myocardial ischaemia caused by muscle bridging. Br Heart J 1995;74:90.

375. Stauffer JC, Sigwart U, Vogt P, et al. Transluminal angioplasty of a single coronary artery. Am Heart J 1991;122:569.

376. Stein PD, Marzilli M, Sabbah HN, et al. Systolic and diastolic pressure gradients within the left ventricular wall. Am J Physiol 1980;238:625.

377. Steinberg I, Holswade GR. Coronary arteriovenous fistula. AJR 1972;116:82.

378. Sundar AS, Fox KA. Anomalous origin of the right coronary artery from the pulmonary artery in association with congenital aneurysm of the sinus of Valsalva: angiographic diagnosis of a rare association. Br Heart J 1992;68:330.

379. Swanton RH, Thomas ML, Coltart DJ, et al. Coronary artery ectasia—a variant of occlusive coronary arteriosclerosis. Br Heart J 1978;40:393.

380. Swaye PS, Fisher LD, Litwin P, et al. Aneurysmal coronary artery disease. Circulation 1983;67:134.

381. Taber RE, Gale MH, Lam CR. Coronary artery-right heart fistulas. J Thorac Cardiovasc Surg 1967;53:84.

382. Takahasi M, Sekiguchi H, Fujikawa H, et al. Multicystic aneurysmal dilatation of bilateral coronary artery fistula. Cathet Cardiovasc Diagn 1994;31:290.

383. Taylor AJ, Byers JP, Cheitlin MD, et al. Anomalous right or left coronary artery from the contralateral coronary sinus: ''high-risk'' abnormalities in the initial coronary artery course and heterogeneous clinical outcomes. Am Heart J 1997;133:428.

384. Taylor AJ, Farb A, Ferguson M, et al. Myocardial infarction associated with physical exertion in a young man. Circulation 1997;96:3201.

385. Taylor AJ, Rogan KM, Virmani R. Sudden cardiac death associated with isolated congenital coronary artery anomalies. J Am Coll Cardiol 1992;20:640.

386. Teno LA, Santos JL, Bestetti RB, et al. Congenital circumflex coronary artery fistula with drainage into the left ventricle. Tex Heart Inst J 1993;20:304.

387. Tingelstad JB, Lower RR, Eldredge WJ. Anomalous origin of the right coronary artery from the main pulmonary artery. Am J Cardiol 1972;30:670.

388. Tio RA, Van Gelder IC, Boonstra PW, et al. Myocardial bridging in a survivor of sudden cardiac near-death: role of intracoronary Doppler flow measurements and angiography during dobutamine stress in the clinical evaluation. Heart 1997;77:280.

389. Tkebuchava T, Von Segesser LK, Vogt PR, et al. Congenital coronary fistulas in children and adults: diagnosis, surgical technique and results. J Cardiovasc Surg 1996;37:29.

390. Topaz O, DeMarchena EJ, Perin E, et al. Anomalous coronary arteries: angiographic findings in 80 patients. Int J Cardiol 1992;34:129.

391. Topaz O, DiSciascio G, Vetrovec GW, et al. Absent left main coronary artery: angiographic findings in 83 patients with separate ostia of the left anterior descending and circumflex arteries at the left aortic sinus. Am Heart J 1991;122:447.

392. Topaz O, DiSciascio G, Goudreau E, et al. Coronary angioplasty of anomalous right coronary arteries: notes on technical aspects. Cathet Cardiovasc Diagn 1990;21:106.

393. Topaz O, Edwards JE. Pathologic features of sudden death in children, adolescents, and young adults. Chest 1985;87:476.

394. Trivellato M, Angelini P, Leachman RD. Variations in coronary artery anatomy: normal versus abnormal. Cardiovasc Dis Bull Tex Heart Inst 1980;7:357.

395. Tuna IC, Bessinger FB, Ophoven JP, et al. Acute angular origin of left coronary artery from aorta: an unusual cause of left ventricular failure in infancy. Pediatr Cardiol 1989;10:39.

396. Ueda K, Saito A, Nakano H, et al. Absence of proximal coronary arteries with pulmonary atresia. Am Heart J 1983;106:596.

397. Upshaw CB. Congenital coronary arteriovenous fistula. Report of a case with an analysis of seventy-three reported cases. Am Heart J 1962;63:399.

398. Urcelay GE, Iannettoni MD, Ludomirsky A, et al. Origin of both coronary arteries from the pulmonary artery. Circulation 1994;90:2379.

399. Urrutia-S CO, Falaschi G, Ott DA, et al. Surgical management of 56 patients with congenital coronary artery fistulae. Ann Thorac Surg 1983;35:300.

400. Vairo U, Marino B, De Simone G, et al. Early congestive heart failure due to origin of the right coronary artery from the pulmonary artery. Chest 1992;102:1610.

401. Van Brussel BL, Van Tellingen C, Ernst SMPG, et al. Myocardial bridging: a cause of myocardial infarction? Int J Cardiol 1984;6:78.

402. van den Brand M, Pieterman H, Suryapranata H, et al. Closure of a

coronary fistula with a transcatheter implantable coil. Cathet Cardiovasc Diagn 1992;25:223.

403. van den Brandhof G, Zijlstra F. Separate origin of a large septal perforator branch. Cathet Cardiovasc Diagn 1992;25:151.

404. Van der Hauwaert L, Dumoulin M, Moerman P. Congenital atresia of the left coronary ostium. Br Heart J 1982;48:298.

405. Vasan RS, Bahl VK, Rajani M. Myocardial infarction associated with a myocardial bridge. Int J Cardiol 1989;25:240.

406. Vavuranakis M, Bush CA, Boudoulas H. Coronary artery fistulas in adults: incidence, angiographic characteristics, natural history. Cathet Cardiovasc Diagn 1995;35:116.

407. Velican D, Petrescu C, Velican C. The branching anatomical pattern of the coronary arteries as a risk factor for coronary heart disease. Med Interne 1981;19:173.

408. Vieweg WVR, Alpert JS, Hagan AD. Caliber and distribution of normal coronary arterial anatomy. Cathet Cardiovasc Diagn 1976;2:269.

409. Virmani R, Chun PKC, Golstein RE, et al. Acute takeoffs of the coronary arteries along the aortic wall and congenital coronary ostial valve-like ridges: association with sudden death. J Am Coll Cardiol 1984;3:766.

410. Virmani R, Patrick K, Kevin R. Anomalous origin of four coronary ostia from the right sinus of Valsalva. Am J Cardiol 1989;63:760.

411. Virmani R, Rogan K, Cheitlin MD. Congenital coronary artery anomalies: pathologic aspects. In: Virmani R, Forman MB, eds. Nonatherosclerotic ischemic heart disease. New York: Raven Press, 1989:153.

412. Vliegen HW, Doornbos J, de Roos A, et al. Value of fast gradient echo magnetic resonance angiography as an adjunct to coronary arteriography in detecting and confirming the course of clinically significant coronary artery anomalies. Am J Cardiol 1997;79:773.

413. Vlodaver Z, Neufeld HN, Edwards JE. Pathology of coronary disease. Semin Roentgenol 1972;7:376.

414. Vlodaver Z, Neufield HN, Edwards JE. Coronary arterial variations in the normal heart and in congenital heart disease. New York: Academic Press 1975:171.

415. Vogelbach KH, Edmiston A, Stenson RE. Coronary artery-left ventricle communications: a report of two cases and review of the literature. Cathet Cardiovasc Diagn 1979;5:159.

416. Vogt PR, Tkebuchava T, Arbenz U, et al. Anomalous origin of the right coronary artery from the pulmonary artery. Thorac Cardiovasc Surgeon 1994;42:125.

417. Voss H, Kupper W, Hanrath P, et al. Clinical correlations, lactate extraction, coronary venous blood flow and thallium-201 myocardial imaging in patients with isolated left anterior descending muscle bridges: normal variant or obstruction? Z Kardiol 1980;69:347.

418. Voudris V, Salachas A, Saounotsou M, et al. Double left anterior descending artery originating from the left and right coronary artery: a rare coronary artery anomaly. Cathet Cardiovasc Diagn 1993;30:45.

419. Vuthoori S, Waisser E, Angelini P. Triple origin of left coronary arteries from right coronary artery: unusual case of single coronary artery. Clin Cardiol 1980;3:67.

420. Wald S, Stonecipher K, Baldwin BJ, et al. Anomalous origin of the right coronary artery from the pulmonary artery. Am J Cardiol 1971;27:677.

421. Waller BF. Five coronary ostia: duplicate left anterior descending and right conus coronary arteries. Am J Cardiol 1983;51:1562.

422. Wang A, Pulsipher MW, Jaggers J, et al. Simultaneous biplane coronary and pulmonary arteriography: a novel technique for defining the course of an anomalous left main coronary artery originating from the right sinus of Valsalva. Cathet Cardiovasc Diagn 1997;42:73.

423. Warren SE, Alpert JS, Vieweg WVR, et al. Normal single coronary artery and myocardial infarction. Chest 1977;72:540.

424. Weinberger I, Rotenberg Z, Fuchs J, et al. Myocardial infarction in young adults under 30 years: risk factors and clinical course. Clin Cardiol 1987;10:9.

425. Wenger NK, Peace RJ. Rudimentary left coronary artery. Am J Cardiol 1961;8:519.

426. Wesselhoeft H, Fawcett JS, Johnson AL. Anomalous origin of the left coronary artery from the pulmonary trunk: its clinical spectrum, pathology, and pathophysiology, based on a review of 140 cases with seven further cases. Circulation 1968;38:403.

427. Wilde P, Watt I. Congenital coronary artery fistulae: six new cases with a collective review. Clin Radiol 1980;31:301.

428. Wilens SL, Plair CM, Henderson DH. Size of the major epicardial

429. coronary arteries at necropsy: relation to age, heart, weight, and myocardial infarction. JAMA 1966;198:1325.

429. Wilkins CE, Betancourt B, Mathur VS. Coronary artery anomalies: a review of more than 10,000 patients from the Clayton Cardiovascular Laboratories. Tex Heart Inst J 1988;15:166.

430. Wilson CS, Weaver WF, Zeman ED, et al. Bilateral nonfistulous congenital coronary arterial aneurysms. Am J Cardiol 1975;35:319.

431. Wilson GJ, Freedom RM, Koike K, et al. The coronary arteries: anatomy and histopathology. In: Freedom RM, ed. Pulmonary atresia with intact ventricular septum. New York: Futura Publishing, 1989:75.

432. Woldow AB, Goldstein S, Yazdanfar S. Angiographic evidence of right coronary bridging. Cathet Cardiovasc Diagn 1994;32:351.

433. Yamagishi M, Haze K, Tamai J, et al. Visualization of isolated conus artery as a major collateral pathway in patients with total left anterior descending artery occlusion. Cathet Cardiovasc Diagn 1988;15:95.

434. Yamabe H, Fujitani K, Mizutani T, et al. Two cases of myocardial infarction with coronary arteriovenous fistula. Jpn Heart J 1983;24:303.

435. Yamanaka O, Hobbs RE. Coronary artery anomalies in 126,595 patients undergoing coronary angiography. Cathet Cardiovasc Diagn 1990;21:28.

436. Yeoh JK, Ling LH, Maurice C. Percutaneous transluminal angioplasty of anomalous right coronary artery arising from the ascending thoracic aorta. Cathet Cardiovasc Diagn 1994;32:254.

437. Zimmerman FH, Cameron A, Fisher LD, et al. Myocardial infarction in young adults: angiographic characterization, risk factors and prognosis (Coronary Artery Surgery Study Registry). J Am Coll Cardiol 1995;26:654.

438. Zumbo O, Fani K, Jarmolych J, et al. Coronary atherosclerosis and myocardial infarction in hearts with anomalous coronary arteries. Lab Invest 1965;14:571.

439. Kolodziej AW, Lobo FV, Walley VM. Intra-atrial course of the right coronary artery and its branches. Can J Cardiol 1994;10:263.

440. Lerer PK, Edwards WD. Coronary arterial anatomy in bicuspid aortic valve. Necropsy study of 100 hearts. Br Heart J 1981;45:142.

441. Krabill KA, Hunter DW. Transcatheter closure of congenital coronary arterial fistula with a detachable balloon. Pediatr Cardiol 1993;14:176.

442. Ramo OJ, Totterman KJ, Harjula AL. Thrombosed coronary artery fistula as a cause of paroxysmal atrial fibrillation and ventricular arrhythmia. Cardiovasc Surg 1994;2:720.

443. Liu PR, Leong KH, Lee PC, et al. Congenital coronary artery-cardiac chamber fistulae: a study of fourteen cases. (Chung Hua i Hsueh Tsa Chih [Taipei])—Chin Med J 1994;54:160.

444. Davis JT, Allen HD, Wheller JJ, et al. Coronary artery fistula in the pediatric age group: a 19-year institutional experience. Ann Thorac Surg 1994;58:760.

445. Millaire A, Goullard L, De Groote P, et al. Congenital high flow coronary cameral fistula in an 81-year-old woman: management problems. Can J Cardiol 1992;8:917.

446. Ludomirsky A, O'Laughlin MP, Reul GJ, et al. Congenital aneurysm of the right coronary artery with fistulous connection to the right atrium. Amer Heart J 1990;119:672.

447. Rosenberg H, Williams WG, Trusler GA, et al. Congenital aortico-right atrial communications. The dilemma of differentiation from coronary-cameral fistula. J Thorac Cardiovasc Surg 1986;91:841.

448. Ryan C, Gertz EW. Fistula from coronary arteries to left ventricle after myocardial infarction. Br Heart J 1977;39:1147.

449. Lin FC, Chang HJ, Chern MS, et al. Multiplane transesophageal echocardiography in the diagnosis of congenital coronary artery fistula. Am Heart J 1995;130:1236.

450. Alkhulaifi AM, Horner SM, Pugsley WB, et al. Coronary artery fistulas presenting with bacterial endocarditis. Ann Thorac Surg 1995;60:202.

451. Santoro G, di Carlo D, Carotti A, et al. Origin of both coronary arteries from the pulmonary artery and aortic coarctation. Ann Thorac Surg 1995;60:706.

452. Berdjis F, Takahashi M, Wells WJ, et al. Anomalous left coronary artery from the pulmonary artery. Significance of intercoronary collaterals. J Thorac Cardiovasc Surg 1994;108:17.

453. Perper JA, Rozin L, Williams KE. Sudden unexpected death following exercise and congenital anomalies of coronary arteries. A report of two cases. Am J Forens Med Pathol 1985;6:289.

454. Alexi-Meskishvili V, Hetzer R, Weng Y, et al. Anomalous origin of

the left coronary artery from the pulmonary artery. Early results with direct aortic reimplantation. J Thorac Cardiovasc Surg 1994;108:354.

455. Koh E, Nakagawa M, Hamaoka K, et al. Congenital atresia of the left coronary ostium: diagnosis and surgical treatment. Pediatr Cardiol 1989;10:159.

456. Maron BJ, Leon MB, Swain JA, et al. Prospective identification by two-dimensional echocardiography of anomalous origin of the left main coronary artery from the right sinus of Valsalva. Am J Cardiol 1991;68:140.

457. Spring DA, Thomsen JH. Severe atherosclerosis in the ''single coronary artery.'' Report of a previously undescribed pattern. Am J Cardiol 1973;31:662.

458. Hackenseller H. Ueber akgessorische, von der arteria pulmonalis abgehende Herzgefaesse und ihre Bedeutung fuer das Verstaendnis der formalen Genese des Ursprunges einer oder beider Coronararterien von der Lungenschlagader. Frankf Z Pathol 1955;66:463.

459. Baird RJ, Manktelow RT, Shah PA, et al. Intramyocardial pressure. A study of its regional variations and its relationship to intraventricular pressure. J Thorac Cardiovasc Surg 1970;59:810.

460. Machado C, Bhasin S, Soulen RL. Confirmation of anomalous origin of the right coronary artery from the left sinus of Valsalva with magnetic resonance imaging. Chest 1993;104:1284.

461. Basso C, Frescura C, Corrado D, et al. Congenital heart disease and sudden death in the young. Hum Pathol 1995;26:1065.

462. Post JC, van Rossum AC, Bronzwaer JG, et al. Magnetic resonance angiography of anomalous coronary arteries. A new gold standard for delineating the proximal course? Circulation 1995;92:3163.

463. McConnell MV, Ganz P, Selwyn AP, et al. Identification of anomalous coronary arteries and their anatomic course by magnetic resonance coronary angiography. Circulation 1995;92:3158.

464. Eguchi S, Nitta H, Asano K, et al. Congenital fistula of the right coronary artery to the left ventricle. The third case in the literature. Am Heart J 1970;80:242.

465. Keeton BR, Keenan DJ, Monro JL. Anomalous origin of both coronary arteries from the pulmonary trunk. Br Heart J 1983;49:397.

466. Galbraith AJ, Werner D, Cutforth RH. Fistula between left coronary artery and superior vena cava. Br Heart J 1981;46:99.

467. Hamilton JR, Mulholland HC, O'Kane HO. Origin of the left coronary artery from the right pulmonary artery: a report of successful surgery in a 3-month-old child. Ann Thorac Surg 1986;41:446.

468. Kirklin JW, Barratt-Boyes BG. Congenital anomalies of the coronary arteries. In: Kirklin JW, Barratt-Boyes BG, eds: Cardiac surgery. New York: Churchill Livingstone, 1993:1179–1189.

469. Mustafa I, Gula G, Radley-Smith R, et al. Anomalous origin of the left coronary artery from the anterior aortic sinus: a potential cause of sudden death. Anatomic characterization and surgical treatment. J Thorac Cardiovasc Surg 1981;82:297.

470. Barthe JE, Benito M, Sala J, et al. Double right coronary artery. Am J Cardiol 1994;73:622.

471. Cafferky EA, Crawford DW, Turner AF, et al. Congenital aneurysm of the coronary artery with myocardial infarction. Am J Med Sci 1969;257:320.

472. Casta A. Hypoplasia of the left coronary artery complicated by reversible myocardial ischemia in a newborn. Am Heart J 1987;114:1238.

473. Piovesana P, Corrado D, Verlato R, et al. Morbidity associated with anomalous origin of the left circumflex coronary artery from the right aortic sinus. Am J Cardiol 1989;63:762.

474. Roberts WC. Anomalous origin of both coronary arteries from the pulmonary artery. Am J Cardiol 1962;10:595.

475. Beretta L, Lemma M, Santoli C. Isolated atresia of the left main coronary artery in an adult. Eur J Cardiothorac Surg 1990;4:169.

476. Nelson-Piercy C, Rickards AF, Yacoub MH. Aberrant origin of the right coronary artery as a potential cause of sudden death: successful anatomical correction. Br Heart J 1990;64:208.

477. Baffa JM, Chen SL, Guttenberg ME, et al. Coronary artery abnormalities and right ventricular histology in hypoplastic left heart syndrome. J Am Coll Cardiol 1992;20:350.

478. Bjork L. Ectasia of the coronary arteries. Radiology 1966;87:33.

479. Murphy ML. Single coronary artery. Am Heart J 1967;74:557.

480. Angelini P. Normal and anomalous coronary arteries: definitions and classification. Am Heart J 1989;117:418.

481. Chu E, Cheitlin MD. Diagnostic considerations in patients with suspected coronary artery anomalies. Am Heart J 1993;126:1427.

482. Smith SC, Taber MT, Robiolio PA, et al. Acute myocardial infarction caused by a myocardial bridge treated with intracoronary stenting. Cathet Cardiovasc Diagn 1997;42:209.

483. Noble J, Bourassa MG, Petitclerc R, et al. Myocardial bridging and milking effect of the left anterior descending coronary artery: normal variant or obstruction? Am J Cardiol 1976;37:993.

484. Raghib G, Bloemendaal RD, Kanjuh VI, et al. Aortic atresia and premature closure of foramen ovale. Myocardial sinusoids and coronary arteriovenous fistula serving as outflow channel. Am Heart J 1965;70:476.

485. Crocker DW, Sobin S, Thomas WC. Aneurysm of the coronary arteries. Am J Pathol 1957;33:819.

486. Cohen LS, Shaw LD. Fatal myocardial infarction in an 11 year old boy associated with a unique coronary artery anomaly. Am J Cardiol 1967;19:420.

487. Harris PN. Aneurysmal dilatation of the cardiac coronary arteries. Am J Pathol 1937;13:89.

488. Nath A, Kennett JD, Politte LL, et al. Anomalous right coronary artery arising from the midportion of the left anterior descending coronary artery—case reports. Angiology 1987;38:142.

489. Barth CW, Bray M, Roberts WC. Sudden death in infancy associated with origin of both left main and right coronary arteries from a common ostium above the left sinus of Valsalva. Am J Cardiol 1986;57:365.

490. Koh KK. Confirmation of anomalous origin of the right coronary artery from the left sinus of Valsalva by means of transesophageal echocardiography. Am Heart J 1991;122:851.

491. Roberts WC, Dicicco BS, Waller BF, et al. Origin of the left main from the right coronary artery or from the right aortic sinus with intramyocardial tunneling to the left side of the heart via the ventricular septum. The case against clinical significance of myocardial bridge or coronary tunnel. Am Heart J 1982;104:303.

492. Fortuin NJ, Roberts WC. Congenital atresia of the left main coronary artery. Am J Med 1971;50:385.

493. Scott DH. Aneurysms of the coronary arteries. Br Heart J 1948;36:403.

494. Thomas D, Salloum J, Montalescot G, et al. Anomalous coronary arteries coursing between the aorta and pulmonary trunk: clinical indications for coronary artery bypass. Eur Heart J 1991;12:832.

495. Fernandes ED, Kadivar H, Hallman GL, et al. Congenital malformations of the coronary arteries: the Texas Heart Institute experience. Ann Thorac Surg 1992;54:732.

496. Sauer U, Gittenberger-de Groot AC, Geishauser M, et al. Coronary arteries in the hypoplastic left heart syndrome. Histopathologic and histometrical studies and implications for surgery. Circulation 1989;80:I168.

496. Partridge JB. High leftward origin of the right coronary artery. Int J Cardiol 1986;13:83.

498. Pollack BD, Belkin RN, Lazar S, et al. Origin of all three coronary arteries from separate ostia in the right sinus of Valsalva: a rarely reported coronary artery anomaly. Cathet Cardiovasc Diagn 1992;26:26.

499. Rakusan K, Flanagan MF, Geva T, et al. Morphometry of human coronary capillaries during normal growth and the effect of age in left ventricular pressure-overload hypertrophy. Circulation 1992;86:38.

500. Line DE, Babb JD, Pierce WS. Congenital aortic valve anomaly. Aortic regurgitation with left coronary artery isolation. J Thorac Cardiovasc Surg 1979;77:533.

501. Kurnik PB, Heymann WR. Coronary artery ectasia associated with hereditary hemorrhagic telangiectasia. Arch Intern Med 1989;149:2357.

502. Liberthson RR. Congenital anomalies of the coronary arteries. Cardiovasc Med 1984;9:857.

503. Goldblatt E, Adams AP, Ross IK, et al. Single-trunk anomalous origin of both coronary arteries from the pulmonary artery. Diagnosis and surgical management. J Thorac Cardiovasc Surg 1984;87:59.

504. Roberts WC, Kragel AH. Anomalous origin of either the right or left main coronary artery from the aorta without coursing of the anomalistically arising artery between aorta and pulmonary trunk. Am J Cardiol 1988;62:1263.

505. James TN. Anatomy of the coronary arteries in health and disease. Circulation 1965;32:1020.

506. Boucek RJ, Morales AR, Romanelli R, et al. Coronary artery disease: pathologic and clinical assessment. Baltimore: Williams & Wilkins, 1984:38.

507. Vollebergh FE, Becker AE. Minor congenital variations of cusp size in tricuspid aortic valves. Possible link with isolated aortic stenosis. Br Heart J 1977;39:1006.

508. Baroldi G, Scomazzoni G. Coronary circulation in the normal heart and the pathologic heart. Washington DC: United States Government Printing Office, 1967.

509. Maseri A. Ischemic heart disease: a rational basis for clinical practise and clinical research. 1st ed. New York: Churchill Livingston, 1995:71.

510. Harrison DG, Bates JN. The nitrovasodilators. New ideas about old drugs. Circulation 1991;87:1461.

511. Hori M, Kitakaze M. Adenosine, the heart, and coronary circulation. Hypertension 1991;18:565.

512. Liang BT. Adenosine receptors and cardiovascular function. Trends Cardiovasc Med 1992;2:100.

513. Van Camp SP, Bloor CM, Mueller FO, et al. Nontraumatic sports death in high school and college athletes. Med Sci Sports Exerc 1995;27:641.

514. Maron BJ, Shirani J, Poliac LC, et al. Sudden death in young competitive athletes: clinical, demographic, and pathological profiles. JAMA 1996;276:199.

515. Corrado D, Thiene G, Nava A, et al. Sudden death in young competitive athletes: clinicopathologic correlations in 22 cases. Am J Med 1990;89:588.

516. Virmani R, Robinowitz M, McAllister HA Jr. Nontraumatic death in joggers: a series of 30 patients at autopsy. Am J Med 1982;72:874.

517. Waller BF, Roberts WC. Sudden death while running in conditioned runners aged 40 years or over. Am J Cardiol 1980;45:1292.

518. Thompson PD, Stern MP, Williams P, et al. Death during jogging or running: a study of 18 cases. JAMA 1979;242:1265.

519. Schlant RC, Blomqvist CG, Brandenburg RO, et al. Guidelines for exercise testing: a report of the Joint American College of Cardiology/American Heart Association Task Force on Assessment of Cardiovascular Procedures (Subcommittee on Exercise Testing). Circulation 1986;74:653A.

520. Corrado D, Basso C, Poletti A, et al. Sudden death in the young: is coronary thrombosis the major precipitating factor? Circulation 1994;90:2315.

521. Mitchell JH, Maron BJ, Epstein SE. 16th Bethesda Conference: cardiovascular abnormalities in the athlete: recommendations regarding eligibility for competition: October 3–5, 1984. J Am Coll Cardiol 1985;6:1186.

522. Suzuki A, Kamiya T, Juwahara N, et al. Coronary arterial lesions of Kawasaki disease: Cardiac catheterization findings of 1100 cases. Pediatr Cardiol 1986;7:3.

523. Kiso I, Itoh T, Morishita M, et al. Blood flow and pressure measurements of right coronary artery to left ventricle fistula. Thorax 1978;33:253.

524. Grollman JH Jr. The fistulous connection: how does it go? Cathet Cardiovasc Diag 1998;43(2):184.

525. Wearn JT, Mettier SR, Klumpp TG, et al. The nature of the vascular communications between the coronary arteries and the chambers of the heart. Am Heart J 1933;9:143.

526. Acierno LJ. The history of cardiology. London: The Parthenon Publishing Group, 1994:3–39.

527. Lo PH, Chang KC, Hung JS, et al. Anomalous origin of left main coronary artery from the noncoronary sinus: an intravascular ultrasound observation. Cathet Cardiovasc Diagn 1997;42:430.

528. Diez JG, Angelini P, Lee VV. Does the anomalous congenital origin of a coronary artery predispose to the development of stenotic atherosclerotic lesions in its proximal segment? Circulation 1997;96(Suppl I):I-154.

529. Ishikawa T, Otsuka T, Suzuki T. Anomalous origin of the left main coronary artery from the noncoronary sinus of Valsalva. Pediatr Cardiol 1990;11:173.

530. Nomina Anatomica, 6th ed. Edinburgh: Churchill-Livingstone, 1989.

531. O'Malley CD, Saunders JB. Leonardo da Vinci on the human body. New York: Greenwich House, 1982:86–142.

532. Mahowald JM, Blieden LC, Coe JI, et al. Ectopic origin of a coronary artery from the aorta: sudden death in 3 of 23 patients. Chest 1986;89:668.

533. Hiraishi S, Misawa H, Horiguchi Y, et al. Effect of suture closure of coronary artery fistula on aneurysmal coronary artery and myocardial ischemia. Am J Cardiol 1998;81:1263.

534. Maron BJ, Thompson PD, Puffer JC, et al. Cardiovascular preparticipation screening of competitive athletes: a statement for health professionals from the Sudden Death Committee (Clinical Cardiology) and Congenital Cardiac Defects Committee (Cardiovascular Disease in the Young), American Heart Association. Circulation 1996;94:850.

Part II

ANGIOGRAPHIC ATLAS
OF CORONARY ANOMALIES

CASE REPORT 4.1

Absent Left Main Trunk

A 68-year-old woman with a previous history of coronary artery disease and mitral regurgitation was admitted with progressive angina. Cardiac catheterization revealed occlusion of the non-dominant RCA, diffuse disease of the LAD (Fig. CR4.1*A*), and a critically stenotic lesion of the proximal circumflex artery (Fig. CR4.1*B*). The left ventricular ejection fraction was normal. The patient underwent successful balloon angioplasty of the proximal circumflex artery, which arose from an independent ostium in the left anterior aortic sinus, adjacent to the separate ostium that gave rise to the LAD (absent left main trunk). ■

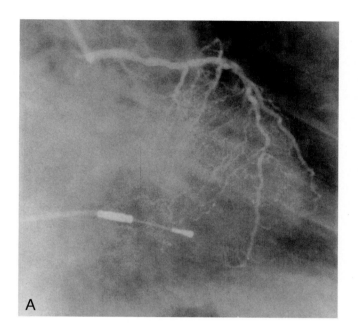 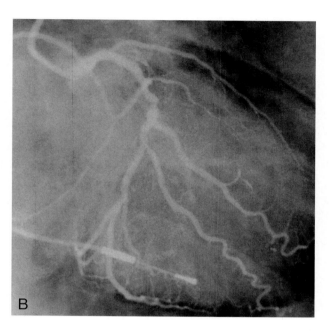

Figure CR4.1. **A.** Angiogram of the LAD in the right anterior oblique projection, showing diffuse coronary disease. **B.** Circumflex artery in the same projection. Note lack of visualization of the other LCA despite reflow of contrast material into the aorta.

CASE REPORT 4.2

Anomalous Location of the Coronary Ostium in the Appropriate Sinus: High Origination of the RCA

A 72-year-old man with diabetes mellitus and hypertension presented with recent-onset angina. The patient was a cigarette smoker and had a family history of coronary artery disease. A myocardial infarction was diagnosed. Cardiac catheterization revealed occlusion of the RCA, which had a high anterior origin

in the right sinus (Fig. CR4.2, A–C). The left coronary system filled the branches of the distal RCA by means of collateral vessels. Submaximal thallium exercise testing showed a nonreversible defect in the inferior ventricular wall. Continued medical treatment was recommended. ■

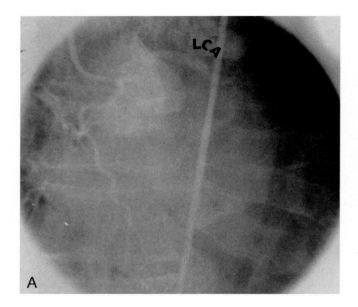

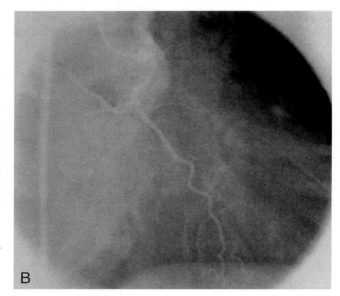

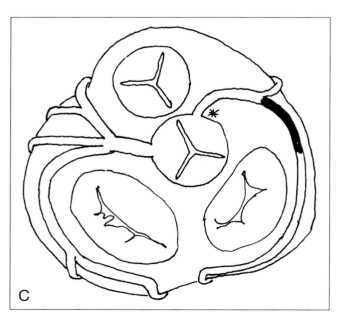

Figure CR4.2. Angiograms of the RCA in the left **(A)** and right **(B)** anterior oblique projections. The ostium has a high anterior origin, close to the anterior commissure. The vessel is totally occluded distal to an anterior ventricular branch. Contrast medium spills over into the left anterior cusp (L), from which the LCA originates. **C.** Schematic diagram of the coronary anomaly (coronal plane). ∗ = Eccentric site of origin of the RCA, close to the anterior commissure.

CASE REPORT 4.3

Anomalous Location of the Coronary Ostium in, or Close to, the Appropriate Sinus: Low Origination of the RCA

A 77-year-old woman with a previous history of coronary artery disease, myocardial infarction, and aortocoronary bypass surgery, presented with recurrent angina. Cardiac catheterization revealed 100% occlusion of the LAD and the RCA, which had a low origin in the right coronary sinus (Fig. CR4.3). Two of the four previous bypass grafts were also occluded. On physical examination, no aortic valve murmur was heard. ■

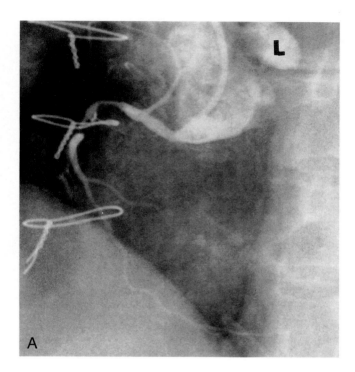

Figure CR4.3. Angiogram of the RCA in the left anterior oblique projection, showing a coronary ostium at the lower end of the coronary sinus. The aortic sinuses may be mildly asymmetric with a diminutive left anterior sinus (L). Figure 4.7 (see main text) shows a schematic diagram of the coronary anomaly.

CASE REPORT 4.4

Anomalous Location of the Coronary Ostium in, or Close to, the Appropriate Sinus: Low Origination of the RCA

A 77-year-old woman presented with a 1-week history of intermittent chest pain that radiated to her left shoulder. The patient was a cigarette smoker with hypertension and severe aortic insufficiency, as well as a 1-year history of dyspnea and fatigue. Cardiac catheterization confirmed the presence of severe aortic insufficiency and normal coronary arteries with low origination of the RCA (Fig. CR4.4, A–B). The aortic regurgitation was assumed to be related to systemic hypertension, with dilation of the aortic annulus. For a diagram of a similar anomaly, see Figure 4.7. ■

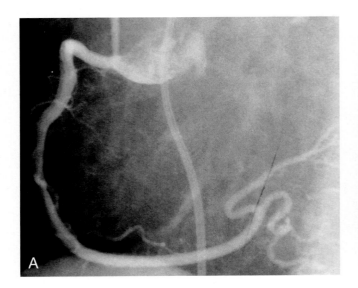 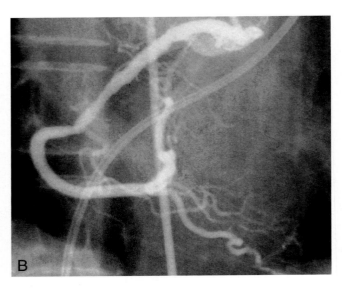

Figure CR4.4. Angiograms of the RCA in the left **(A)** and right **(B)** anterior oblique projections (see text).

CASE REPORT 4.5

Anomalous Location of the Coronary Ostium in the Appropriate Sinus: Commissural Origination of the RCA

A 59-year-old woman with hypertension and coronary artery disease was admitted with Canadian Heart Association functional class-III angina. Cardiac catheterization showed a critical lesion in the LAD (at the site of previous percutaneous transluminal coronary angioplasty) and a dominant RCA, which had a com-

missural origin (Fig. CR4.5, *A–C*). Interestingly, the patient had ST-segment elevation and angina during selective catheterization and contrast injection at the RCA. It is likely that the ectopic RCA had a tangential proximal trunk with enhanced spasticity. Coronary vasodilator therapy was recommended. ∎

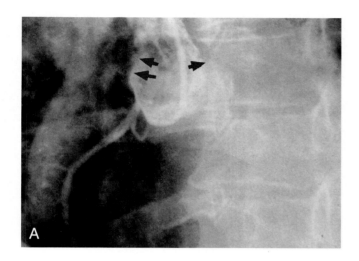

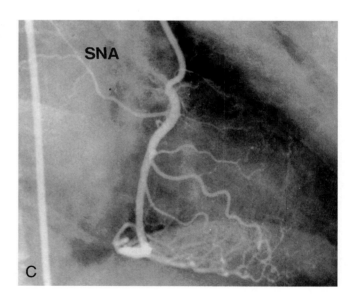

Figure CR4.5. A. Angiogram of the RCA in the left anterior oblique projection. A Judkins right coronary catheter could not selectively cannulate the ectopic artery but did reveal the ostium's unusual location in the posterior-most portion of the right anterior sinus. Single arrow = anterior commissure of the right anterior sinus of Valsalva; double arrows = posterior-right commissures of the right anterior sinus of Valsalva. **B** and **C.** After the angina resolved, selective angiograms of the RCA in the posteroanterior **(B)** and right anterior oblique **(C)** projections showed a normal luminal size. Selective catheterization was achieved with an Amplatz-I right coronary catheter. Initial attempts to cannulate the RCA with a noncoaxial catheter may have resulted in ostial spasm (not documented on cineangiography). SNA = sinus node artery.

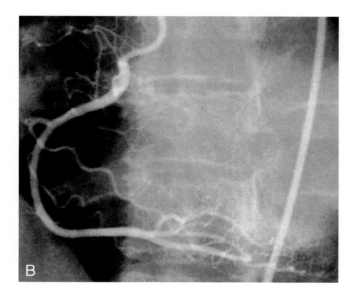

CASE REPORT 4.6

Anomalous Location of the Coronary Ostium in, or Close to, the Appropriate Sinus: Commissural Origination of the RCA

A 41-year-old man presented with new-onset angina and abnormal thallium stress test results indicating an inferior, reversible defect. On physical examination, no heart murmur was heard. Cardiac catheterization revealed "absence" of the LAD, as well as commissural origination of the RCA and the right aortic arch (Fig. CR4.6, *A–C*). The stress test was deemed false positive, and medical treatment was continued. ■

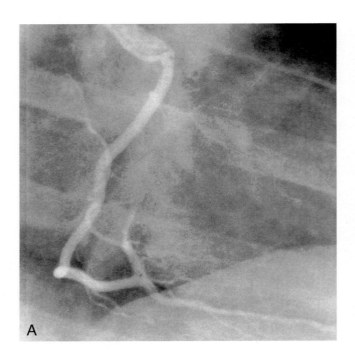

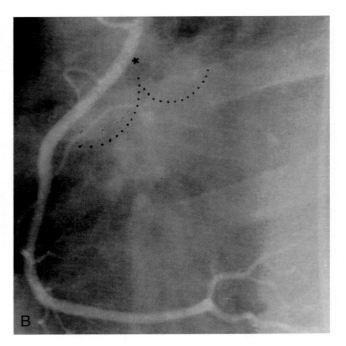

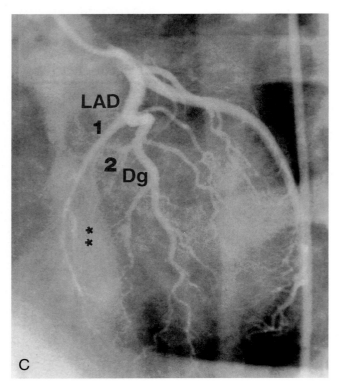

Figure CR4.6. Angiogram of the RCA, in the right **(A)** and left **(B)** anterior oblique projections, showing the ostium located above the commissure, between the right and left anterior sinuses. The right sinus seems larger than the left one, but no specific study was carried out to confirm the presence of asymmetry. In view **A**, the RCA pursues a direct course down to the right atrioventricular groove, and spilled-over contrast material fills the neighboring right coronary sinus. Both features suggest commissural (versus left sinus) origination of the RCA. In view **B**, the asterisk indicates the peak of the anterior commissure, and the dotted lines indicate the intercuspal space or triangle. **C.** Angiogram of the LCA in the left anterior oblique projection. The LAD is present only as far as the bifurcation of the second septal branch. The LAD continues into a large epicardial vessel (Dg), which lies lateral to the anterior interventricular groove (asterisks), and should be called the diagonal artery (absent distal epicardial LAD). 1 = first septal branch; 2 = second septal branch.

CASE REPORT 4.7

Anomalous Location of the Coronary Ostium in, or Close to, the Appropriate Sinus: High Posterior Origination of the LCA

A 53-year-old man with hypertension and obesity was admitted for exertional epigastric discomfort and dyspnea. Cardiac catheterization showed diffuse coronary ectasia but no obstructive coronary artery disease (Fig. CR4.7, A–F). The left ventricular ejection fraction was normal. Continued medical treatment was recommended. ▶

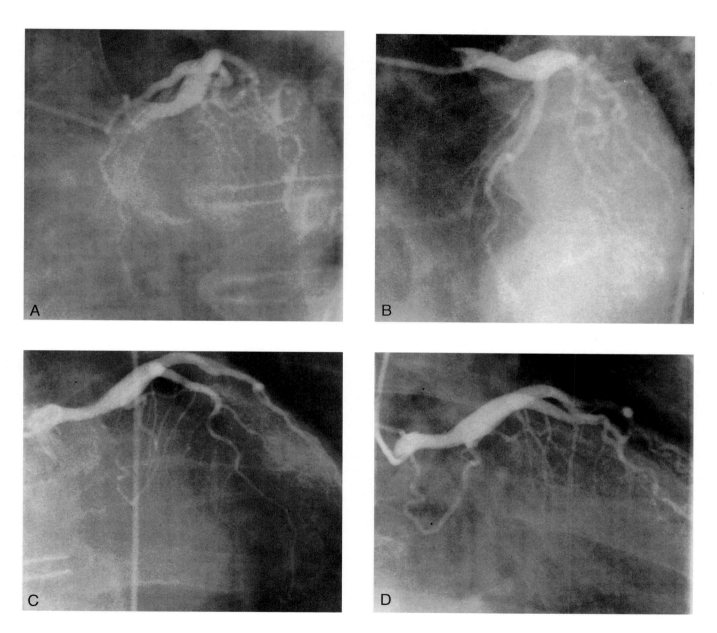

Figure CR4.7. Angiograms of the LCA in the caudal left anterior oblique **(A)**, cranial left anterior oblique **(B)**, posteroanterior **(C)**, and right anterior oblique **(D)** projections. (continued)

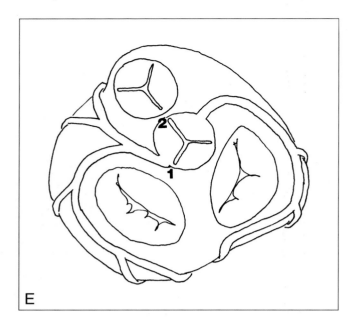

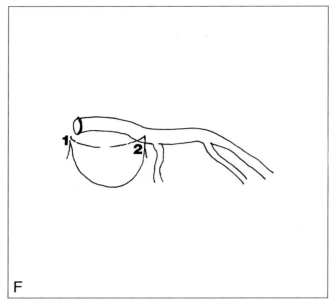

Figure CR4.7. (Continued) **E.** In this schematic diagram, imaged in the coronal plane, the LCA originates close to the posterior commissure (1) of the coronary sinus and away from the anterior commissure (2). **F.** This schematic diagram, imaged in the sagittal plane, shows the ostial location in its vertical relationship to the left coronary sinus.

CASE REPORT 4.8

Anomalous Location of the Coronary Ostium Outside the Normal "Coronary" Sinuses: LCA Origination From the Right Posterior ("Noncoronary") Sinus and RCA Origination From the Left Anterior Sinus

A 61-year-old man with hypertension and dilated cardiomyopathy was admitted to our institution for evaluation. Cardiac catheterization showed that the LCA originated from the posterior sinus and the RCA originated from the left anterior sinus (Fig.

CR4.8, A–C). On physical examination, no heart murmur was heard. The coronary anomalies were considered to be unrelated to the cardiomyopathy, and continued medical treatment was recommended. ■

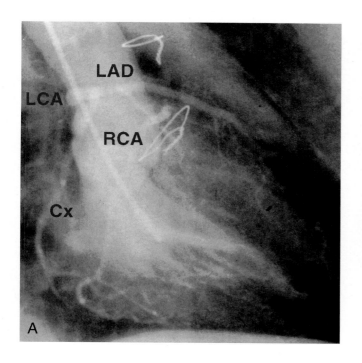

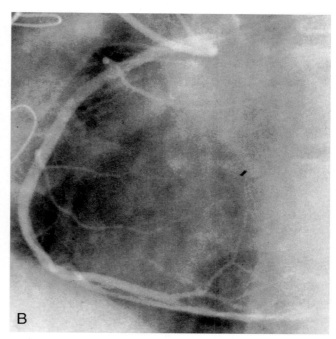

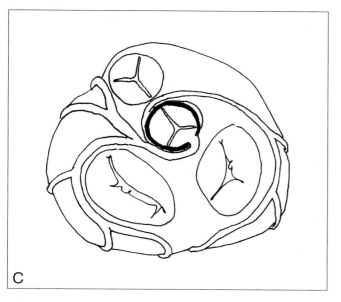

Figure CR4.8. A. Left ventriculogram, in the right anterior oblique projection, showing the anomalous coronary morphology: the proximal LCA originates posterior to the aorta, above the aortic sinus level, and the RCA originates lower, from the left anterior sinus. Cx = circumflex artery; LAD = left anterior descending artery. A selective left coronary angiogram (not shown) confirmed the origination of the LCA from a site above the noncoronary sinus. **B.** Selective angiogram of the RCA, showing associated ectopy of the LCA, which originates from the left coronary sinus. **C.** In this schematic diagram of the anomaly, both coronary arteries, at their origins, seem to be rotated 120° counterclockwise with respect to normal. The LCA originates above the usual level inside the aortic root. The dark circle above the aortic valve represents the sinotubular junction.

CASE REPORT 4.9

Anomalous Location of the Ectopic Coronary Ostium Outside the Normal "Coronary" Sinuses: Origination of the Circumflex Artery From the Right Posterior ("Noncoronary") Sinus and Absent Left Main Trunk

A 70-year-old man with hypertension, hyperlipidemia, and a previous myocardial infarction presented with progressive angina. Cardiac catheterization showed triple-vessel coronary obstructive disease and diffuse hypokinesia (Fig. CR4.9, A and B). The circumflex artery originated separately and anomalously from the posterior aortic sinus (Fig. CR4.9, C). The LAD originated independently from the left aortic sinus, so this case involved an absent left main trunk. Aortocoronary artery bypass surgery was successfully carried out. ∎

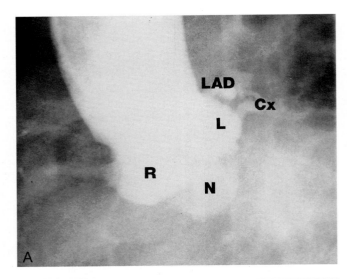

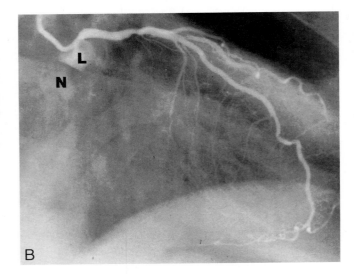

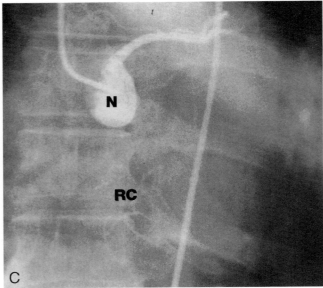

Figure CR4.9. A. Aortogram in the left anterior oblique projection. This image suggests, but does not prove, the absence of a left main trunk. The aortic sinuses are grossly equal in size. Cx = circumflex artery; L = left; LAD = left anterior descending artery; N = noncoronary sinus; R = right sinus. **B.** Selective angiogram of the LAD, in the right anterior oblique projection, showing the artery's isolated origination from the left coronary sinus (L). N = noncoronary sinus. **C.** Nonselective angiographic visualization of the circumflex artery, in the posteroanterior projection, showing that this artery originates from the noncoronary sinus (N), independently of the LAD. The distal RCA (RC) is filled via collateral vessels from the circumflex artery.

CASE REPORT 4.10

Anomalous Location of the Coronary Ostium in the Ascending Aorta

A 70-year-old man with diabetes mellitus was admitted because of exertional angina that was relieved by rest. Cardiac catheterization showed that the RCA originated ectopically from the ascending aorta, some 4 cm above the left coronary sinus (Fig. CR4.10, A–D). It also showed nonobstructive plaques in the proximal LAD. Left ventricular systolic function was normal. The patient's angina improved with beta-blocking drugs. ■

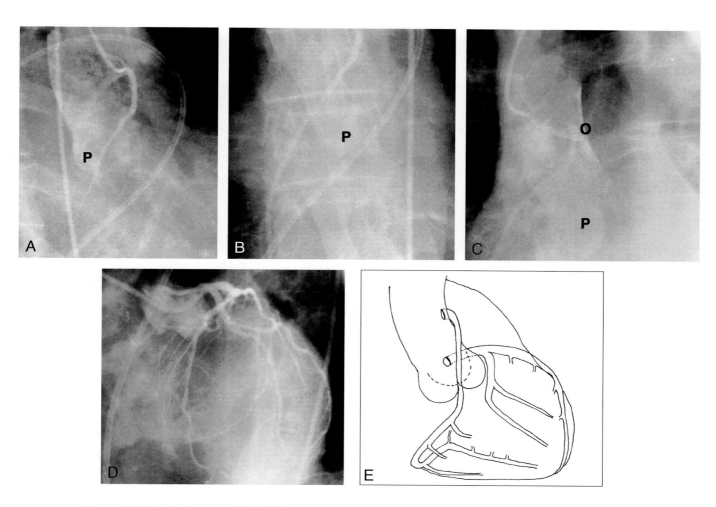

Figure CR4.10. Angiograms of the RCA in the right anterior oblique **(A)**, posteroanterior **(B)**, and left anterior oblique **(C)**, projections, showing origination of the RCA from the ascending aorta, some 4 cm above the left coronary sinus (P = posterior sinus; O = coronary ostium). **D.** Angiogram of the LCA in the left anterior oblique projection, showing normal angiographic features. **E.** Diagrammatic representation of the coronary anomaly (right anterior oblique view).

CASE REPORT 4.11

Anomalous Location of the Coronary Ostium Outside the Normal "Coronary" Sinuses: Origination of the LCA From the Pulmonary Artery

A 26-year-old woman with dyspnea and atypical chest pain was admitted for cardiac evaluation. Physical examination disclosed a continuous murmur at the left sternal border. Transesophageal Doppler echocardiography showed a dilated RCA, with an abnormal vessel showing a high-velocity flow signal and draining into the pulmonary artery. Moderate, diffuse left ventricular hypokinesia (ejection fraction, 35%) was also present. Catheterization showed that the LCA originated anomalously from the posterior sinus of the pulmonary artery; a significant oxygen step-up was present, with a calculated pulmonary-to-systemic flow ratio of 1.9:1. The LCA was reimplanted directly into the aortic root, and the pulmonary artery was repaired with an expanded polytetrafluoroethylene patch. ▶

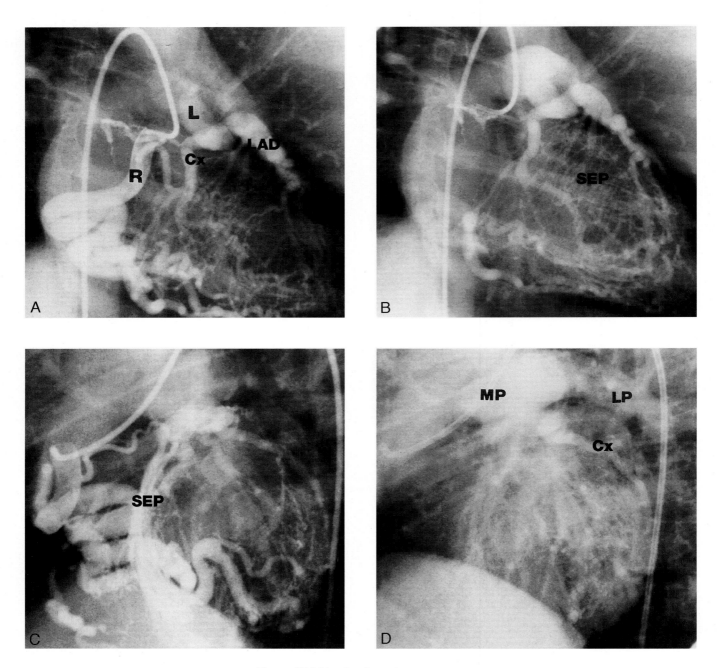

Figure CR4.11. See legend on next page

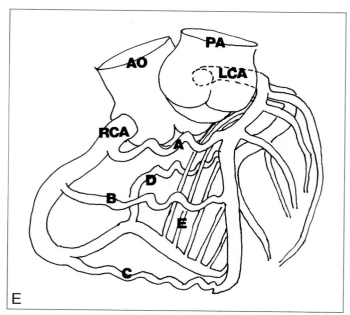

Figure CR4.11. **A** and **B.** Angiograms of the RCA: photograms obtained during the early **(A)** and late **(B)** phases of contrast injection in the posteroanterior projection. The proximal RCA is highly tortuous (see also views **C** and **D**) and exhibits diffuse (disorderly) ectasia. Filling of the left coronary system quickly occurs, mainly via a highly developed septal penetrating network (SEP). The left coronary artery (LCA), LAD, and circumflex (Cx) trunks are aneurysmatically dilated. The LCA drains into the posterior sinus of the pulmonary artery. **C** and **D.** Simultaneous photograms of the RCA, in the lateral projection. Cx = circumflex artery; L = left main artery; LP = left pulmonary artery; MP = main pulmonary artery; SEP = septal network; R = right coronary artery. **E.** Diagrammatic representation of the collateral circles in this anomaly: A = infundibular; B = anterior right ventricular; C = acute marginal to apical LAD; D = distal RCA to circumflex; E = septal. AO = aorta; PA = pulmonary artery.

CASE REPORT 4.12

RCA Arising From the Left Anterior Sinus: "Single Left Coronary System" with the RCA Arising From the Distal Circumflex Artery and Following a Posterior Course

A 29-year-old man, with a history of insulin-dependent diabetes mellitus and cigarette smoking, was admitted for exertional angina, diaphoresis, and dyspnea. At age 5 years, he had undergone surgical repair of a patent ductus arteriosus and pulmonic stenosis. During the present admission, echocardiography revealed an atrial septal defect, mild pulmonary hypertension, and moderate pulmonary insufficiency. Cardiac catheterization confirmed these findings and showed that the LCA was anomalous

(it indeed had a mixed proximal trunk) because it produced not only the LAD and the circumflex arteries but also all of the right coronary branches, including the posterior descending artery and the anterior infundibular (terminal) branches (Fig. CR4.12, A and B). The RCA arose from the distal circumflex artery and followed a posterior course. Elective closure of the atrial septal defect was recommended but has not yet been carried out. ∎

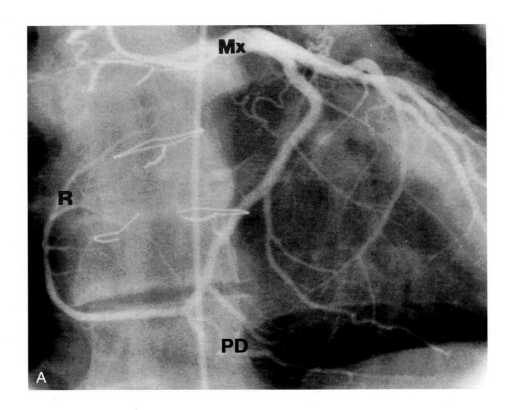

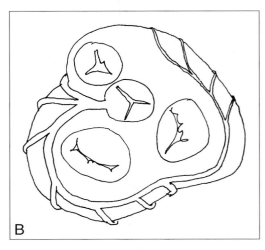

Figure CR4.12. A. Angiogram of the LCA in the posteroanterior projection (see text). Mx = mixed proximal trunk; PD = posterior descending artery; R = terminal RCA branches. **B.** Schematic diagram of the coronary anomaly (coronal plane).

CASE REPORT 4.13

Single Coronary Artery: RCA Arising From the Distal Circumflex Artery and Following a Posterior Course

A 48-year-old woman underwent coronary angiography for atypical chest pain. Treadmill exercise testing had yielded inconclusive results. Coronary angiography (Fig. CR4.13, A–C) revealed a single coronary artery that originated in the left anterior aortic sinus; the RCA arose as a continuation of the left circumflex artery in the right atrioventricular groove. The anterior right ventricular artery originated from the proximal LAD and coursed anterior to the pulmonary infundibulum, representing an anomaly in itself. The RCA's terminal branch was the sinus node artery. Continued medical treatment was recommended. ■

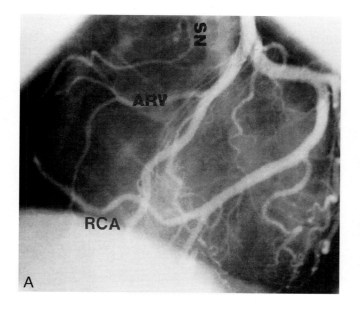

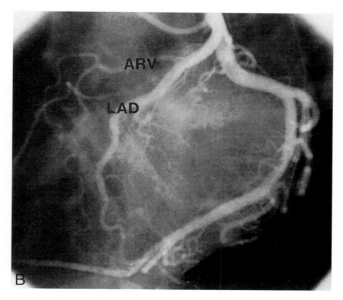

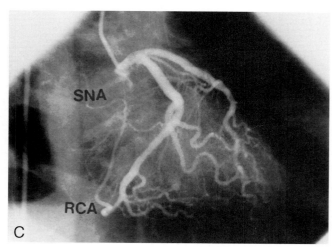

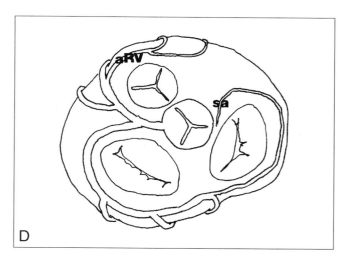

Figure CR4.13. Angiograms of the left coronary artery in the cranial left anterior oblique **(A)**, left anterior oblique **(B)**, and right anterior oblique **(C)** projections (see text). The anterolateral free wall of the right ventricle is supplied essentially by LAD-originating branches (ARV): Is this a case of split RCA? The distal circumflex extends to the right of the posterior descending branch and terminates in the sinus node artery (SNA). **D.** Diagrammatic representation of the anomaly in the coronal plane. aRV = anterior right ventricular branch; sa = sinus node artery.

CASE REPORT 4.14

Anomalous Location of the Coronary Ostium in the Opposite Sinus: Circumflex Artery Arising From the Right Anterior Sinus (Mixed Trunk) and Following a Retrocardiac Course Behind the Atrioventricular Valves

A 70-year-old man, with a history of hypertension, cigarette smoking, diabetes mellitus, and coronary artery disease, presented with unstable angina. Cardiac catheterization revealed nonobstructive plaques in the LAD and the diagonal artery; the LAD was the only vessel to originate from the left sinus (Fig. CR4.14A). The territories of the circumflex and obtuse marginal arteries were supplied by terminal branches of the "RCA:" the

proximal coronary artery, which arose from the right sinus, was actually a mixed trunk (producing the RCA and the circumflex artery) until it passed the cardiac crux and the posterior descending artery (Fig. CR4.14, *B* and *C*). After that point, it became an anomalous circumflex artery with two large obtuse marginal branches. Continued medical treatment was recommended. ■

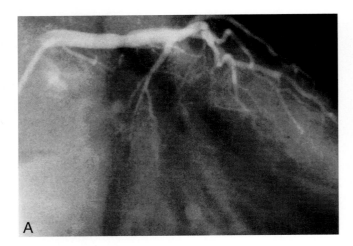

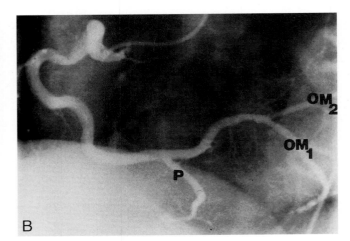

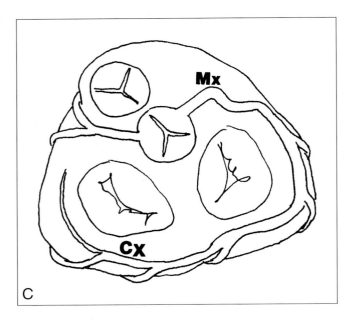

Figure CR4.14. A. Angiogram of the LAD in the right anterior oblique projection. **B.** Angiogram of the right-sided coronary vessel in the left anterior oblique projection. This highly dominant vessel produces not only the posterior descending artery (P) but also two obtuse marginal (OM) branches. The implication is that the circumflex artery is the terminal branch of a mixed trunk, composed of the RCA and the circumflex. **C.** Schematic diagram of the coronary anomaly (coronal plane). cx = circumflex artery; Mx = mixed proximal trunk.

CASE REPORT 4.15

Anomalous Location of the Coronary Ostium in the Opposite Sinus: Circumflex Artery Arising From the Right Anterior Sinus and Following a Retroaortic Path

A 45-year-old man with a history of hypertension, smoking, hyperlipidemia, and chronic angina presented with unstable angina. The patient had a family history of coronary artery disease. Cardiac catheterization showed nonobstructive plaques in the proximal circumflex artery, which originated from the right coronary sinus and had a dominant pattern (Fig. CR4.15, A and B). An obtuse marginal branch also had a significant lesion. The RCA was

nondominant, essentially serving only the free wall of the right ventricle (Fig. CR4.15, C). The left coronary ostium provided flow only to the large diagonal (ramus) branch (Fig. CR4.15, D and E). The LAD was totally occluded at its origin from the left-sided artery, and filling occurred via collateral vessels. Aortocoronary bypass surgery was recommended. ►

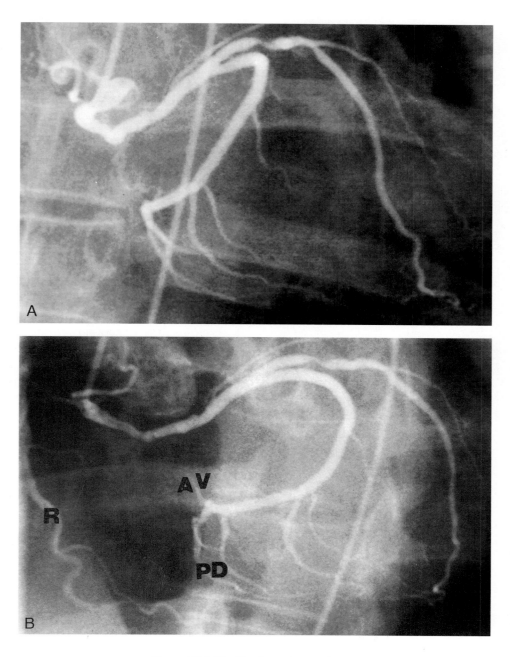

Figure CR4.15. See legend on next page.

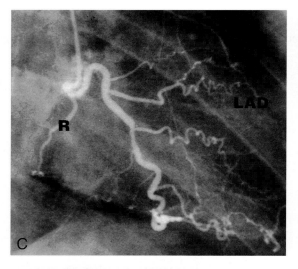

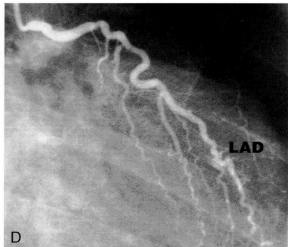

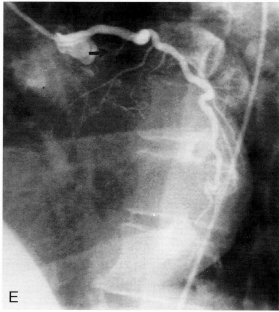

Figure CR4.15. Angiograms of the circumflex artery in the posteroanterior **(A)** and left anterior oblique **(B)** projections, showing origination of the posterior descending (PD) and atrioventricular node (AV) arteries from the distal vessel. The RCA (R), which has an adjoining ostium, is also visible. **C.** On selective injection, the RCA (R) appears as a small, nondominant vessel in the atrioventricular groove; a large anterior right ventricular branch also provides collaterals to the LAD. Right **(D)** and left **(E)** anterior oblique views of the left-sided artery, showing a stump of the LAD (view **D;** arrow, view **E**) and a large diagonal (ramus) branch.

CASE REPORT 4.16

Anomalous Location of the Coronary Ostium in the Opposite Sinus: Circumflex Artery Arising From the Right Anterior Sinus

A 72-year-old man with hypercholesterolemia and a recent myocardial infarction was admitted for postinfarction angina. Electrocardiography showed sinus bradycardia, with tall R waves in leads V_1 to V_3 that suggested a posterior infarct. Coronary angiography indicated that the circumflex artery arose independently from the right anterior sinus and contained a 95% proximal stenosis (Fig. CR4.16, A); this artery supplied obtuse marginal branches 1 and 2. Angioplasty of the circumflex artery resulted

in moderate improvement (Fig. CR4.16, B). Use of an 8F multipurpose catheter tended to cause ostial spasm and wedging. The circumflex artery supplied obtuse marginal branches 1 and 2.

Comment: In general, use of a catheter with side holes does not prevent catheter-induced spasm; moreover, the side holes allow monitoring only of the aortic pressure, not of the pressure at the tip of the guiding catheter. ∎

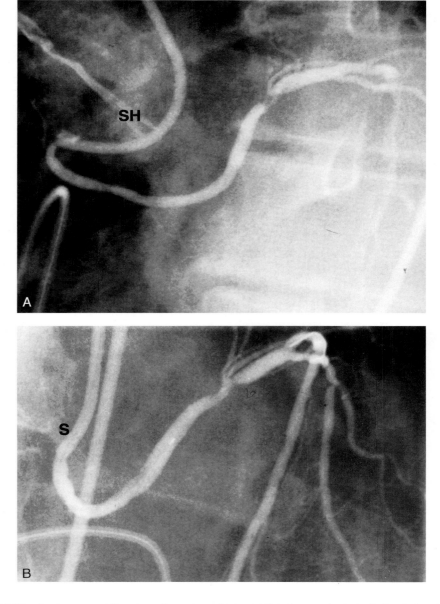

Figure CR4.16. Angiograms of the circumflex artery obtained **(A)** before angioplasty (left anterior oblique view) and **(B)** after angioplasty (right anterior oblique view) (see text). Both views show ostial spasm and wedging. S, SH = side-hole catheter.

CASE REPORT 4.17

Anomalous Location of the Coronary Ostium in the Opposite Sinus: Circumflex Artery Arising From the Right Anterior Sinus and Following a Retroaortic Path

A 34-year-old man with a history of hypertension was admitted for the evaluation of atypical nonexertional chest pain. A resting nuclear scan showed a defect in the inferoposterior portion of the left ventricle. At cardiac catheterization, no coronary artery disease was present, but the circumflex artery originated abnormally from the right coronary sinus and followed a retroaortic path; there was no left main trunk proper (Fig. CR4.17, A–D).

The patient had evidently had a false positive nuclear stress test in the presence of normal coronary circulation. The hypothesis that he had had a previous myocardial infarction related to the anomalous path of the circumflex artery could not be supported by the clinical history, the electrocardiogram, or ventricular function studies. No intervention was necessary. ■

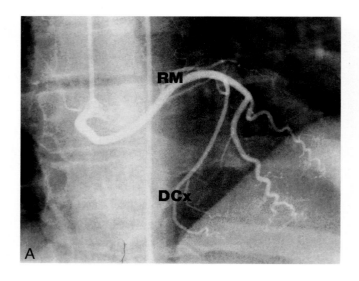

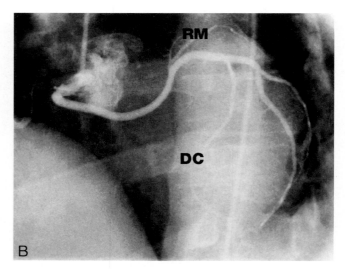

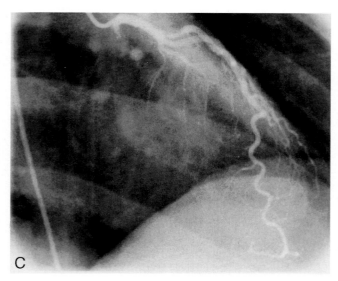

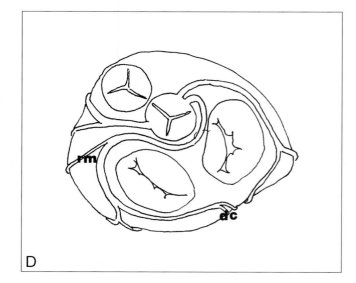

Figure CR4.17. Angiograms of the anomalous circumflex artery in the posteroanterior **(A)** and left anterior oblique **(B)** projections. The artery follows the posterior aortic annulus as far as the origin of the first branch, the ramus intermedius (RM). Also visible is the distal circumflex (DCx) and codominant (circumflex-right) pattern. **C.** Angiogram of the LAD in the right anterior oblique projection. In cases of this type, there is no left main trunk proper. **D.** Schematic diagram of the coronary anomaly (coronal plane). RM = ramus intermedius; DCx = distal circumflex.

CASE REPORT 4.18

Anomalous Location of the Coronary Ostium in the Opposite Sinus: Circumflex Artery Arising From the Right Anterior Sinus and Following a Retroaortic Path

A 55-year-old woman, with a history of rheumatic heart disease and mitral valve replacement, presented with a significant paravalvular leak, as diagnosed by transesophageal echocardiography. Preoperative cardiac catheterization (Fig. CR4.18, A–C)

showed that the circumflex artery arose from the right coronary sinus and confirmed that significant mitral insufficiency was present. The patient underwent successful repeat mitral valve replacement. ∎

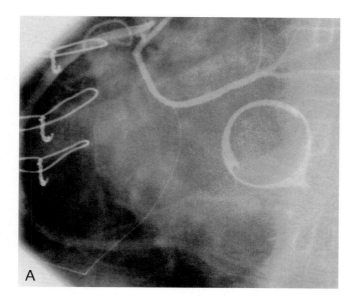

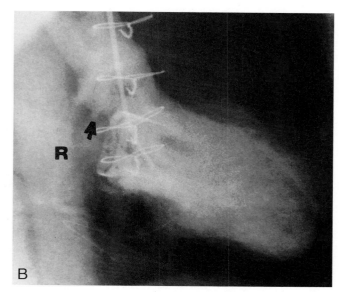

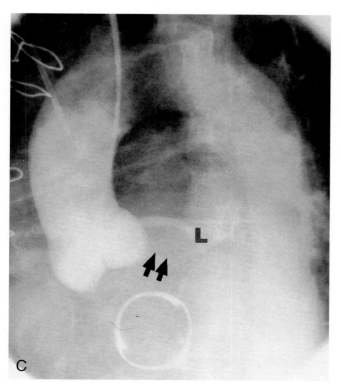

Figure CR4.18. A. Angiogram of the RCA and circumflex artery, in the left anterior oblique projection, showing adjoining ostia in the right anterior sinus. The circumflex artery is relatively small. **B.** Left ventriculogram, in the right anterior oblique projection, showing the relationship between the aortic and mitral valves; the anomalous circumflex artery exhibits a "nipple," or "dot," sign (arrow). **C.** Aortogram, in the left anterior oblique projection, showing normal origination of the LAD from the left sinus. The anomalous circumflex artery (arrowheads) is barely visible at the bottom of the left sinus. L = LCA.

CASE REPORT 4.19

Anomalous Location of the Coronary Ostium in the Opposite Sinus: Circumflex Artery Arising From the Right Anterior Sinus (Right Mixed Trunk) and Following a Retroaortic Path

A 68-year-old woman with a history of hypertension, cigarette smoking, and hyperlipidemia was admitted for the evaluation of frequent severe chest pain. On cardiac catheterization, the small LAD was the only vessel seen to originate from the left sinus (Fig. CR4.19, A–D). The dominant RCA arose jointly with the circumflex artery, which followed a retroaortic path. Mild prolapse of the mitral valve was noted, but no coronary obstructive disease was present. Medical treatment was recommended. ■

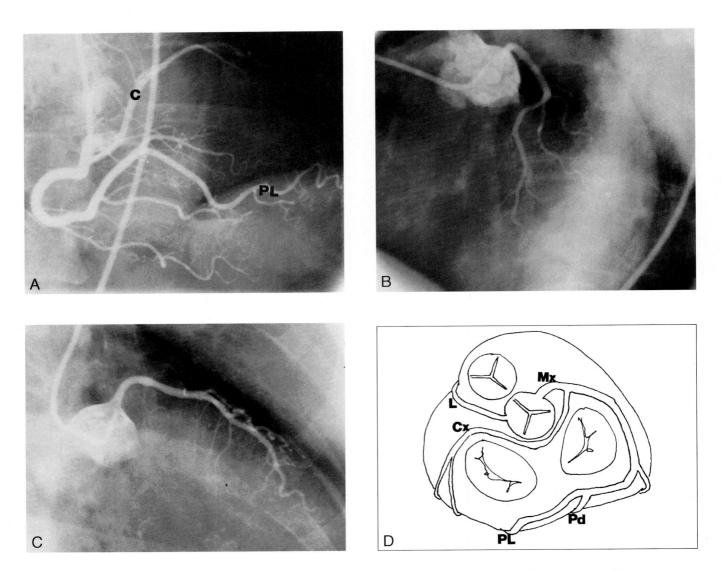

Figure CR4.19. **A.** Angiogram of the RCA in the posteroanterior projection, showing anomalous origination of the circumflex (Cx) artery from the proximal RCA. The distal RCA provides a large posterolateral branch (PL) that partially nourishes territory normally served by the circumflex artery. The circumflex artery itself is rather small. **B** and **C.** Left coronary angiograms in the left **(B)** and right **(C)** anterior oblique projections, showing that only the small LAD arises from the left sinus. **D.** Schematic diagram of the coronary anomaly (coronal plane). Cx = circumflex artery; L = LAD; Mx = mixed proximal trunk; Pd = posterior descending artery; PL = posterolateral branch.

CASE REPORT 4.20

Anomalous Location of the Coronary Ostium in the Opposite Sinus: Circumflex Artery Arising From the Right Anterior Sinus (Right Mixed Trunk) and Following a Retroaortic Path

A 51-year-old man with a history of hyperlipidemia and angina was admitted because of worsening exertional angina. The patient had had a myocardial infarction 15 years earlier. Cardiac catheterization showed significant disease in all three major coro- nary arteries (not illustrated). The circumflex artery originated from a right mixed trunk and coursed behind the aorta (Fig. CR4.20). Surgical treatment of the coronary obstructive disease was successfully carried out. ∎

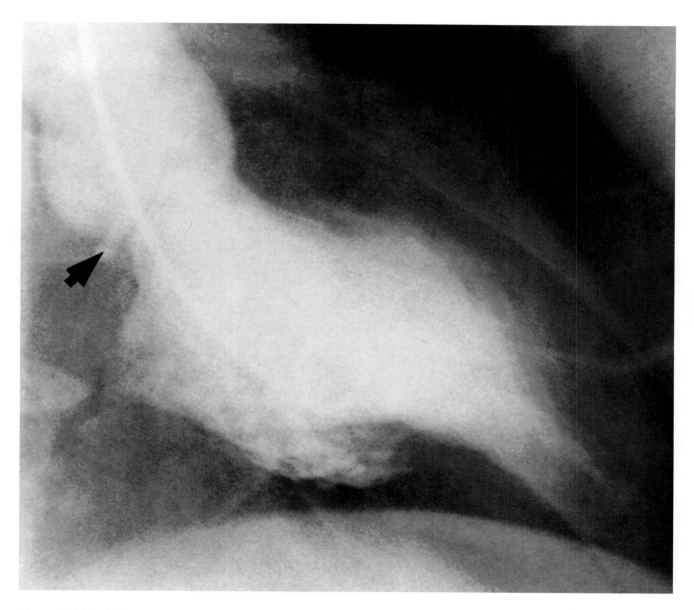

Figure CR4.20. Left ventriculogram in the right anterior oblique projection, showing the "nipple," or "dot," sign (arrow) that indicates a retroaortic circumflex artery. This angiographic sign is particularly consistent and pathognomonic, because the anomalous circumflex is seen longitudinally (with enhanced density of contrast material) in the right anterior oblique projection.

CASE REPORT 4.21

Anomalous Location of the Coronary Ostium in the Opposite Sinus: Circumflex Artery Arising From the Right Anterior Sinus (Right Mixed Trunk) and Following a Retroaortic Path

A 38-year-old woman, who had had an "innocent" cardiac murmur since childhood, presented with a 1-year history of exertional dyspnea and mild cyanosis. Physical examination revealed a harsh 4/6 pansystolic murmur at the left sternal border. Cardiac catheterization showed a large ventricular septal defect and infundibular stenosis (anatomically, because the pulmonary valve was normal, the patient did not have tetralogy of Fallot; physiologically, however, she had a mild form of that anomaly). Coronary angiography revealed anomalous origination of the circum-

flex artery and the ramus medianus (RM), which arose with a common trunk from the right anterior sinus jointly with the RCA and followed a retroaortic path (Fig. CR4.21, A&B). The left anterior aortic sinus gave rise to only a small LAD artery (Fig. 4.21C) that did not reach the cardiac apex (dominant RCA with terminal branches wrapped around the apex). The patient underwent successful surgical correction of the congenital heart defect. ∎

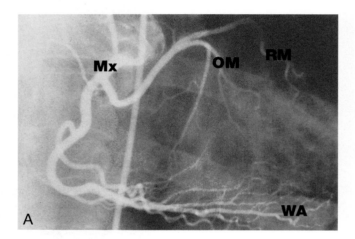

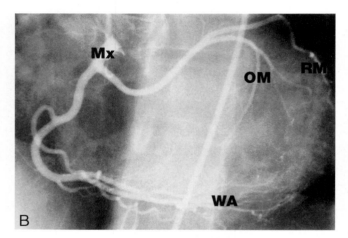

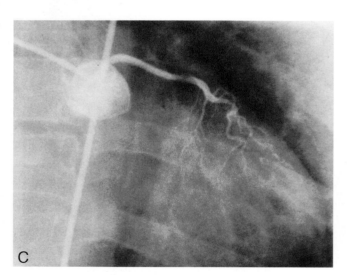

Figure CR4.21. Angiograms of the right anterior sinus artery in the posteroanterior **(A)** and left anterior oblique **(B)** projections. The initial common, mixed trunk (Mx) subdivided into a retroaortic circumflex/ramus artery (RM) and a dominant RCA. Note the unusual extent of the distal RCA, whose posterior descending branches wrap around the apex (WA). At the right cusp, the mixed trunk covers a larger territory than the normal left main trunk in the usual coronary pattern. In clinical practice, the term "left main equivalent" is used for this unusual pattern. OM = obtuse marginal branch. **C.** Solitary LAD arising from the left sinus.

CASE REPORT 4.22

Anomalous Location of the Coronary Ostium in the Opposite Sinus: Circumflex Artery Arising From the Right Anterior Sinus (Mixed Trunk) and Following a Retroaortic Path

A 73-year-old man with new-onset typical exertional angina underwent an electrocardiographic treadmill test that was positive for coronary artery disease. His risk factors included hypertension, hyperlipidemia, and a family history of coronary artery disease. Coronary angiography revealed critical disease of an artery that originated from the left anterior aortic sinus. The artery did not supply the circumflex territory but only the LAD system (Fig. CR4.22, A and B). A large, trifurcated diagonal artery gave

rise to the ramus medianus. The right anterior aortic sinus had a single coronary ostium, which produced both a dominant RCA and an anomalous small circumflex artery that followed a retroaortic path (mixed initial trunk) (Fig. CR4.22, C and D). The circumflex artery had critical lesions in its proximal and mid portions. The patient underwent successful aortocoronary bypass of the LAD and diagonal arteries, but the circumflex artery was too small for a bypass graft. ▶

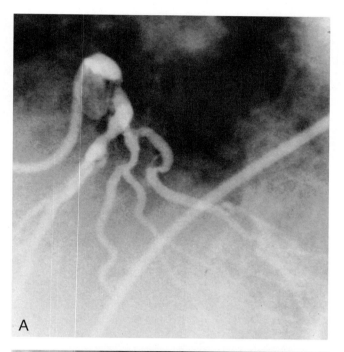

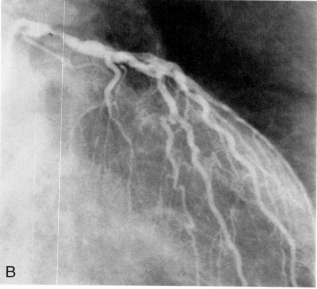

Figure CR4.22. See legend on next page

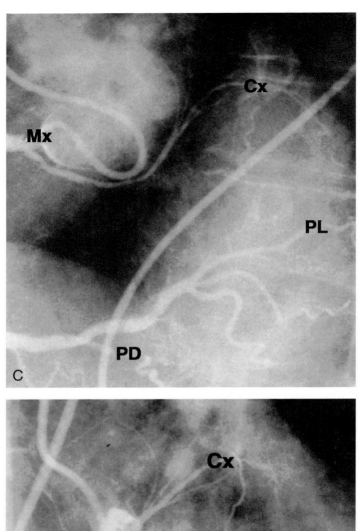

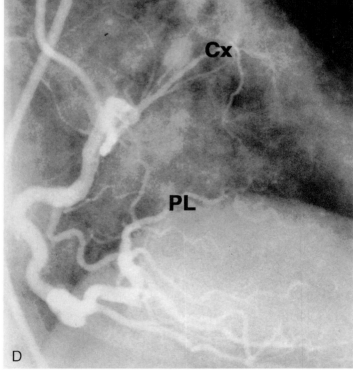

Figure CR4.22. Angiograms of the LAD in the left **(A)** and right **(B)** anterior oblique projections. Angiograms of the right coronary sinus, in the cranial left **(C)** and right **(D)** anterior oblique projections, showing a mixed trunk that arises from the right sinus. The posterolateral (PL) branch of the RCA supplies a larger territory around the obtuse marginal artery than does the circumflex artery (Cx) proper, which may be considered split. Mx = mixed proximal trunk; PD = posterior descending artery.

CASE REPORT 4.23

Anomalous Location of the Coronary Ostium: RCA Arising From the Left Anterior Sinus and Following a Retroaortic Path ("Single LCA")

A 56-year-old woman presented with recent-onset typical angina and exertional dyspnea 4 years after having an unconfirmed acute myocardial infarction. Electrocardiographic treadmill testing was negative for coronary artery disease. Coronary angiography revealed no significant coronary obstructive disease. Left ventricular angiography showed a normal volume and normal wall motion (Fig. CR4.23, A). The RCA arose from the left ante-

rior sinus, by way of a mixed trunk that was shared with the left coronary system (single coronary artery arising from the left anterior sinus) (Fig. CR4.23, B–E). The RCA followed a retroaortic path (Fig. CR4.23, A, double arrows). No coronary artery was observed in the right anterior sinus. Continued medical treatment was recommended. ▶

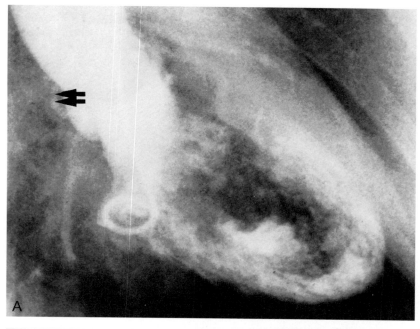

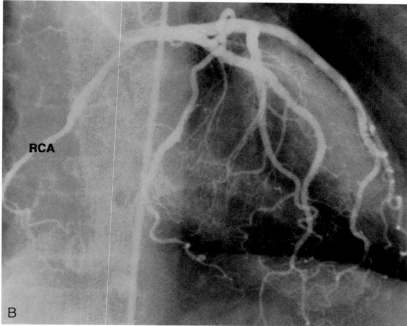

Figure CR4.23. See legend on next page

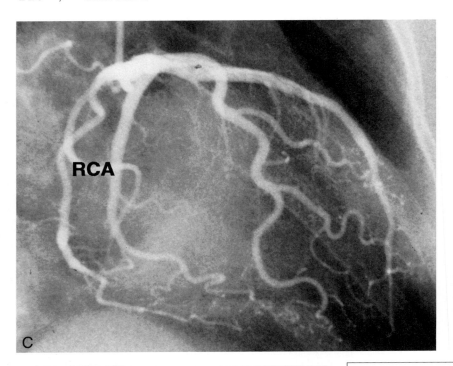

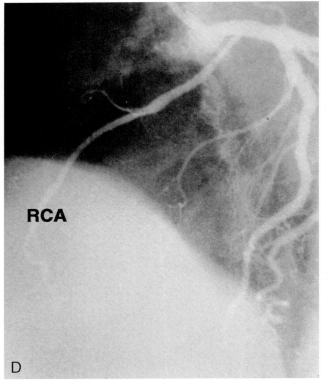

Figure CR4.23. A. Left ventriculogram in the right anterior oblique projection. The RCA (arrows) courses behind the aortic root. Coronary angiograms in the posteroanterior (B), right anterior oblique (C), and left anterior oblique (D) projections show that the circumflex artery is dominant and the RCA relatively small. E. Schematic diagram of the coronary anomaly (coronal plane).

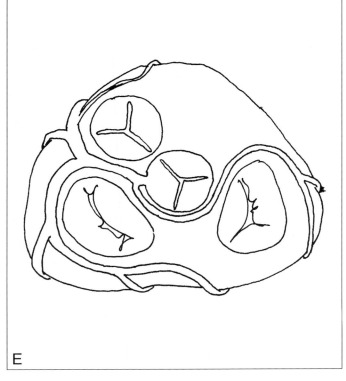

CASE REPORT 4.24

RCA Arising From the Left Anterior Sinus and Coursing Anomalously "Between the Aorta and Pulmonary Artery" (Preaortic Path)

A 42-year-old man with hypertension and a family history of heart disease was admitted because of an acute anteroseptal infarction. During the preceding few weeks, the patient had had effort-related angina. Echocardiography revealed an ejection fraction of 45%, with akinesia of the mid and distal portions of the septum. Coronary angiography showed a subtotal stenosis of the LAD. The RCA, which was totally occluded, shared a common mixed trunk with the LCA, arising from the left anterior sinus

and coursing between the aorta and pulmonary artery (Fig. CR4.24, *A–E*). The patient underwent successful aortocoronary bypass surgery.

Comment: In this case, a coronary anomaly that had the potential for causing sudden death was discovered during assessment of acquired atherosclerotic disease at a site remote from the anomalous path. ▶

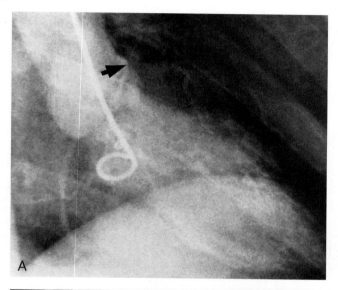

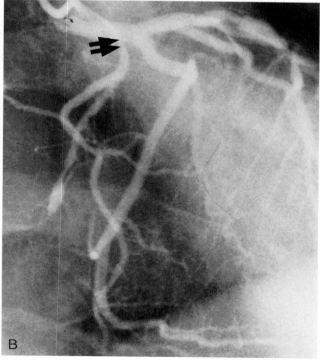

Figure CR4.24. See legend on next page

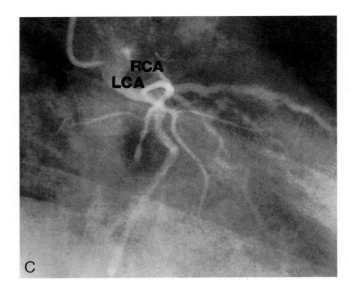

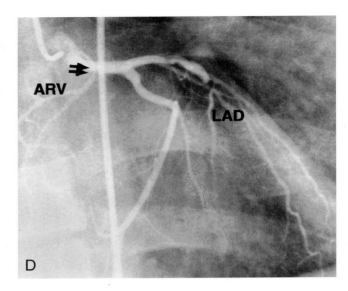

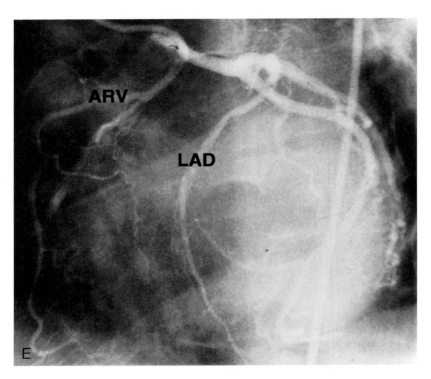

Figure CR4.24. **A.** Left ventriculogram in the right anterior oblique projection, showing inferoapical akinesia and suggesting that the RCA has an anomalous path anterior to the aortic root (arrow). Angiograms of the left coronary trunk in the straight **(B)** and caudal **(C)** right anterior oblique projections show early splitting of the left mixed trunk. A long, eccentric stenotic lesion appears to lie against the aortic wall (view **B**, arrows) in the concavity of the RCA. **D** and **E.** Angiograms of the left coronary ostium in the posteroanterior **(D)** and left anterior oblique **(E)** projections. In the RCA, an occlusion is present, distal to the initial eccentric lesion (view **D**, arrows) and the origin of the large anterior right ventricular branch (ARV). LAD = left anterior descending artery.

CASE REPORT 4.25

Anomalous Location of the Coronary Ostium in the Opposite Sinus: RCA Arising From the Left Sinus and Following a Preaortic Path

A 48-year-old man with hypertension and exertional angina underwent thallium stress testing, which revealed ischemia of the inferior left ventricular wall. Cardiac catheterization showed multiple nonobstructive plaques in the LCA (Fig. CR4.25, A). The

RCA arose independently from the left coronary sinus, coursed between the aorta and the pulmonary artery, and had a 60% proximal eccentric stenotic lesion (Fig. CR4.25, B and C). Surgical treatment was recommended. ■

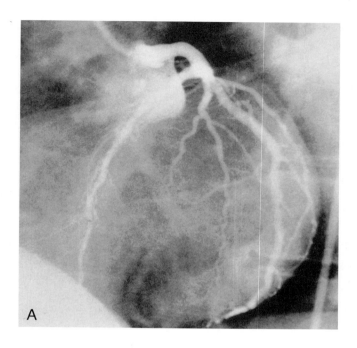

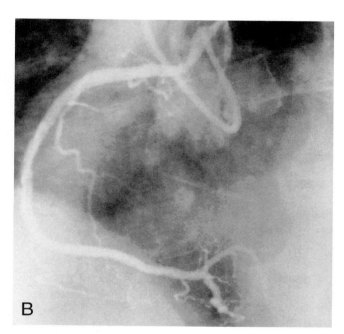

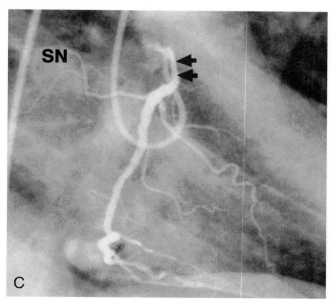

Figure CR4.25. A. Normal angiogram of the LCA in the left anterior oblique projection. Angiograms of the RCA in the left **(B)** and right **(C)** anterior oblique positions, showing the artery's ectopic origination and course. The ostium is located high above the left coronary sinus and features a proximal, tangential tract with an eccentric, stenotic lesion that is best visualized in the right anterior oblique view (**C**, arrows). SN = sinus node artery.

CASE REPORT 4.26

Anomalous Location of the Coronary Ostium in the Opposite Sinus: RCA Arising From the Left Sinus (Left Mixed Trunk) and Following a Preaortic Path ("Single LCA")

A 77-year-old hypertensive male smoker presented with a history of dyspnea, angina, and near syncope. Echocardiography revealed a critical aortic stenosis. Cardiac catheterization showed no significant coronary obstructive lesions, but the RCA arose anomalously from a left mixed trunk and followed a preaortic path (Fig. CR4.26, A–D). The patient underwent successful aortic valve replacement and prophylactic aortocoronary venous by-

pass grafting of the RCA. The anatomopathology of the aortic valve suggested a congenital bicuspid anomaly rather than rheumatic valve disease. This case is another example of "single LCA." The indication for a "prophylactic" RCA bypass is not well established, but such a surgical procedure is clearly justified in a patient who requires cardiac surgery for other reasons (in this case, aortic valve replacement). ■

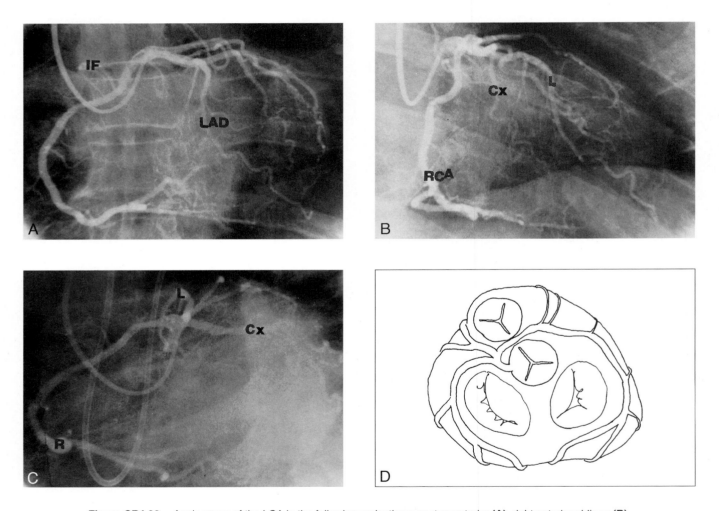

Figure CR4.26. Angiograms of the LCA in the following projections: posteroanterior **(A)**, right anterior oblique **(B)**, and left anterior oblique with a slight caudal tilt **(C)**. The dominant RCA takes off from the proximal common (mixed) trunk at a 90° angle and immediately pursues a normal course in the right atrioventricular groove, as shown by the origination of the infundibular branches (IF). **(D)** Schematic diagram of the coronary anomaly (coronal plane). Cx = circumflex artery; L = LAD; R = RCA.

CASE REPORT 4.27

LAD Arising From the Right Anterior Sinus and Following an Intraseptal Path (Split LAD)

A 64-year-old man with early-stage cutaneous T-cell lymphoma was admitted for unstable angina. The patient had multiple risk factors for coronary artery disease and had previously undergone repair of an abdominal aortic aneurysm. Coronary angiography showed proximal occlusion of the RCA and circumflex artery, as well as severe stenosis of the left main vessel (Fig. CR4.27, A–E). The LAD arose from the right anterior sinus, next to the stump of the RCA, and followed an intraseptal path, supplying the mid and distal portions of the anterior left ventricular wall.

The LAD also supplied collateral circulation to the posterior descending artery of the RCA and obtuse marginal branches of the circumflex. The patient underwent aortocoronary bypass grafting of the RCA, LAD, and diagonal and obtuse marginal branches. This case is another example of a split LAD. It could also be termed "anomalous origination of the LAD from a septal branch," since the proximal vessel that originates from the right sinus predominantly has the features of a septal branch (with respect to its course and the majority of its branches). ▶

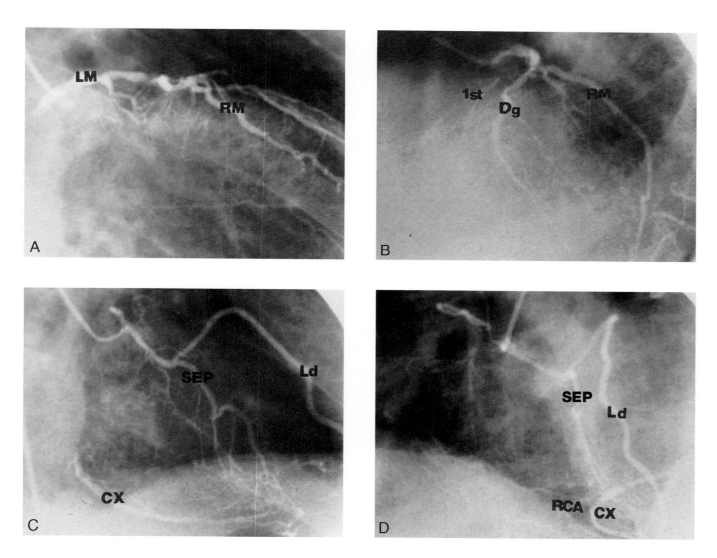

Figure CR4.27. Angiograms of the LCA in the right **(A)** and left **(B)** anterior oblique projections. The LAD is not totally absent from the left side: the proximal anterior trunk (LM) soon subdivides into a first septal (1st) and a large diagonal branch (Dg) and a ramus (RM). The circumflex artery is totally occluded but shows a dominant pattern when it fills via collateral vessels from the ectopic LAD. Angiograms of the right anterior sinus, in the right **(C)** and left **(D)** anterior oblique projections, reveal a totally occluded proximal RCA, which arises from a single niche shared with the ectopic LAD. The LAD courses lower than is usual in similar anomalies (see Case Report 4.28): it descends into the left ventricular septum and gives rise to a large septal branch (SEP) (which supplies most of the septum) before resurfacing in the proximal anterior interventricular groove. Cx = circumflex artery. continued

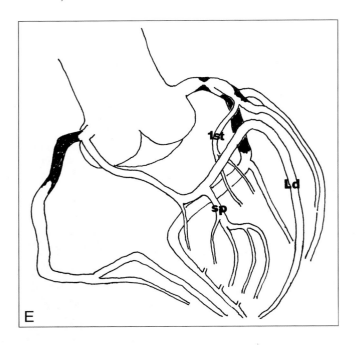

Figure CR4.27. (continued) **E.** Schematic diagram of the coronary anomaly (frontal plane); 1st = first septal branch; Ld = left anterior descending; sp = septal.

CASE REPORT 4.28

Anomalous Location of the Coronary Ostium in the Opposite Sinus: LCA Arising From the Right Anterior Sinus and Following an Intraseptal Path

A 74-year-old man, with hypertension, hyperlipidemia, and a family history of coronary artery disease, presented with acute severe chest pain that occurred on mild exertion and was associated with diaphoresis. The patient's cardiac enzyme levels were elevated, suggesting a non–Q-wave acute myocardial infarction.

Cardiac catheterization showed a critical stenosis in the mid RCA and minimal plaques in the LCA, which arose from the right coronary sinus (Fig. CR4.28, A–D). Medical treatment was recommended. ■

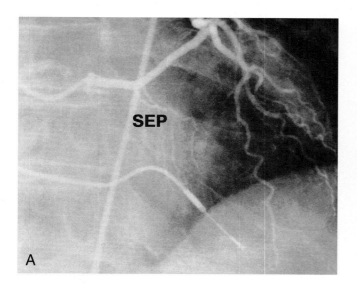

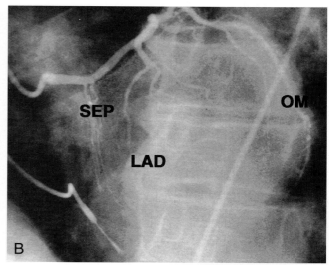

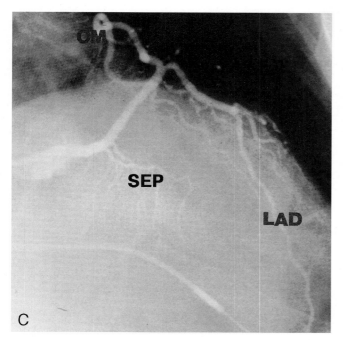

Figure CR4.28. Angiograms of the LCA in the posteroanterior **(A),** left anterior oblique **(B),** and cranial right anterior oblique **(C)** projections. The artery's ostium is located in the right anterior sinus, adjacent to the right coronary ostium. The left main trunk produces a large septal vessel (SEP) as its first ramification, soon after the left main trunk enters the ventricular septum, before terminating in the LAD and the circumflex/obtuse marginal (OM) artery.

CASE REPORT 4.29

LCA Arising From the Right Anterior Sinus and Following an Intraseptal Course

A 59-year-old man had a history of mild dyspnea on exertion. Because an echocardiographic workup revealed left ventricular dysfunction, the patient underwent heart catheterization. Left ventricular angiography revealed a left ventricular ejection fraction of 30%, with a diffuse, even pattern of hypokinesia (Fig. CR4.29, *A*). Selective coronary angiography failed to show a coronary ostium in the left anterior sinus; this absence was confirmed by means of aortography (Fig. CR4.29, *B*). The LCA arose adjacent to the right coronary ostium, in the right anterior sinus (Fig. CR4.29, *C–F*). The left main trunk was initially considered to run ''between the aorta and pulmonary artery,'' but further analysis indicated an intraseptal course. No significant coronary obstructive lesions were seen. Medical treatment was continued; prophylactic bypass of the left coronary system was seriously considered but was not performed.

Comments: This case involved an intriguing association between a coronary anomaly and a severe left ventricular myopathy of unknown etiology. Whereas preaortic coursing of the LCA is known to be associated with left ventricular myopathy, intraseptal coursing of that artery does not seem to have such an association, although the subject remains open to investigation. A review of the angiographic literature suggests that the preaortic, intraseptal, and prepulmonic courses are best differentiated from each other in the right anterior oblique projection (Fig. CR4.29, *F–G*). The anomalous preaortic left main trunk (coursing between the aorta and the pulmonary artery) assumes a slightly superoposterior path and reaches the left main stem usual site before separating into the circumflex artery and the LAD (as shown in the literature[435]). In our experience, most of the cases labeled as preaortic in clinical practice have actually turned out to be intraseptal on critical analysis. ▶

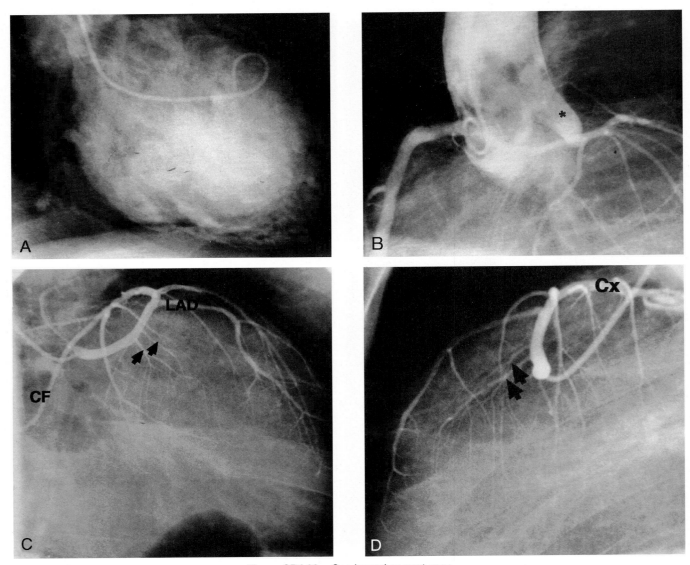

Figure CR4.29. See legend on next page

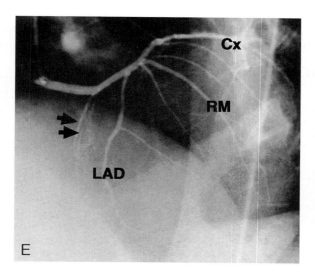

E

Figure CR4.29. A. Left ventricular angiogram in the right anterior oblique projection (systolic frame), showing diffuse, severe hypokinesia and cavitary dilation. **B.** Aortogram of the ascending aorta in the left anterior oblique projection, showing the absence of a normally located left coronary ostium at the left anterior sinus (asterisk) This sinus appears to be somewhat smaller than the other two sinuses. The anomalous origin of the LCA is clearly demonstrated, suggesting an intraseptal path (which is lower than the aortic root), as discussed in the Comments Section. **C–E.** Selective angiograms of the LCA in the right anterior oblique **(C)**, lateral **(D)**, and caudal left anterior oblique **(E)** projections, showing the LCA branches (arrowheads = septal branches; RM = ramus; Cx = circumflex artery. The left main trunk is considered to follow an intraseptal path, because it turns anteriorly and slightly interiorly (view **D**), gives off septal branches (arrows), and reaches the proximal LAD before the circumflex artery (Cf). **F** and **G.** Diagrams of differential angiographic features of the left main coronary artery in the right **(F)** and left **(G)** anterior oblique projections, showing the artery's three different "anterior" paths as it originates anomalously from the right sinus: 1, prepulmonic; 2, preaortic; 3, intraseptal, and 4, expected site of left coronary ostium. Only the preaortic course seems to be clearly associated with an unfavorable prognosis (see also Types of Pathophysiologic Mechanisms and Clinical Implications, pages 63–69). if = infundibular branch; sp = septal branches.

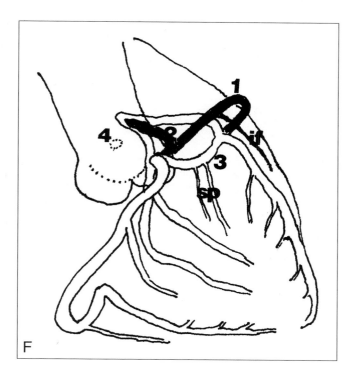

F

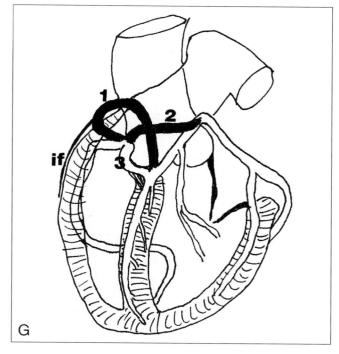

G

CASE REPORT 4.30

Anomalous Location of the Coronary Ostium in the Opposite Sinus: LAD Arising From the Right Anterior Sinus and Following an Intraseptal Path

A 49-year-old woman with diabetes mellitus and a history of angina had an acute inferior myocardial infarction that was treated with thrombolytic agents. Cardiac catheterization revealed occlusion of the proximal RCA, with inferior akinesia and a mildly decreased ejection fraction. The LAD originated from the right coronary sinus and followed an intraseptal path. The patient re-fused to undergo coronary artery bypass surgery. Interestingly, a follow-up examination 2 years later showed that her coronary disease had progressed to involve the proximal circumflex, ramus intermedius, and LAD (at the ostium). The patient later succumbed to sudden death. ►

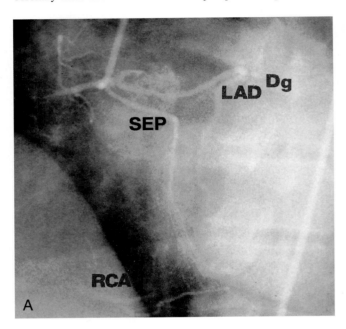

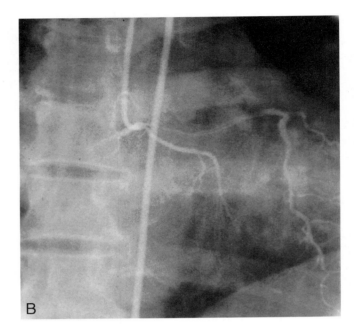

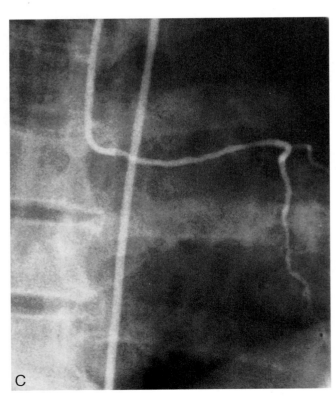

Figure CR4.30. Angiograms of the RCA in the left anterior oblique **(A)** and posteroanterior **(B,C)** projections. (continued)

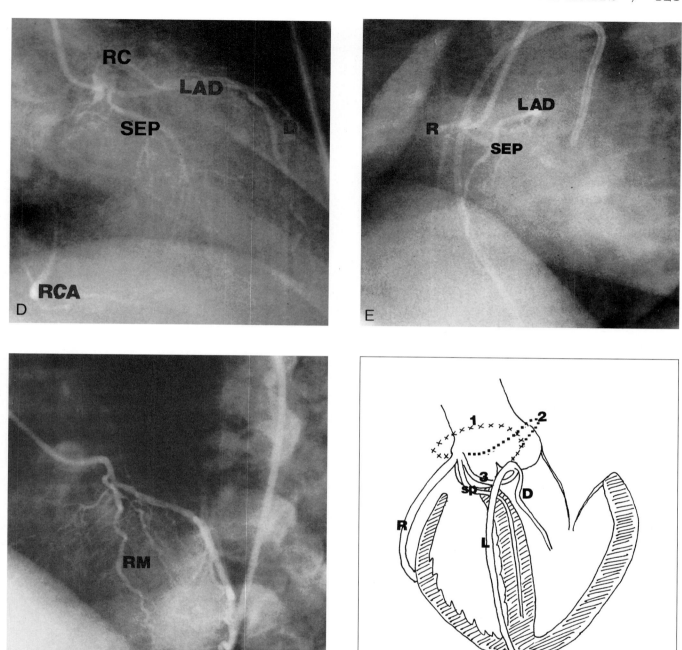

Figure CR4.30. (Continued) D,E. Angiograms of the RCA in the right anterior oblique **(D)**, and lateral **(E)** projections. The short, mixed trunk arising from the right cusp presents early splitting into the RCA (which has a totally occluded proximal segment, R), the LAD, the diagonal branch (D), and a large septal artery (SEP). The paths of the two anomalous vessels (LAD and SEP) are parallel to each other and are clearly intraseptal, running posterior to the pulmonary artery, as best seen in the lateral projection **(E)**, where a catheter is visible in the pulmonary artery. RC (view **D**) = right conal branch; RM (view **F**) = ramus medianus. **F.** Angiogram of the LCA, in the left anterior oblique projection, showing that the ostium in the left coronary sinus leads only to the circumflex artery and the ramus intermedius (RM). **G.** Schematic diagram of this case in the left anterior oblique projection. The three possible "anterior" anomalous courses of an LCA originating from the right sinus are superimposed for comparison (1, prepulmonic = crosses; 2, preaortic = squares; 3, intraseptal course, as seen in this case). D = diagonal artery; L = LAD; R = RCA; sp = septal artery.

CASE REPORT 4.31

RCA Arising From the Left Anterior Sinus and Following a Precardiac (or Prepulmonic) Path

A 40-year-old hypertensive man with typical exertional angina underwent a treadmill electrocardiographic test that was negative for coronary artery disease. Coronary angiography revealed multiple significant lesions in the LAD. The nondominant RCA arose from the LAD and followed a precardiac path (Fig. CR4.31, A–C). The circumflex artery was the dominant vessel, but it stopped at the posterior descending artery (PDA) (Fig. CR4.31, C). The patient underwent successful balloon angioplasty of the LAD. ∎

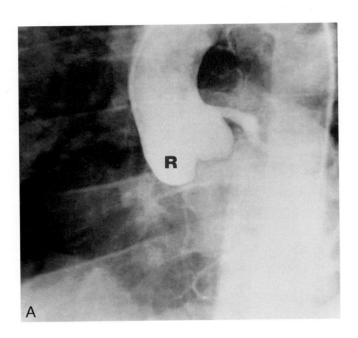

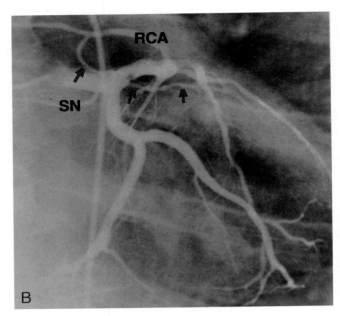

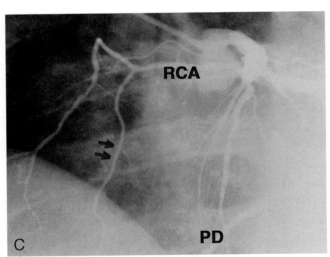

Figure CR4.31. A. Aortogram in the left anterior oblique projection, confirming that the right anterior sinus (view **A,** R) has no coronary ostia. Left coronary artery angiograms, in the posteroanterior **(B)** and left anterior oblique **(C)** projections, showing the RCA's anomalous origin and path. The sinus node artery (SN) originates from the mixed main trunk. The fact that the anomalous RCA's path is prepulmonic (not intraseptal) is indicated by both the anterior and the superior course and by the presence of a proximal infundibular (and anterior right ventricular) branch instead of a septal one (arrows). PD = posterior descending artery.

CASE REPORT 4.32

Anomalous Location of the Coronary Ostium in the Opposite Sinus: LAD Arising From the Right Sinus (via a Mixed Trunk) and Following a Prepulmonary (or Precardiac) Path

A 49-year-old man with hypertension, hyperlipidemia, and coronary artery disease was admitted because of angina at rest. Cardiac catheterization revealed two LAD arteries (split LAD): one that arose from the left sinus and had a 90% stenotic lesion, and the other (RAD) that arose from the right mixed trunk ("RCA")

and was free of disease (Fig. CR4.32, *A–D*). The circumflex artery originated anomalously from the proximal RCA and followed a retroaortic path. The patient underwent successful rotablation/angioplasty of the diseased LAD. ∎

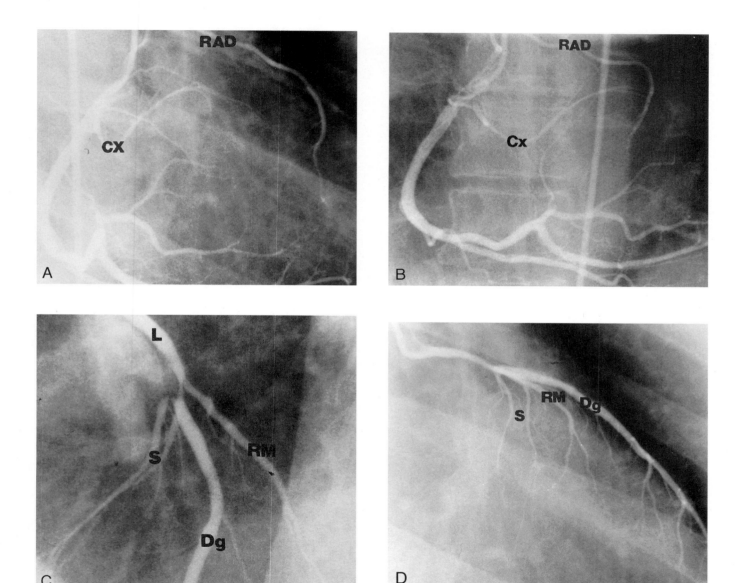

Figure CR4.32. Angiograms of the RCA, in the right anterior oblique **(A)** and posteroanterior **(B)** projections, showing a small "LAD" that arises from the RCA and supplies the lower interventricular septum. The RCA proper is dominant. Cx = circumflex artery; RAD = right anterior descending artery. **C** and **D.** Angiograms of the LCA, in the left **(C)** and right **(D)** anterior oblique projections. The main vessel (L) leads to two branches that serve the upper septum (S), a ramus medianus (RM) and a large diagonal (Dg) branch. Because the diagonal and septal branches belong to the LAD, the vessel should be labeled split LAD (with components from both the right and left coronary sinuses).

CASE REPORT 4.33

Anomalous Location of the Coronary Ostium in the Opposite Sinus: LCA Arising From the Right Sinus (via a Mixed Trunk) and Following a Prepulmonary Path ("Single Coronary Artery")

A 37-year-old male smoker presented with severe atypical chest pain associated with inversion of the inferior electrocardiographic T wave. Cardiac catheterization showed marked mitral valve prolapse. The LCA arose from a right-sided mixed trunk (so-called "single RCA") and followed a prepulmonary path (Fig. CR4.33, A–F). Medical treatment was recommended. ▶

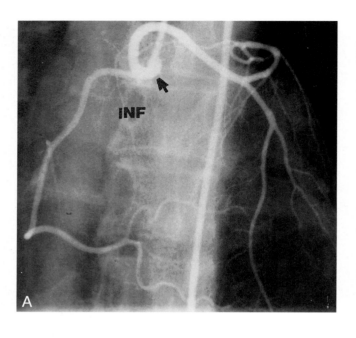
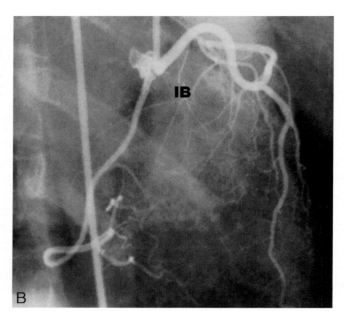
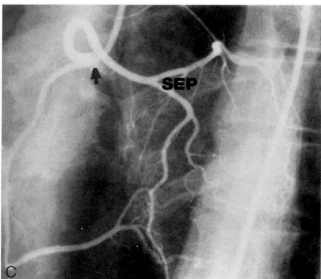
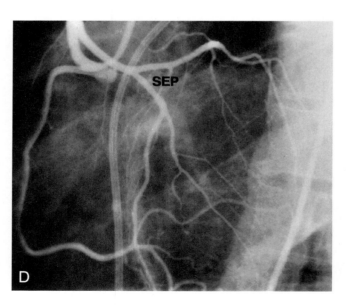

Figure CR4.33. Angiograms of the single coronary artery, in the posteroanterior **(A),** mildly cranial right anterior oblique **(B),** left anterior oblique **(C),** mildly cranial left anterior oblique **(D),** and lateral **(E)** projections. The undivided LCA trunk runs just in front of the expected site of the pulmonary valve (see view **E,** pulmonary catheter), and gives rise only to a small infundibular branch (INF, IB). The short, mixed trunk (single coronary ostium) is clearly evident (arrow). The proximal portion of the circumflex artery produces a septal branch (SEP). (continued)

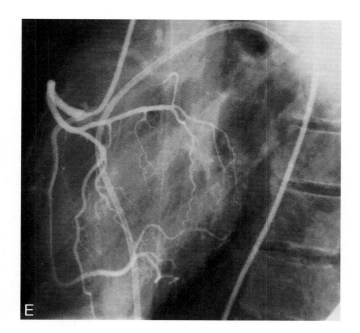

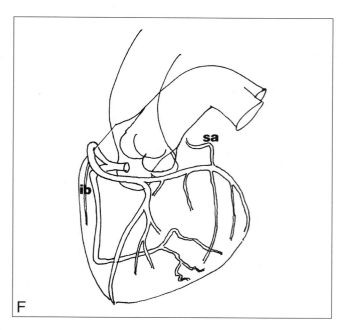

Figure CR4.33. (Continued) **E.** See legend on previous page. **F.** Schematic interpretation in the lateral projection. The sinus node artery (sa) originates from the circumflex artery at the origin of the obtuse marginal branch. ib = infundibular branch.

CASE REPORT 4.34

Atresia of the LAD Ostium Versus Origination of the LAD From the RCA/Posterior Descending Artery

A 60-year-old male smoker with hypercholesterolemia and diabetes mellitus had a family history of sudden cardiac death. For several months, the patient had been experiencing fatigue and shortness of breath on moderate exertion. He had had no clinical or electrocardiographic evidence of a myocardial infarction. During the present admission, treadmill testing was terminated within less than 5 minutes because of dyspnea, but no electrocardiographic changes were observed. Cardiac catheterization revealed a significant stenosis of the proximal RCA (Fig. CR4.34, A). Atresia or occlusion of the proximal LAD was also documented; the rest of the LAD could be visualized only from the

RCA via its end-to-end anastomosis with the posterior descending artery (Fig. CR4.34, B and C). The patient underwent successful balloon angioplasty, followed by stenting of the proximal RCA (which may constitute a mixed trunk or a left main "equivalent" as classified by Roberts et al[326]).

Comment: The fact that, in this case, the LAD shows a single angiographic origin from the posterior descending artery, in the presence of normal left ventricular function, suggests that the proximal LAD interruption is a case of congenital atresia (prenatal) origin, not an acquired occlusion. ▶

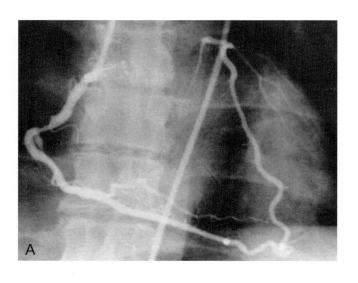

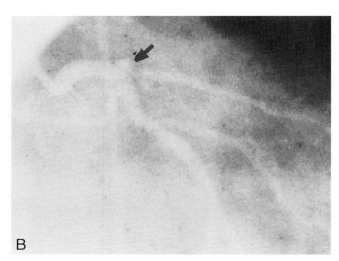

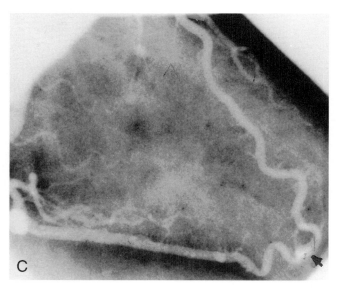

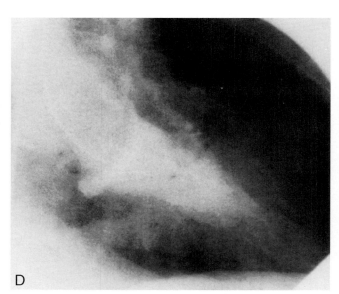

Figure CR4.34. See legend on next page

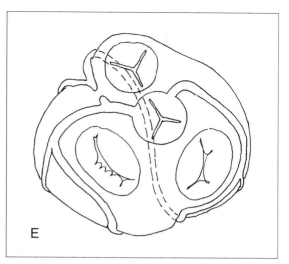

E

Figure CR4.34. **A.** Angiogram of the RCA, in the posteroanterior projection, revealing stenosis in the proximal portion of the RCA (equivalent to stenosis of the left main coronary artery) and a single communication between the posterior descending artery and the distal LAD. **B.** Angiogram of the LCA, in the right anterior oblique projection, showing a "nipple" that suggests the site of anatomic origin of the LAD (arrow), and an absence of homolateral collaterals to the LAD. **C.** Magnified angiogram of the RCA, in the right anterior oblique projection, showing continuity (arrow) between the RCA and the LAD without a change in diameter (as is usually seen in cases of acquired collaterals). **D.** Left ventricular angiogram in the right anterior oblique projection, revealing a normal end-systolic contour (without anteroseptal hypokinesia). **E.** Diagrammatic representation of the anomaly in the coronary plane.

CASE REPORT 4.35

Coronary (Pseudo) Hypoplasia

A 40-year-old man with hypertension, hypercholesterolemia, and diabetes mellitus, had an abnormal baseline electrocardiogram. Exercise thallium scintigraphy suggested the presence of antero-lateral ischemia. Cardiac catheterization revealed a '' hypoplastic'' distal LAD system, featuring a large diagonal branch and a dominant RCA whose posterior descending branch wrapped around the cardiac apex (Fig. CR4.35, *A–C*). Medical treatment was continued.

Comment: This abnormal coronary pattern is probably congenital and benign (not associated with ischemia or an increased risk of myocardial infarction). In this case, it did not appear to be responsible for the abnormal nuclear scintigram. In cases of acquired coronary artery disease, the LAD would not be by-passable. ■

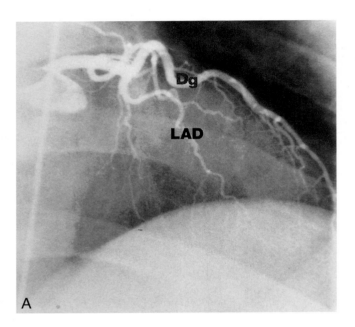

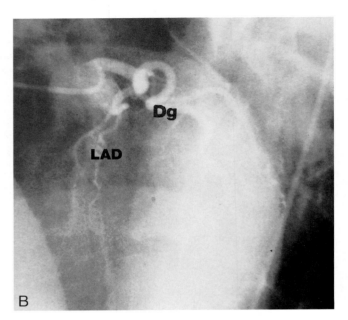

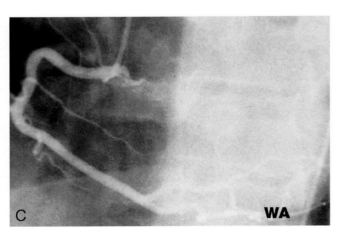

Figure CR4.35. Angiograms of the LCA, in the posteroanterior **(A)** and left anterior oblique **(B)** projections, showing a large diagonal branch (Dg) and a small postdiagonal LAD. **C.** Angiogram of the RCA, in the left anterior oblique projection, showing a large posterior descending branch that wraps around the cardiac apex (WA).

CASE REPORT 4.36

Intramural Coronary Artery (Muscular Bridge)

A 67-year-old hypertensive woman underwent coronary angiography because of atypical chest pain and increased risk factors for coronary artery disease. The study showed an intramural proximal-to-mid LAD segment, or muscular bridge, without signifi-

cant fixed obstructive disease (Fig. CR4.36, A–F). The left ventricle was moderately hyperkinetic (Fig. CR4.36G). The patient continued to undergo medical treatment for hypertension. ▶

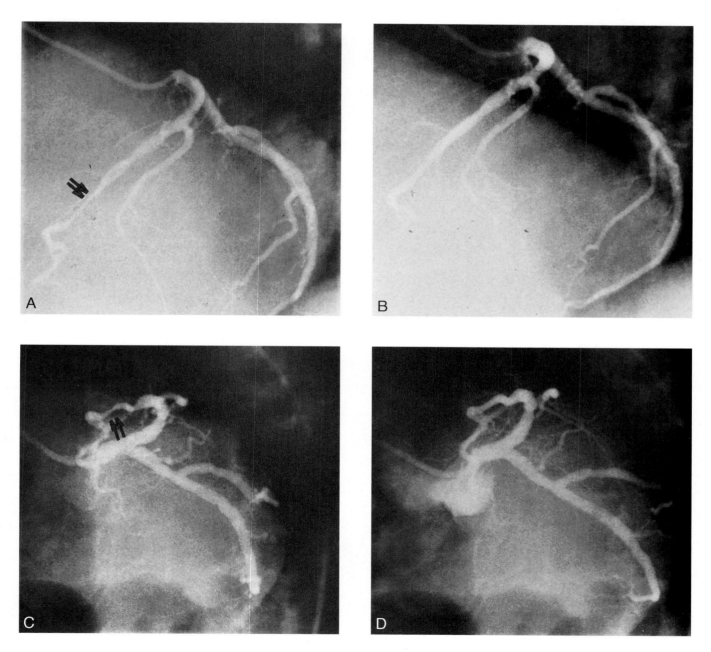

Figure CR4.36. Angiograms of the LCA, in the cranial left anterior oblique projection, during systole **(A)** and diastole **(B). C** and **D.** Angiograms of the LCA, in the caudal left anterior oblique projection, during systole **(C)** and diastole **(D).** continued

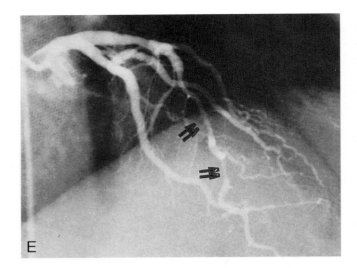

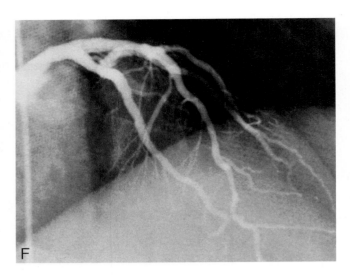

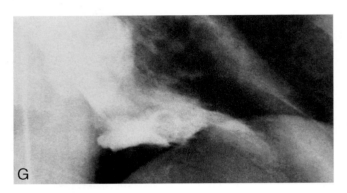

Figure CR4.36. (Continued) **E** and **F.** Angiograms of the LCA, in the right anterior oblique projection, during systole **(E)** and diastole **(F). G.** Left ventricular angiogram, in the right anterior oblique projection, showing a hyperkinetic left ventricle during end-systole. The systolic narrowing of the LAD's midsection is severe (80%), involving a relatively long segment of this artery (arrows, views **A, C,** and **E**).

CASE REPORT 4.37

Epicardial Crossing

A 59-year-old woman, with significant risk factors for coronary artery disease, presented with unstable angina. Selective angiography showed no critical fixed coronary obstructive lesions. The second obtuse marginal branch appeared to have a relatively large (2-mm diameter) branch that abnormally crossed the first obtuse marginal branch (Fig. CR4.37, A–C). ■

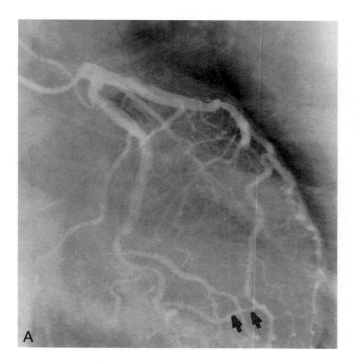 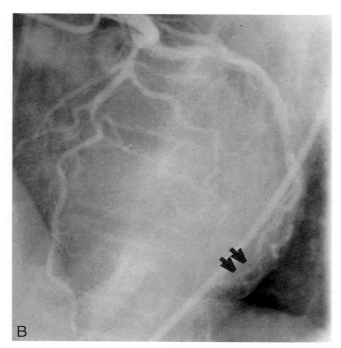

Figure CR4.37. Angiograms of the LCA in the right anterior oblique **(A)** and left anterior oblique **(B)** projections. The abnormally crossing, obtuse marginal branches (arrows) appear to be in the subepicardial space.

CASE REPORT 4.38

"Absent Posterior Descending Branch" (Split RCA)

An 81-year-old man was admitted with a history of prolonged chest pain at rest. The pain had begun a few weeks earlier. Cardiac catheterization revealed occlusion of the mid LAD (not shown), with a mildly to moderately decreased ejection fraction. The RCA showed no significant coronary disease, but it had two posterior descending branches (split RCA) (Fig. CR4.38). A rest-stress nuclear left ventricular performance study was significant only for mild inferior hypokinesia at peak stress, without changes in the LAD's territory. The patient was discharged from the hospital on a medical regimen. ∎

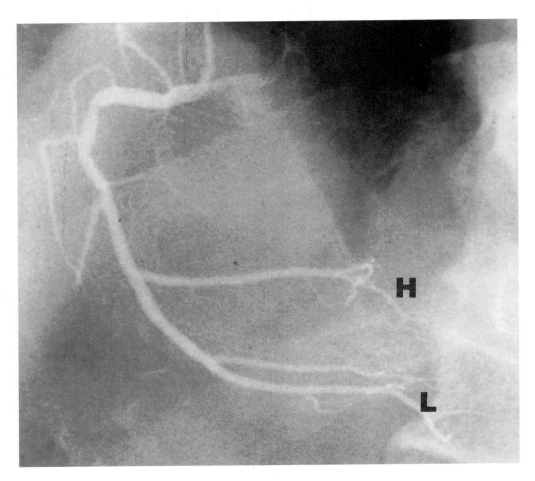

Figure CR4.38.   Angiogram of the RCA in the cranial left anterior oblique projection. The high (H) posterior descending branch originates from the RCA, which courses in the distal atrioventricular groove. The low (L) posterior descending branch arises as the continuation of an abnormally large acute marginal branch and supplies the infero-apical portion of the ventricular septum.

CASE REPORT 4.39

"Absent Posterior Descending Branch" (Split RCA)

A 49-year-old man with diabetes mellitus and hypertension presented with a 1-month history of effort-related angina. Treadmill exercise testing showed borderline ischemia. Cardiac catheterization revealed that the proximal segment of the RCA split into two major branches, both supplying the posterior interventricular septum (Fig. CR4.39, A–C). In addition, left coronary angiography showed a significant lesion in the diagonal branch (not shown). The patient underwent successful angioplasty of the lesions in the two distal branches of the RCA. ∎

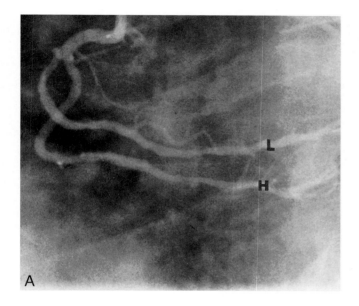

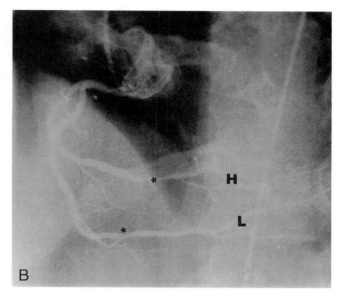

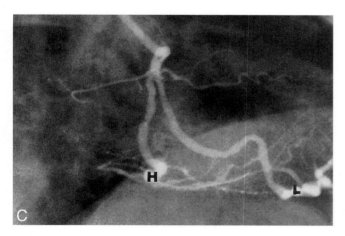

Figure CR4.39. Angiograms of the RCA in the caudal left anterior oblique **(A)**, cranial left anterior oblique **(B)**, and right anterior oblique **(C)** projections. The proximal segment of the artery splits into two major branches, both of which have significant focal lesions (view **B**, asterisks). The infero-basal portion of the ventricular septum is supplied by the high branch (H), located at the atrioventricular groove, as far as the crux. The infero-apical portion of the septum is supplied by the low branch (L) located at the lateral wall of the right ventricle, as far as the peri-apical posterior interventricular groove.

CASE REPORT 4.40

"Absent"/Split LAD: One LAD Originating From the LCA and the Other Originating From the RCA

A 62-year-old woman with a history of aortic valve replacement underwent cardiac catheterization before having elective redo aortic valve surgery. Her RCA produced an epicardial vessel that coursed in the mid and distal portions of the anterior interventricular groove, and the proximal LAD ended prematurely in the proximal groove (Fig. CR4.40, A–C). The circumflex artery originated anomalously from the proximal RCA and followed a retroaortic course. Echocardiography revealed normal left ventricular function. At the time of redo aortic valve surgery, no intervention was carried out on the anomalous coronary artery (no infarction was noted at the apex). ■

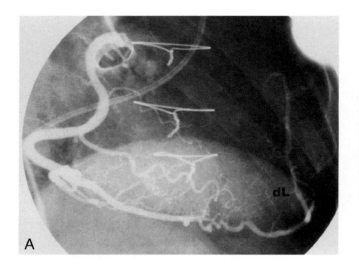

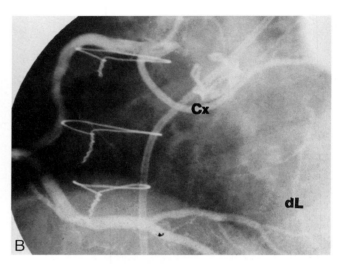

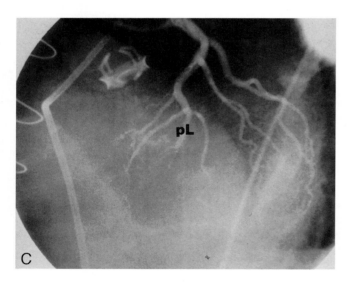

Figure CR4.40. Angiograms of the RCA in the right **(A)** and left **(B)** anterior oblique projections. The anomalous circumflex (Cx) and distal LAD (dL) arteries clearly originate from the proximal "RCA" (right mixed trunk) and the posterior descending artery, respectively. In view **B**, note the close proximity between the anomalous circumflex artery and the aortic prosthesis. **C.** Angiogram of the LCA, in the cranial left anterior oblique projection, showing the proximal LAD's unusually short length (pL): beyond the origin of the second septal branch, the LAD ends in three small terminal branches. No collaterals are seen between the proximal LAD and the distal LAD. It is possible that the interruption of the LAD was caused by an acquired condition (not a congenital one); nevertheless, the absence of collaterals from the proximal LAD and the continuation of the posterior descending artery into the anterior (distal) descending artery, with gradual tapering as it ascends the anterior interventricular groove, in the absence of anterio-apical scarring, support the theory that this was indeed a congenital variant (see also Case Report 4.34).

CASE REPORT 4.41

"Absent" Coronary Artery (LAD with Large Septal and Diagonal Branches)

A 55-year-old man with hyperlipidemia was admitted because of atypical chest pain and an abnormal treadmill test result. Selective coronary angiography showed a peculiar LAD pattern: the first septal branch was quite large and provided most of the anterior septal perforating branches (Fig. CR4.41, *A* and *B*); the diag-

onal artery was also large, reaching the apex with its terminal branch. No significant coronary obstruction was detected. The RCA (not shown) was dominant and normal. This coronary pattern fulfills the criteria for a "split LAD." No intervention was considered necessary. ■

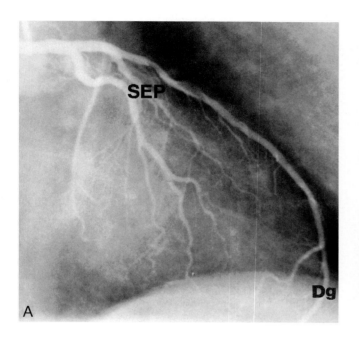

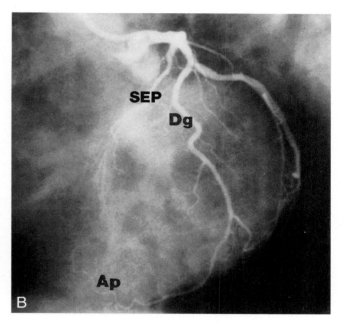

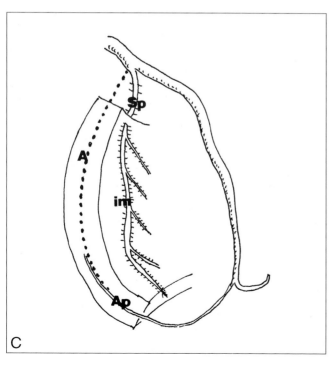

Figure CR4.41. Angiograms of the LCA, in the right **(A)** and left **(B)** anterior oblique projections. A large first septal branch (SEP) is present, but no anterior interventricular groove artery can be identified. The large diagonal artery (Dg) produces an apical branch (Ap). **C.** Diagrammatic representation of the anomaly. The dotted line represents the expected location of the "missing" LAD at the anterior interventricular groove. The area of the septum normally supplied by the LAD is in this case supplied by the large first septal branch and a recurrent apical branch of the large diagonal artery. A = expected site of epicardial LAD; im = intramural location; Sp = first septal branch.

CASE REPORT 4.42

Coronary Artery Fistula to the Right Ventricle

A 32-year-old policeman presented with recent-onset chest pain associated with diaphoresis. A treadmill thallium test showed mild anterolateral stress-induced ischemia and mild left ventricular dilation. At ages 7 and 12 years, the patient had undergone cardiac catheterization for a continuous precordial murmur, and a coronary fistula had been diagnosed. At that time, medical treatment was recommended because of the absence of symptoms and the evidence of a mild left-to-right shunt (1.1:1 pulmonary-to-systemic flow ratio). Cineangiograms obtained when the patient was 12 years old showed a fistula that arose from the proximal LAD and drained into the right ventricular outflow tract (Fig. CR4.42, A and B). Distal to the fistula, the LAD was small but patent. Left ventricular systolic function was normal.

On the present admission, physical examination was significant for a continuous murmur at the anterior precordium. Cardiac catheterization revealed significant left-to-right shunting (Qp:Qs = 1:1.25) at the level of the right ventricular outflow tract. Left ventricular angiography indicated that systolic function was diffusely impaired, with an ejection fraction of 40%. The proximal left main coronary artery had a mild, but definite, ostial stenosis related to the presence of a membrane-like structure (Fig. CR4.42C, arrows). The proximal trunk of the LAD showed a large aneurysmatic dilation (of the same diameter as the left anterior sinus), which ended in a short fistulous connection with the right ventricular outflow tract (Fig. CR4.42, D and E). AN = aneurysm; FS = fistula; PA = pulmonary artery; RVOT = right ventricular outflow tract. On left coronary angiography, the distal branches of the LCA were poorly filled, and the distal LAD and circumflex arteries were filled by means of collateral vessels (COLL) from the RCA (Fig. CR4.42F). These collaterals had not been seen on the angiogram obtained at age 12 (Fig. CR4.42B). The pressure in the proximal LAD was obtained by advancing a left coronary Amplatz-II guiding catheter over a 0.001-inch guidewire. The pressure looked ventricularized, with a diastolic value of about 20 mm Hg. Figure CR4.42G shows a schematic diagram of the coronary anomaly.

At corrective surgery, the LAD aneurysm was entered to ligate the fistulous tract to the right ventricle. A 1-mm probe could not be passed into the small distal portion of the LAD. Therefore, the left internal mammary artery was implanted into the distal LAD (1-mm diameter), and a vein graft was inserted between the aorta and the ramus medianus (2.5-mm diameter). The circumflex artery was entered with a 1-mm probe but was not bypassed. An ostial ridge on the aortic left coronary ostium was resected.

The patient recovered uneventfully but, 1 month after surgery, he presented with an episode of prolonged chest pain, accompanied by electrocardiographic T-wave changes and mild creatine phosphokinase elevation. New angiograms (Fig. CR4.42, H–L) showed the disappearance of the earlier left main ostial membrane, filling of the small circumflex system, and distal obstructive disease of the obtuse marginal branch (view H). This disease was interpreted as evidence of recent distal clot embolization, probably from the aneurysmatic left main trunk. The vein graft to the ramus medianus was patent (view I), but the left internal mammary artery implant had a critical stenosis (arrow) at the distal anastomosis (views J and K). The distal LAD had a much larger diameter than on the preoperative angiogram, and multiple new collateral vessels connected the LAD with the lower left pulmonary artery. Angiography of the RCA (view L) revealed an absence of collaterals (arrows), and the RCA had a normal diameter.

The patient underwent angioplasty of the distal left internal mammary artery anastomosis with a 2.5-mm balloon catheter, followed by insertion of a 3.0-mm stent (NIR ON; SCIMED, Boston Scientific, Boston, Massachusetts, USA).

This case clearly illustrates the possible complications that may be associated with the natural course of a medium-sized coronary artery fistula: aneurysmatic dilation (with the potential for distal embolization of mural thrombus before and after repair of the fistula) and distortion of the coronary anatomy resulting from different rates of growth of the different coronary segments (see the ostial obstructions of the left main coronary artery and distal branches). ▶

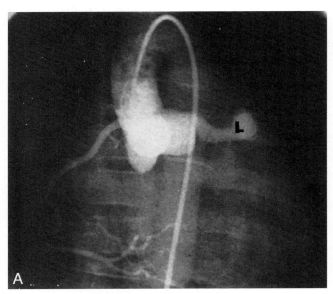
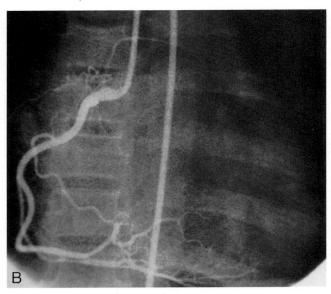

Figure CR4.42. **A.** Posteroanterior aortogram obtained at age 12 years, showing the ectasic left main and proximal LAD arteries, with a poorly visualized (in this photo) fistula from the LAD (L) to the right ventricular infundibulum. **B.** Angiogram of the RCA in the posteroanterior projection, obtained at age 12 years, showing no ectasia or collateral flow to the LCA. (continued)

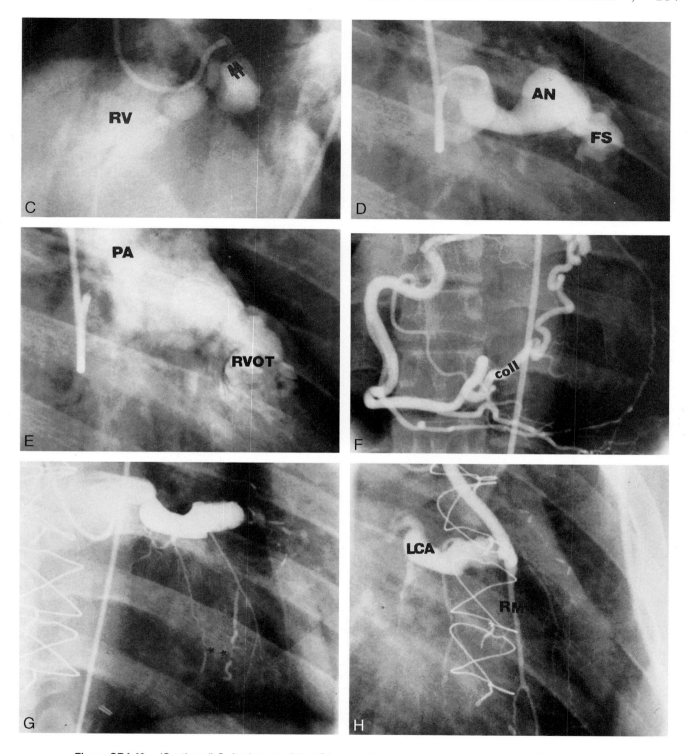

Figure CR4.42. (Continued) **C.** Angiogram of the LCA at age 32 years, in the cranial left anterior oblique projection, showing the ostial membrane-like stenosis and the LAD to right ventricular (RV) fistula. **D** and **E.** Angiogram of the LCA in the right anterior oblique projection, clearly showing the fistulous tract (FS) in the early phase **(D)** and the right ventricular outflow tract (RVOT) in the late phase **(E)** of the injection. AN = aneurysm; FS = fistulous orifice; PA = pulmonary artery. **F.** Angiogram of the RCA in the posteroanterior projection, showing diffuse ectasia and a rich collateral network to the circumflex (COLL) and LAD. **G.** Angiogram of the LCA in the right anterior oblique projection, showing persistent ectasia and poor runoff into the diminutive circumflex system, which contains newly apparent distal stenoses (asterisks) with sluggish runoff. **H.** Ramus medianus (RM) vein graft, in the right anterior oblique projection, showing good runoff and backup filling of the LCA. (continued)

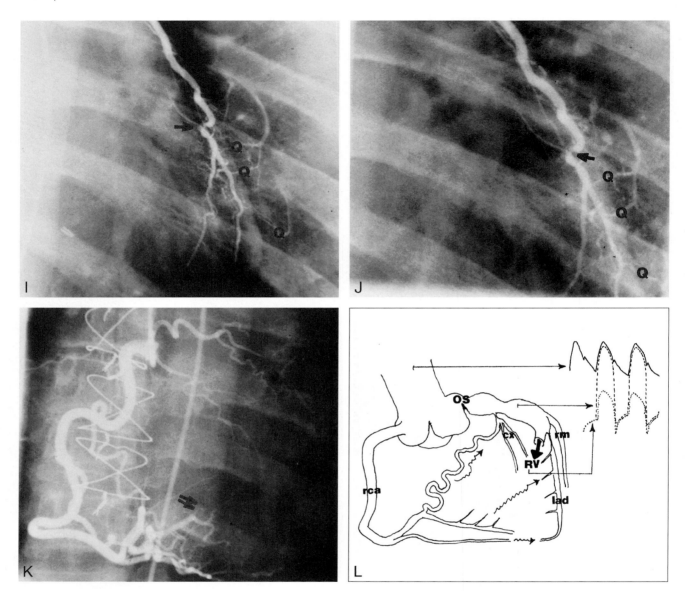

Figure CR4.42. (Continued) **I** and **J.** Left internal mammary artery graft to the LAD, in the right anterior oblique projection, showing distal anastomotic stenosis (arrow) and multiple newly formed collaterals (Q) leading from the LAD to branches of the left-lower-lobe pulmonary artery. **K.** Angiogram of the RCA in the posteroanterior projection, showing the absence of collateral filling of LCA branches (arrows). The size of the RCA has decreased since preoperative angiography. **L.** Diagram of the preoperative coronary anatomy and physiology, with a simulated rendering of the pressure tracings obtained at the following sites proximal and distal to the fistulous tract (arrow): aorta (driving source), LAD (direct source), and RCA (receiving cavity). Abbreviations as above; OS = ostial stenosis.

CASE REPORT 4.43

Coronary Ectasia with Multiple Coronaro-Cameral Fistulas

A 64-year-old man, who had previously had a myocardial infarction and a transient ischemic attack, presented as a candidate for repair of an abdominal aortic aneurysm. Cardiac catheterization showed coronary ectasia, occlusion of the distal circumflex artery, and extensive coronaro-cameral fistulas to the right ventricle (Fig. CR4.43, A–E). The patient had diffuse proximal coronary ectasia that appeared excessive with respect to the amount of fistulous flow, although it was certainly related to such flow. It is possible that the distal circumflex was also originally involved in the fistulous communications but eventually became thrombosed. The obtuse marginal artery is the only branch without fistulous involvement. Medical treatment was continued after the patient underwent uncomplicated repair of the abdominal aortic aneurysm. ▶

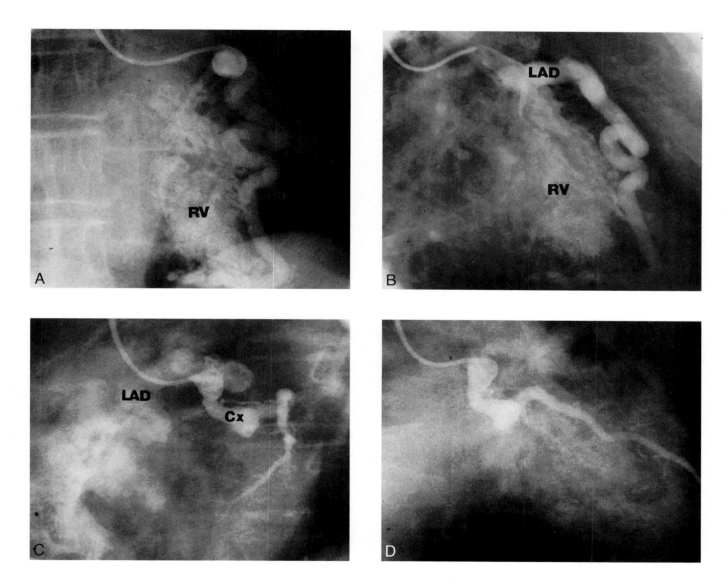

Figure CR4.43. Selective angiograms of the LAD in the posteroanterior **(A)** and right anterior oblique **(B)** projections. RV = right ventricle. Because of the very short left main trunk and the severe diffuse coronary ectasia, subselective catheterization of both major left arteries (the circumflex and LAD) was necessary. **C** and **D.** Selective angiograms of the circumflex artery (Cx) in the left **(C)** and right **(D)** anterior oblique projections (see text above). (continued)

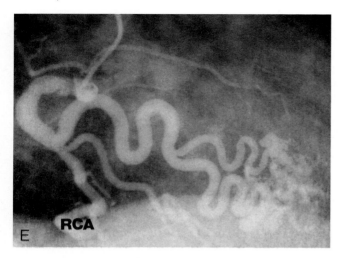

Figure CR4.43. (Continued) **E.** Angiogram of the RCA, in the right anterior oblique position, showing that the large anterior right ventricular branch and the proximal RCA are quite ectatic and carry most of the fistulous flow, while the distal RCA seems to have a normal luminal size.

CASE REPORT 4.44

RCA to Right Ventricular Fistulas Secondary to Multiple Right Ventricular Biopsies

A 55-year-old man, who had had an orthotopic heart transplant because of ischemic cardiomyopathy, underwent an annual post-transplant cardiac catheterization procedure. Right coronary angiography showed a coronary-to-right ventricular fistula that had not been present on the first posttransplant angiogram. Postoperatively, the patient had had several right ventricular biopsies, which resulted in the acquired fistula. No intervention was necessary for this acquired coronary anomaly.

Comment: The fact that an acquired fistula causes coronaro-cameral drainage from adjoining coronary branches may suggest that collateral branches have been activated by the right ventricular (low-pressure) run-off. This phenomenon might be relevant for interpreting the frequent angiographic finding of multiple souces (by neighboring coronary branches) also for coronaro-cameral fistulas of congenital origin. ■

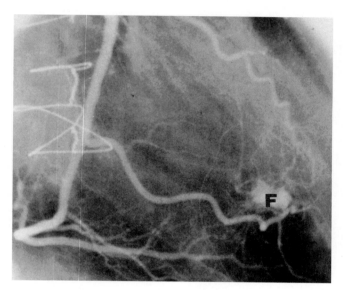

Figure CR4.44. Angiogram of the RCA in the right anterior oblique projection. A small coronary to right ventricular fistula (F) is clearly seen to fill from a proximal and a distal right ventricular branch.

CASE REPORT 4.45

Double Coronary Artery Fistulas to the Coronary Sinus

A 51-year-old man was evaluated for cardiovascular disease after experiencing acute dyspnea, diaphoresis, and atypical chest pain. A heart murmur was detected, and cardiac catheterization revealed two fistulas (Fig. CR4.45, A–C), one arising from the circumflex artery and the other arising from the RCA, both of which drained into the coronary sinus. The patient was treated with coumadin. Because his exertional dyspnea worsened, he sought a second opinion 6 months after the first evaluation. Physical examination was significant for a 2/6 systolic ejection murmur and a 1/6 diastolic murmur at the left sternal border. Echo-cardiography showed a dilated coronary sinus, with an increased flow velocity across the coronary sinus into the right atrium. The right atrium and right ventricle were mildly dilated, and the pulmonary artery pressure was normal. The pulmonary-to-systemic flow ratio was calculated at between 1.8 and 2.1. Coronary angiography confirmed the presence of circumflex artery and RCA fistulas that drained jointly into the coronary sinus (Fig. CR4.45, D). A sestamibi treadmill test was negative for ischemia or myocardial scarring. The patient underwent successful elective ligation of both distal feeding arteries. ∎

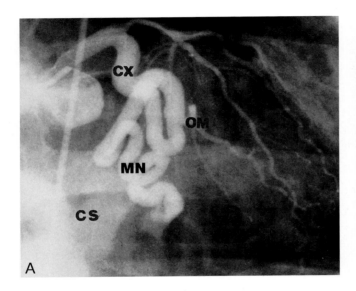

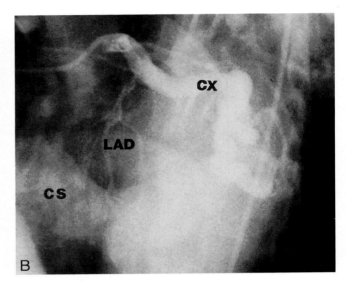

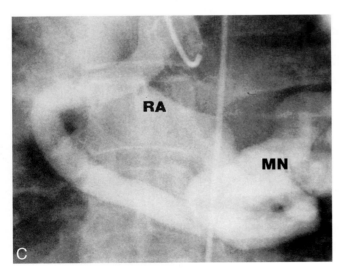

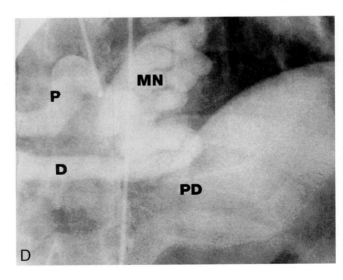

Figure CR4.45. Angiograms of the LCA in the posteroanterior **(A)** and left anterior oblique **(B)** projections, showing the greatly enlarged (6- to 8-mm) left main and circumflex arteries, as well as meandering (MN) tortuosity (view **A,** *) of the distal circumflex (Cx) artery before its entry into the coronary sinus (CS). The LAD (view **B**) and the obtuse marginal (view **A,** OM) branch are somewhat smaller than average. Early **(C)** and late **(D)** angiograms of the RCA, in the posteroanterior projection, show aneurysmatic dilation of the entire artery, which ranged from 10 to 12 mm in diameter; the artery followed a meandering, tortuous distal course before draining into the coronary sinus next to the fistulous termination in the circumflex artery. In view **C,** the right atrium (RA) is well visualized. MN = meandering tortuosity of the RCA. In view **D,** the posterior descending artery (PD) appears smaller than expected. D = distal RCA; P = proximal RCA.

CASE REPORT 4.46

Coronary Artery Fistula to the Coronary Sinus

A 36-year-old woman had an orthotopic heart transplant because of ischemic cardiomyopathy. At her first annual postoperative evaluation, right-sided cardiac pressures were within normal limits, with no step-up in oxygen saturation. Coronary angiography showed an aneurysmal RCA with a moderate-sized fistula that drained into the coronary sinus (Fig. CR4.46, *A*). The posterolateral branch of the RCA was occluded, and it filled from the left coronary system (Fig. CR4.46, *B*). At the coronary sinus, the ostium of the fistula seemed partially obstructed. Left ventricular function was normal. Medical treatment was recommended.

Comment: This fistula was apparently not noted by the transplant surgeons, nor was it accompanied by a continuous murmur. Most likely, earlier in the donor patient's life, the fistula was probably larger, and it eventually underwent a spontaneous process of distal obliteration, possibly during the transplant procedure. Alternatively, the fistulous tract was indeed acquired and a sign of inadvertent surgical trauma, although this is unlikely. ■

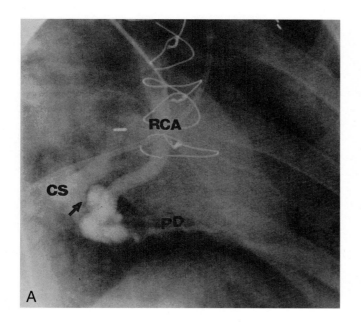 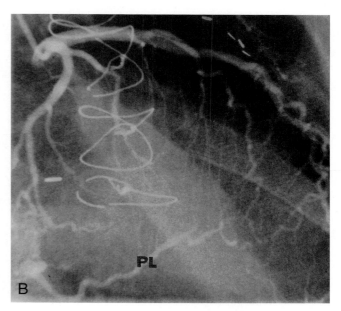

Figure CR4.46. **A.** Angiogram of the RCA, in the right anterior oblique projection, showing a patent posterior descending branch (PD), as well as a membrane-like stenosis (arrow) that partially obstructs the fistula's ostium in the coronary sinus (CS). **B.** Angiogram of the LCA, in the right anterior oblique projection, showing the posterolateral (PL) branch of the RCA, which fills from collaterals that connect with the circumflex artery.

CASE REPORT 4.47

Acquired LCA to Pulmonary Artery Fistula

A 67-year-old man underwent coronary artery bypass surgery, with placement of a left internal mammary artery graft to the LAD. Eight years postoperatively, follow-up angiography showed that the graft was patent, but abnormal neovasculariza-tion was noticed (Fig. CR4.47, *A–C*). The neovessels originated from a diagonal branch and fed a fistula to a left pulmonary arterial branch. The lesion was considered unimportant clinically, and medical treatment was recommended. ■

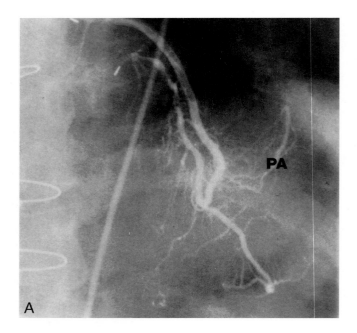

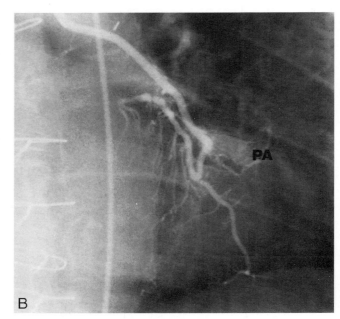

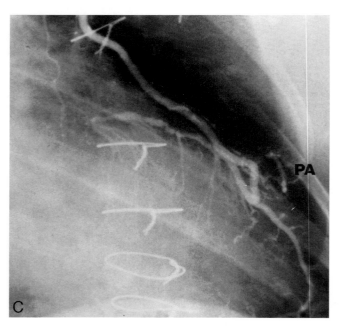

Figure CR4.47. Angiograms of the left internal mammary artery graft in the right anterior **(A)**, posteroanterior **(B)**, and left anterior oblique **(C)** projections. Abnormal neovessels (not present before coronary artery bypass surgery) fed a left pulmonary artery branch (PA).

CASE REPORT 4.48

LCA to Pulmonary Artery Fistula

A 61-year-old man with exertional chest pain underwent coronary angiography, which failed to reveal coronary artery disease but showed a small, short coronary to pulmonary artery fistula (Fig. CR4.48, *A* and *B*). Medical treatment was recommended. ∎

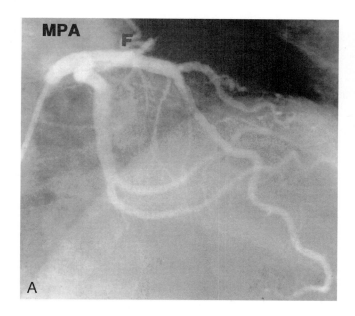
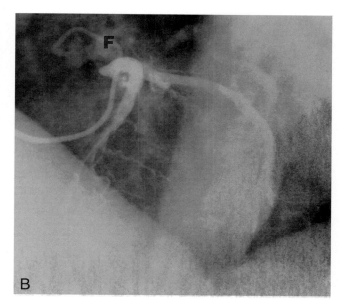

Figure CR4.48. Angiograms of the LCA in the right **(A)** and left **(B)** anterior oblique projections. A small fistula (F) arises from the proximal LAD artery and shows faint evidence of filling the main pulmonary artery (view **A, MPA**).

CASE REPORT 4.49

LCA to Left Ventricular Fistulas

A 57-year-old man with a history of hypertension and increasingly frequent episodes of angina underwent selective coronary angiography, which failed to indicate fixed coronary obstructive disease. All the coronary main branches were connected to the left ventricle by means of extensive microfistulas. A nuclear stress test yielded negative results. Medical treatment was continued. ∎

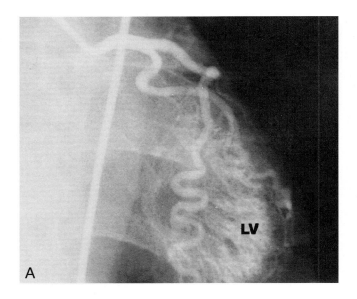

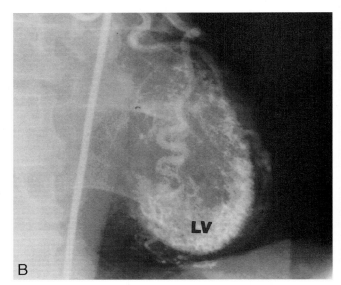

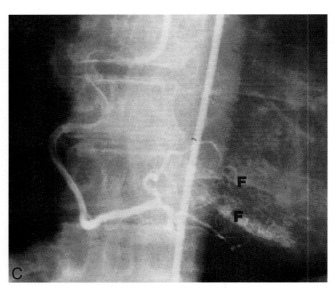

Figure CR4.49. Early (A) and late (B) angiograms of the LCA in the right anterior oblique projection, showing the diffuse, "systematic" nature of the patient's multiple small fistulas. In view **B,** which was obtained at end-diastole, a full ventriculogram becomes apparent. LV = left ventricle. **C.** Right coronary angiogram, in the posteroanterior projection, showing that the left (but not the right) ventricular branches of the RCA also had microfistulas (F).

CASE REPORT 4.50

Spasm and Coronary Anomalies: A Case of Prinzmetal's Angina and an LAD Muscular Bridge

A 53-year-old man with no history of constitutional risk factors presented with recent-onset chest and jaw pain that occurred at rest and occasionally during exercise; he had been able to continue with a regular exercise program (brisk walking/jogging for 1 hour a day). Nevertheless, treadmill testing was interrupted at 5 minutes because of chest/jaw pain and sudden ST-segment elevation (Fig. CR4.50, A and B) followed by nonsustained polymorphic ventricular tachycardia. The symptoms resolved soon after the administration of sublingual nitroglycerin. Although the patient was treated with a calcium antagonist and a topical nitroglycerin patch, follow-up Holter monitoring continued to show periods of asymptomatic and mildly symptomatic ST-segment changes. Echocardiography showed normal left ventricular function and morphology. Heart catheterization was carried out during pharmacologic withdrawal. Selective coronary angiography (Fig. CR4.50, C and D) revealed a 20% lesion in the RCA and a strictly systolic phasic narrowing (muscular bridge) of the mid LAD. Intravenous ergonovine (0.05 mg) quickly caused reproduction of the patient's symptoms, including electrocardiographic changes (inferior ST-segment elevation and ventricular tachycardia), hypotension, and profuse perspiration. Left coronary angiography revealed an intense fixed LAD stenosis proximal to the area of phasic systolic narrowing (Fig. CR4.50, E and F). Intracoronary nitroglycerin (200 μg) quickly resolved the symptoms, as well as the electrocardiographic changes and LAD

fixed stenosis (Fig. CR4.50, A–C). Intravascular ultrasound examination of the LAD revealed a systolic concentric narrowing (muscular bridge) of the mid LAD (Fig. CR4.50, G–I) and spasm of the proximal LAD (Fig. CR4.50, J–N). The patient refused to undergo redo ergonovine testing to visualize the RCA, which was the most likely culprit for the ST-segment elevation (inferior leads). He was treated with increased amounts of calcium antagonists and nitrates, which resulted in adequate clinical suppression of the syndrome of Prinzmetal's angina.

This case clearly illustrates the relationship between a congenital coronary anomaly (muscular bridge of the LAD) and a possible mechanism with clinical consequences: coronary spasm. Although the patient indeed had coronary spasm, it was elicited by the ergonovine test not at the site of the LAD muscular bridge but rather at a proximal site, as demonstrated angiographically and by intravascular ultrasound (passage of the device may cause mechanical stimulation at the proximal systolic bend). A site remote from the muscular bridge (the RCA) was actually the culprit for most of the patient's symptoms. More studies are needed to rule out direct involvement of the muscular bridge in Prinzmetal's angina. Interestingly, the site of the LAD spasm in this patient is the site reported in the literature as commonly featuring a fixed stenosis (atherosclerotic proximal LAD muscular bridge). ▶

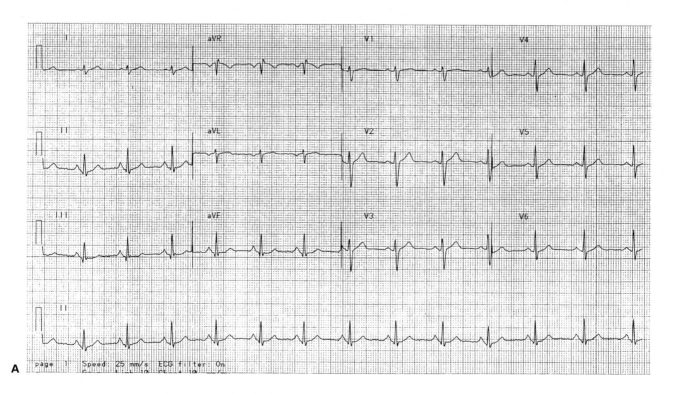

Figure CR4.50. (A) Electrocardiogram at rest (systolic frame). (continued)

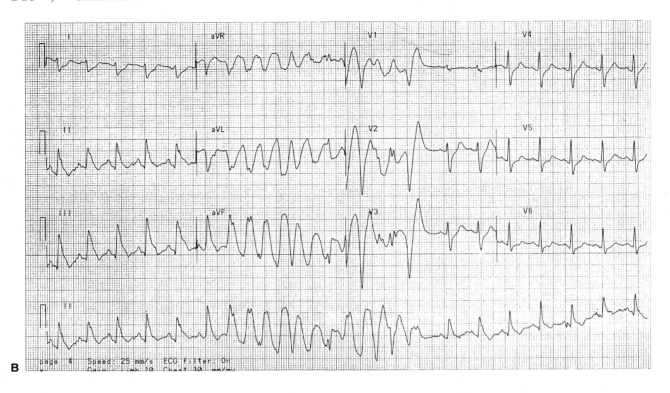

B

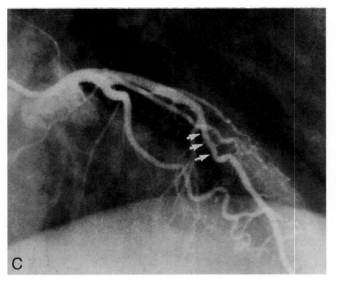

C

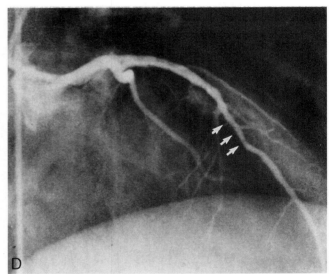

D

Figure CR4.50. (Continued) **(B)** Electrocardiogram at the end of treadmill exercise (diastolic frame), when ST-segment elevation in the inferior leads was severe and an episode of nonsustained polymorphic ventricular tachycardia was recorded. **C** and **D.** Initial angiograms of the LCA in the right anterior oblique projection during pharmacologic withdrawal. The muscular bridge is indicated by arrows. (continued)

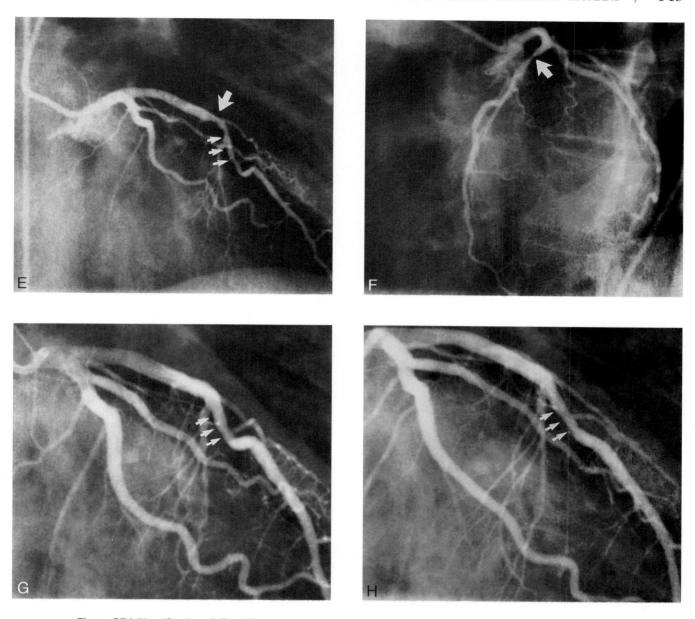

Figure CR4.50. (Continued) **E** and **F.** Angiograms of the LCA obtained 3 minutes after ergonovine administration. **E.** Systolic frame in the right anterior oblique projection. **F.** Diastolic frame in the left anterior oblique projection. Spasm is indicated by the large arrow; muscular bridge-related systolic narrowing is indicated by small arrows. **G–H.** Systolic and diastolic angiographic frames of the LCA in the right anterior oblique projection, showing total resolution of spasm and the persistence of systolic narrowing at the muscular bridge. (continued)

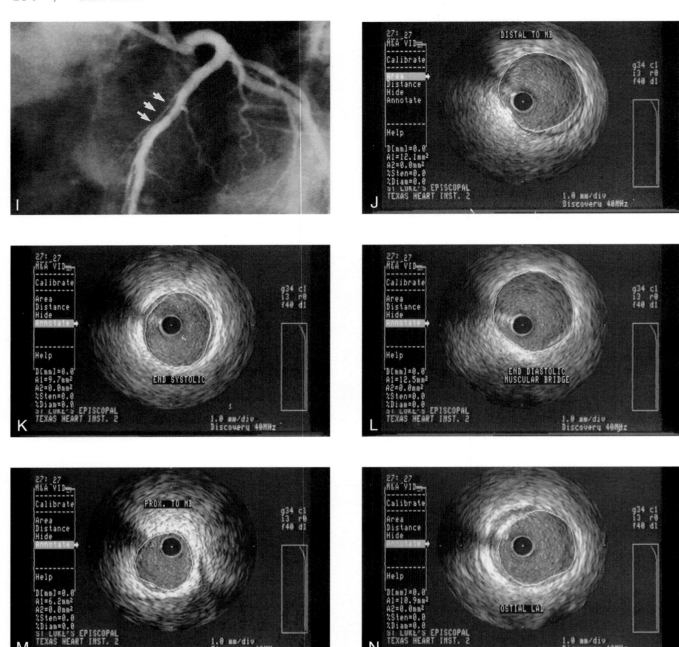

Figure CR4.50. (Continued) **I.** Diastolic angiographic frame in the left anterior oblique projection, showing total resolution of spasm and the persistence of systolic narrowing at the muscular bridge. **J–N.** Intracoronary ultrasound images of the LAD, after intracoronary nitroglycerin administration, at the following sites: distal to the muscular bridge **(J)**; at the muscular bridge (end-systole) **(K)**; at the muscular bridge (end-diastole) **(L)**; at the bend, proximal to the muscular bridge **(M)**; and at the LAD ostium (just distal to the circumflex separation) **(N)**. Note that passage of the ultrasound catheter caused spasm at the proximal LAD bend (view **M**), most likely because of mechanical stimulation. Area calculations are indicated in each view.

Coronary Artery Anomalies: A Comprehensive Approach, edited by P. Angelini.
Lippincott Williams & Wilkins, Philadelphia © 1999.

CHAPTER 5

Coronary Artery Anomalies in Pediatric Patients

Thomas E. Fagan, Alexis Palacios-Macedo, Michael R. Nihill,
Charles D. Fraser, Jr., and Denton A. Cooley

Congenital anomalies of the major coronary arteries or their main branches are fairly common, especially in patients with congenital heart disease. In most cases, the myocardium is perfused by the systemic circulation and, in the absence of acquired coronary artery disease, patients with coronary anomalies are hemodynamically stable (anomalies of this type are discussed in Chapter 4). Rare congenital coronary anomalies may result in poor myocardial perfusion and myocardial ischemia in children. The two most common congenital lesions that place the myocardium at risk for ischemia are anomalous origination of the left coronary artery from the pulmonary artery (ALCAPA) and coronary artery fistula. This chapter discusses these two forms of ischemic congenital heart disease in the pediatric patient.

ANOMALOUS ORIGINATION OF THE LEFT CORONARY ARTERY FROM THE PULMONARY ARTERY

The anatomy and blood flow pattern of ALCAPA was first defined in 1886 by Brooks.[13] In 1908, Abbott[1] observed this anomaly in a 60-year-old woman who died accidentally. Bland, White, and Garland[11] provided the first clinical description of the infantile presentation in 1933, establishing the eponym ''Bland-White-Garland syndrome'' for the designation of ALCAPA. Gouley[39] described the physiology of ALCAPA in asymptomatic adults. In 1955, Paul and Robbins[79] reported the first surgical treatment, which involved pericardial poudrage.

Accounting for 0.24% of congenital cardiac anomalies, ALCAPA occurs in approximately 1 in 300,000 live births.[51] It is seen in 18% of patients younger than 2 years of age who present with congestive heart failure.[47] Although ALCAPA is often fatal, it may be surgically corrected if diagnosed early. Therefore, it should be considered in all young

patients, especially infants, who present with congestive heart failure.

Anatomy

The anomalous left coronary artery may originate anywhere along the pulmonary artery, but it most commonly originates from that artery's left sinus (Fig. 5.1). Other possible sites of origin include the pulmonary artery's right sinus, the pulmonary trunk, and the branch pulmonary arteries (usually the right).

Although typically an isolated cardiac lesion, ALCAPA may be seen with other congenital cardiac lesions such as ventricular septal defect, atrioventricular canal, tetralogy of Fallot, truncus arteriosus, and aortic valve stenosis.[4,31,41,83] The clinical presentation of patients with associated malformations depends on the effect of other lesions on the cardiac physiology and the extent of myocardial ischemia produced by ALCAPA.

Embryology (see Chapter 2)

Experimental studies in quail and chick embryos have shown that formation of the coronary arteries involves three developmental phases during which nutrients are delivered to the embryonic myocardium. In the first phase, a network of intratrabecular sinusoids forms and extends from the ventricular cavity.[106] In the second phase, endothelial-lined vascular channels form within the subepicardium. These channels penetrate the myocardium of the atrial and ventricular walls, and some of them communicate with the sinusoidal capillary network. The vascular channels develop at sites with the most abundant subepicardial matrix, such as the atrioventricular, sinoatrial, and interventricular sulci.[103] Finally, in the third phase, the developing vascular channels

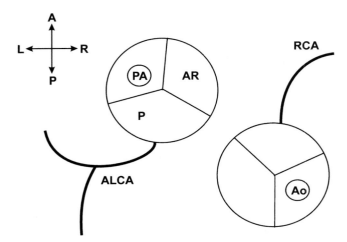

FIGURE 5.1. The most common site of anomalous origination of the left coronary artery is the left sinus of the pulmonary artery. ALCA = anomalous left coronary artery; Ao = aortic root; AR = right sinus of the pulmonary artery; P = left sinus of the pulmonary artery; PA = pulmonary artery root; RCA = right coronary artery.

coalesce into muscular arteries that are continuous with the proximal right and left coronary arteries.[97]

A capillary plexus forms around the truncus arteriosus and communicates with the proximal coronary arteries. This plexus organizes to form single large proximal coronary vessels that penetrate the aortic wall at the aortic sinuses.[106]

Two theories have been proposed to explain how the left coronary artery arises from the pulmonary artery during embryonic development.[43] In the first theory, conotruncal septation occurs abnormally. Under normal circumstances, when the conotruncal septum divides the great arteries, the proximal coronary arteries penetrate the aortic wall at the root of the ascending aorta. If the conotruncal septum divides the great vessels abnormally, the left coronary artery may penetrate at the root of the pulmonary artery. In the second theory, the conotruncal septum develops normally, but the proximal left coronary artery penetrates abnormally into the conotruncal wall at a site destined to become part of the pulmonary artery. Despite these theories, the exact mechanism of anomalous origination is unknown.

Pathophysiology

Because myocardial tissue can efficiently extract oxygen from the coronary circulation, low oxygen tension is tolerated within broad limits, as in patients with cyanotic congenital heart disease. In contrast, low perfusion pressure and low flow rates are not tolerated. In patients with ALCAPA, the myocardium becomes ischemic because of low perfusion pressure.

Before birth, the pulmonary arterial pressure equals the systemic pressure because the ductus arteriosus connects the pulmonary artery to the aorta. Therefore, in the presence of an anomalous left coronary artery, myocardial perfusion is normal, but oxygen tension is decreased. Because the perfusion pressure is normal, intracoronary collateral vessels are not well developed (Fig 5.2A). After birth, the pulmonary artery pressure decreases; coupled with the increasing intramural pressure of the left ventricle, this decrease leads to a reduction in left ventricular perfusion. As the diastolic pressure in the pulmonary arteries falls, decreased coronary perfusion leads to myocardial ischemia, which results in varied pathophysiologic responses.[5,18,27,111]

In children with ALCAPA, the decline in pulmonary resistance is often gradual. As myocardial perfusion of the left ventricle decreases, the function of the ventricle deteriorates, leading to an increased left ventricular end-diastolic pressure. In turn, the increased diastolic pressure causes the left atrial pressure to rise, producing an increase in the pulmonary artery pressure. This secondary pulmonary hypertension improves perfusion through the anomalous left coronary artery and slows the process of myocardial ischemia. By 6 to 8 weeks after birth, however, the pulmonary pressure usually falls to a critical level that results in a low myocardial perfusion pressure. Some patients then become symptomatic with the infantile form of ALCAPA.

In other patients, an extensive intramyocardial collateral network develops and establishes adequate circulation from the right to the left coronary system, initially improving perfusion. In this situation, the left coronary system fills by means of retrograde blood flow. Because the left ventricular transmural pressure is higher than the pulmonary artery pressure, however, oxygenated blood in the left coronary artery will drain into the lower-pressure pulmonary system. This

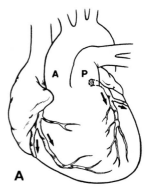
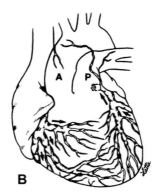

FIGURE 5.2. Physiology of anomalous origination of the left coronary artery. **A.** Elevated pulmonary artery pressure in the newborn. Deoxygenated blood from the pulmonary artery fills the anomalous artery in prograde fashion. **B.** The pulmonary artery pressure decreases with increased age. Collateral vessels develop from the right coronary artery to the anomalous artery. Oxygenated blood then fills the anomalous artery in retrograde fashion. A pulmonary steal develops when blood flows from the anomalous left coronary artery into the pulmonary artery. A = aorta; P = pulmonary artery.

pulmonary artery "steal phenomenon" reduces myocardial perfusion (Fig. 5.2*B*). Nevertheless, if the myocardium receives sufficient blood flow, patients can reach adulthood before developing symptoms of low-grade, progressive myocardial ischemia, or the adult form of ALCAPA. Brooks,[13] who first postulated the steal phenomenon in 1886, suggested that the anomalous artery not only fails to supply blood to the myocardium but also diverts oxygenated blood from the heart to the pulmonary artery (left-to-right shunt). His hypothesis was later supported by postmortem studies carried out by Sabiston and colleagues[89] and by Edwards.[28]

Pathology

Because the myocardium is poorly perfused in ALCAPA, the left ventricle becomes ischemic and dilated. The weight of the heart significantly increases because of hypertrophy, which develops secondary to an augmented preload and myocardial ischemia. In turn, hypertrophy increases myocardial ischemia, resulting in progressive fibrosis and deteriorating myocardial function. Both new and old myocardial infarctions may be found in the inner third to inner half of the left ventricle. The spectrum of scarring ranges from areas of subendocardial fibrosis to complete calcification; in addition, secondary endocardial fibroelastosis and aneurysmal dilation of the left ventricular apex may occur.[108]

The course of the dilated right coronary artery becomes tortuous. On gross examination, a well-developed network of intercoronary collateral vessels is usually seen.

Patients with ALCAPA who present with congestive heart failure often have mitral valve dysfunction. The mitral annulus and the papillary muscles are often affected by ischemic changes. The anterior papillary muscle is usually involved, but both papillary muscles may have areas of infarction and scarring. This scarring, combined with calcification and shortening of the chordae tendineae, leads to mitral insufficiency. In addition, endocardial fibrosis may develop in the adjacent myocardial tissue and reduce the function of the mitral valve.

Clinical Manifestations

In 1968, Wesselhoeft and coauthors[108] developed a system for classifying ALCAPA on the basis of the patient's initial presentation. Although no longer used clinically, this system is helpful in describing the clinical manifestations of the disease. Wesselhoeft and colleagues reviewed 140 cases of ALCAPA, 82% involving presentation in infancy and 18% involving presentation in childhood or adulthood. The patients were divided into four groups. The first and largest group comprised patients between the ages of 6 weeks and 4 months who had tachypnea, wheezing, and failure to thrive. Other symptoms typically associated with feeding included angina-like episodes, sudden irritability, and pallor or an ashen-gray appearance. In addition, cardiomegaly was present. Without surgery, this group had a mortality of 90% in

TABLE 5.1. *ALCAPA: Clinical presentation*

Infantile ALCAPA (poorly developed collateral system)
  Congestive heart failure
  Angina-like episodes
  Respiratory distress
Adult ALCAPA (well-developed collateral system)
  Asymptomatic until the third decade of life
  Angina
  Shortness of breath
  Sudden death

the first year of life. In the second group, patients presented before age 4 months with a murmur of mitral insufficiency; the risk of mortality or left ventricular dysfunction during the first year of life was significantly less than in the first group, but all group-2 patients developed congestive heart failure by late adolescence or adulthood. In contrast, the third group was small and relatively asymptomatic, ranging in age from 3 to 9 years. Their most common symptom was angina. (In such patients, a continuous murmur produced by left coronary artery flow into the pulmonary artery was usually mistaken for a patent ductus arteriosus.) The fourth group ranged in age from 16 to 60 years and presented with sudden death. No patient had had previous cardiac symptoms, and all deaths occurred on physical exertion.

Currently, classification of ALCAPA patients is based on the degree of intercoronary collateral development (Table 5.1). Patients with the infantile form of the disease have poorly developed collateral vessels and present, as newborns, with congestive heart failure, angina-like episodes, and respiratory distress. The mortality of infantile ALCAPA may be as high as 90% during the first year of life.[73,108] Patients with the adult form of the disease have a well-developed collateral network that supplies nutrients to the left ventricular myocardium. Although relatively asymptomatic, these patients are at high risk of sudden death. By a mean age of 35 years, their risk may be as high as 80 to 90%.[31] Sudden death may be related to acute ischemia resulting from pulmonary artery steal, progressive stenosis of the intercoronary collaterals, or ventricular arrhythmias.

Certain anatomic and physiologic variants may improve survival. As already stated, a well-developed intercoronary collateral system from the right to the left coronary artery enhances survival. In addition, survival is improved when the right coronary artery is dominant and directly supplies a large portion of the myocardium, so that a smaller percentage of tissue is at risk for ischemia. An elevated pulmonary artery pressure helps maintain perfusion pressure in the left coronary artery and thus improves survival. In the setting of suprasystemic pulmonary hypertension, desaturated blood is supplied to the left ventricle; because the capacity for oxygen uptake in cardiac tissue is high, an adequate flow of desaturated blood is tolerated better than a decreased perfusion pressure (and flow). Finally, patients with ALCAPA may have stenosis at the origin of the left coronary artery, which increases survival by limiting pulmonary steal from the left coronary artery. However, these patients are still at risk for ischemia and sudden death because of unreliable flow through the intercoronary collateral network.

Physical Examination

As a result of ALCAPA's variable clinical focus of presentation, the condition produces a multiplicity of physical signs. Physical examination may elicit the following findings:

- Failure to thrive, with body weight lower than normal
- Dyspnea, with an increased respiratory rate, intercostal retractions, rales, or a full-blown pattern of acute pulmonary edema
- Hepatomegaly
- Peripheral cyanosis and/or hypoperfusion signs secondary to pulmonary congestion and/or low cardiac output
- Continuous murmur in the precordium (that becomes more obvious after infancy)
- Gallop extra tones (S_3 and S_4 sounds)
- Systolic murmur of mitral regurgitation (which may change dramatically with the onset of myocardial ischemic spells). Diastolic mitral inflow from the left to right shunt and mitral regurgitation are present
- Cardiomegaly, which at times may be quite dramatic

Diagnostic Evaluation

Radiographic findings are nonspecific in patients with ALCAPA. The predominant finding is cardiac enlargement produced by left atrial and ventricular dilation. Left atrial dilation may be especially obvious in patients with significant mitral insufficiency.

The electrocardiogram almost always indicates a recent or old anterolateral myocardial infarction (Fig. 5.3). In 80% of patients, characteristic Q waves or ST-segment elevations appear in leads I, aV_L, and V_{4-6}.[108] In 1995, Johnsrude and coworkers[47] reported specific electrocardiographic measurements useful for differentiating ALCAPA from myocarditis and dilated cardiomyopathy. Using multiple logistic regression, they developed a highly sensitive and specific equation that incorporates the width of the Q wave in lead I and the depth of the Q wave and the height of the ST-segment elevation in lead aV_L.

The first reports concerning the use of echocardiography in the evaluation of patients with ALCAPA were published in the early 1980s.[16,32,49] In initial reports, the anomalous origin of the left coronary artery was seen at the pulmonary artery on two-dimensional echocardiography. When the anomalous origin cannot be visualized, ALCAPA can be suspected because of the large right coronary artery. If the left coronary artery is seen to originate from the aorta, ALCAPA can obviously be excluded. The sole use of two-

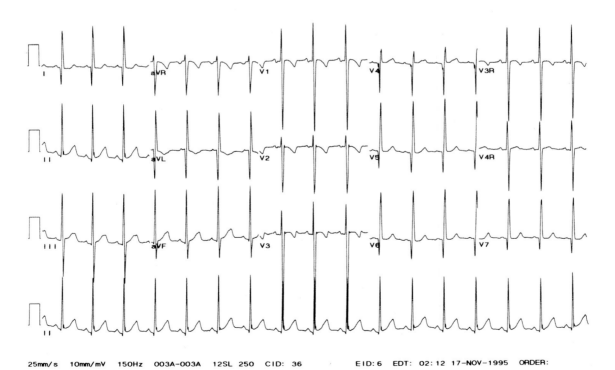

25mm/s 10mm/mV 150Hz 003A-003A 12SL 250 CID: 36   EID: 6 EDT: 02: 12 17-NOV-1995 ORDER:

FIGURE 5.3. Electrocardiogram from a 2-year-old patient with ALCAPA. Deep Q waves in leads I and aV_L and in the left precordial leads indicate an anterolateral infarction.

dimensional or Doppler echocardiography is associated with relatively high false-positive and false-negative rates. A false-positive diagnosis may result when the normal origin of the left coronary artery cannot be seen for technical or anatomic reasons (such as ectopic origination from the right cusps). In contrast, a false-negative diagnosis may result from the appearance of an "echo-free space" at the left sinus of Valsalva.[88] This false interpretation is often related to the appearance of the transverse sinus of the pericardium (which runs between the aortic root and the left atrium). Doppler studies are important in this regard.

Echocardiographic diagnosis of ALCAPA is greatly facilitated by Doppler color-flow mapping.[48,50] With this technique, a continuous-flow jet may be present in the pulmonary artery arising from the ectopic ostium of the left coronary artery. This finding, in conjunction with retrograde flow in two of the three major segments of the left coronary system (the left main, left anterior descending, and circumflex arteries), is diagnostic of ALCAPA. With the advent of Doppler color-flow mapping and other sophisticated technologies, echocardiography has become an essential adjuvant in the screening and diagnostic evaluation of this anomaly.

Cardiac catheterization is the most accurate, illustrative procedure for diagnosing ALCAPA. Although this condition can sometimes be diagnosed on the basis of echocardiographic and other noninvasive studies, cardiac catheterization and cineangiography (the gold standard for diagnosis) should be performed in the presence of any uncertainty regarding cardiac anatomy or hemodynamics.

A "step-up" of more than 4% in the percentage of oxygen saturation from the right ventricle to the pulmonary artery is a typical finding during cardiac catheterization of ALCAPA patients. This increase in oxygen saturation results from the left-to-right shunt, in which fully saturated blood enters the pulmonary artery via the anomalous left coronary artery. Moreover, this step-up in oxygen saturation can be used to calculate the degree of left-to-right shunting.[101] A large increase in oxygen saturation indicates a large shunt from the left coronary artery to the pulmonary artery. In the absence of other structural heart defects, this shunt measures the amount of fistulous flow in ALCAPA. The left ventricular end-diastolic and left atrial pressures are increased as a result of poor left ventricular function, mitral insufficiency, or both. The cardiac output and cardiac index may be low, depending on the severity of left ventricular dysfunction.

Cineangiography provides a clear picture of the cardiac anatomy and aids in assessing left ventricular and mitral valve function. ALCAPA is usually diagnosed after injection of contrast dye into the aortic root or right coronary artery. The dilated and tortuous right coronary artery quickly fills with contrast material (Fig. 5.4, A and B). Collateral vessels of various sizes originate from the right coronary artery and communicate with the left coronary system. That system fills in a retrograde manner, the extent of filling depending on the predominant sites of intercoronary collateral communication. If the ectopic ostium of the left coronary artery is not severely stenosed, contrast dye will enter the pulmonary arteries (Fig. 5.4, C and D). Inability to selectively inject contrast material into the left coronary artery from a retrograde aortic approach does not, by itself, prove the diagnosis of ALCAPA but, rather confirms that diagnosis. Injection of contrast material into the pulmonary artery rarely causes filling of the anomalous origin of the left coronary artery; a negative contrast "washout" from the anomalous origin of the left coronary artery may be seen, but this finding should not be the sole criterion for diagnosis. Pulmonary angiography with temporary distal pulmonary artery balloon occlusion may help visualize the anomalous coronary artery. Left ventricular cineangiography can be used to assess the extent of ventricular dilation and left ventricular systolic dysfunction, the presence of a ventricular aneurysm and areas of dyskinesia or akinesis, and the presence and severity of mitral valve insufficiency.

Differential Diagnosis

The spectrum of differential diagnoses of ALCAPA is broad because the clinical presentation varies (Table 5.2). In patients with a dilated, poorly functioning left ventricle, ALCAPA can be difficult to distinguish from acute myocarditis or dilated cardiomyopathy of any etiology. If the predominant finding is mitral regurgitation, primary congenital mitral valve disease and rheumatic pancarditis must be considered. In patients with a continuous murmur and cardiomegaly, ALCAPA mimics patent ductus arteriosus or coronary artery fistula. Atherosclerotic heart disease should be excluded in older patients with angina or sudden death.

Medical Management

Patients with ALCAPA usually seek medical attention after having myocardial ischemia and infarction. For successful treatment, an adequate oxygen and blood supply must be restored to the myocardial tissue, and the demand for oxygen must be reduced. Medical strategies are directed toward improving contractility, reducing congestion, and decreasing the patient's energy expenditure. To preserve myocardial function, treatment strategies should be adjusted on

TABLE 5.2. *ALCAPA: Differential diagnosis*

Cardiomegaly
  Myocarditis
  Cardiomyopathy (all types)
Mitral regurgitation
  Primary mitral valve disease (e.g., cleft mitral valve)
  Rheumatic pancarditis
Continuous murmur
  Patent ductus arteriosus
  Coronary artery fistula
Angina or sudden death
  Atherosclerotic coronary disease
  Congenital coronary ostial stenosis or atresia

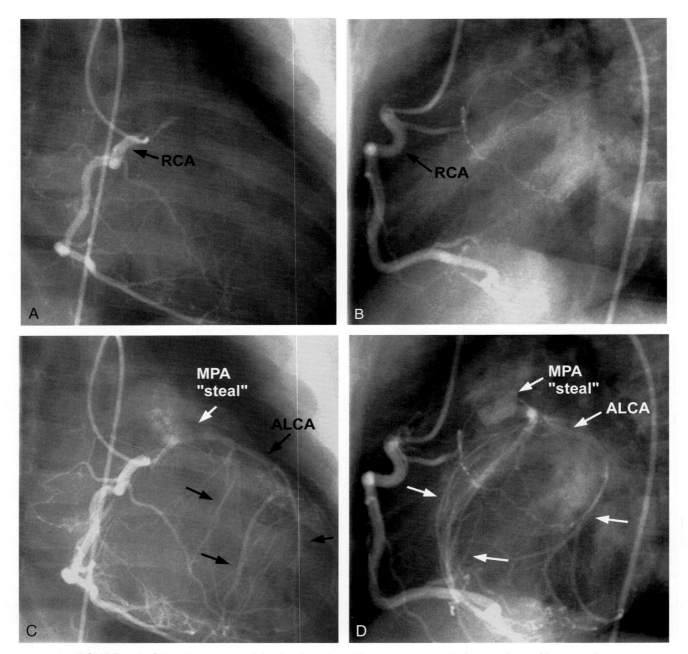

FIGURE 5.4. Selective contrast injection into the right coronary artery in a patient with anomalous origination of the left coronary artery. In the early phases of the angiogram (anteroposterior **[A]** and lateral **[B]** projections), a dilated, tortuous right coronary artery (RCA) is seen. In the later phases (anteroposterior **[C]** and lateral **[D]** projections), multiple intercoronary collateral vessels (arrows) opacify and fill the anomalous left coronary artery (ALCA) in retrograde fashion. A main pulmonary artery (MPA) steal is present, with contrast material entering the pulmonary artery from the anomalous artery.

the basis of clinical status and response. Additional modification may be necessary, depending on whether early or late surgical intervention is being considered. The current trend is to operate early, so the goal of medical therapy is to improve and preserve the hemodynamic status.

Although several agents can augment myocardial contractility in these patients, the cardiac glycosides are the mainstay of inotropic therapy. Digoxin improves cardiac function directly by acting on cardiac muscle to increase contractility and indirectly by acting on the autonomic nervous system to decrease the heart rate.[52] Whereas the increase in contractility improves cardiac output and perfusion, the decrease in heart rate reduces the myocardial oxygen demand. Although useful for treating symptoms of congestive heart failure, digoxin may trigger ventricular and supraventricular dysrhythmias in hearts with ischemic injury and should be used with caution.[96] The safest route for administering digoxin is enteral; therefore, in patients who are severely symptomatic and cannot tolerate enteral therapy, other agents should be considered. Dobutamine, a parenterally administered synthetic sympathomimetic amine, has powerful inotropic effects but only modest chronotropic effects. Its inotropic potency results from stimulation of myocardial beta- and alpha-receptors.[53,66] Because of its limited effect on the heart rate and peripheral vasculature, dobutamine is particularly useful in children. The phosphodiesterase inhibitors (amrinone and milrinone) are a relatively new class of inotropic agents. Inhibition of cyclic AMP (cAMP) phosphodiesterases eventually leads to an increase in the concentration of cytoplasmic cAMP, which, in turn, leads to improved heart muscle contractility. In contrast, increased levels of cytoplasmic cAMP in vascular smooth muscle lead to vasodilation. The combination of improved cardiac function and afterload reduction improves cardiac output and reduces myocardial consumption of oxygen. However, phosphodiesterase inhibitors have an unpredictable vasodilatory effect on pulmonary vessels. In patients with ALCAPA, a decrease in pulmonary vascular resistance could lead to an increase in the left-to-right shunt and a subsequent decrease in myocardial perfusion. Therefore, the use of phosphodiesterase inhibitors in patients with ALCAPA is not routinely recommended.

The loop diuretics are generally used to treat congestive heart failure in children. The goal of diuretic therapy is to reduce pulmonary edema, the ventricular preload, and ventricular wall stress, thereby decreasing the myocardial oxygen demand. Furosemide can be administered enterally or parenterally in patients who are severely symptomatic or who do not respond adequately to enteral therapy. The loop diuretics can be used alone or in combination with other diuretics.

In patients with ALCAPA who have severe symptoms or significantly impaired ventricular function, aggressive therapy may be necessary to increase the myocardial oxygen supply and decrease the myocardial workload. Oxygen supplementation should be given to all patients who have symptoms or suspected ongoing ischemia. In those with respiratory distress or profound acidosis, endotracheal intubation and artificial respiration (with or without muscle relaxation) significantly reduces the total energy expenditure and cardiovascular demand. Parenteral nutrition may be required by patients with gastrointestinal edema and feeding intolerance. Ventricular arrhythmias secondary to poor cardiac function and ischemia are often seen. Close patient monitoring and appropriate use of antiarrhythmic agents are essential.

In treating ALCAPA patients, deciding the appropriate time for surgical intervention can be very difficult. Although many reports have been published regarding the indications and timing of surgery,[4,15,25,31,82] recommendations differ. A significant confounding variable in these studies is that patients with the worst ventricular function can benefit the most from surgery; however, these patients also have the highest risk of surgical complications and death. Therefore, a selection bias is difficult to avoid in studies of clinical outcomes. In one study, infants with severely reduced ventricular function (ejection fraction <20% on angiography) had a poor outcome with either medical or surgical intervention.[25] In the same study, patients with an ejection fraction of >20% survived regardless of which treatment regimen was used. The clinical condition of the patient and the expertise of the treatment team should be considered when formulating a treatment plan.

Surgical Treatment

General Considerations

Several surgical approaches have been used to treat patients with ALCAPA; however, the current consensus is that restoration of a two-vessel coronary artery system is desirable when possible. In one of the first surgical attempts to palliate ALCAPA, Potts and associates in 1953 created an aortopulmonary anastomosis in hopes of increasing oxygen saturation in the anomalous coronary artery.[57] In the same year, Mustard[75] reported performing an end-to-end anastomosis between the left carotid artery and the anomalous coronary artery. Although the first successful treatment of ALCAPA involved ligation of the anomalous artery (see next section),[76,90] this approach is successful only in patients who have an extensive collateral system. However, most patients have the infantile form, in which the primary blood supply to the left ventricle is via the anomalous artery. Although different techniques for establishing a two-vessel coronary system have been described, left coronary transfer is the preferred method.[3,22,104]

After such correction of ALCAPA, myocardial function improves markedly. The probable reason for this improvement is that ischemic, but viable, myocardial cells are scattered throughout the scarred ventricle. Therefore, surgical excision of left ventricular myocardium is not recommended.[63] Similarly, mitral valve dysfunction, a common finding that results from left ventricular dilation and ischemic damage of the papillary muscles, improves significantly after surgery. For this reason, routine primary surgical repair of the valve is not advisable, because repair during infancy can be difficult and can increase the operative risk. Moreover, even moderate to severe mitral insufficiency is not associated with an increased postoperative risk.

When cardiopulmonary bypass is used during any technique for correcting ALCAPA, the left and right pulmonary arteries should be occluded with either atraumatic vascular clamps or tourniquets to prevent the coronary steal that would otherwise occur in the decompressed pulmonary trunk.

Ligation of the Anomalous Artery

The first successful surgical treatment of ALCAPA, which involved ligating the anomalous artery, was reported in 1960 by Sabiston and colleagues.[90] This technique increased the pressure in the ectopic artery, diverted collateral blood flow to the left coronary system, and confirmed the existence of a steal phenomenon.[90] Although ligation of the anomalous artery is easily performed through a left thoracotomy without cardiopulmonary bypass, several reports regarding long-term follow-up have shown a higher mortality with this procedure than with those that establish a two-coronary system.[7,15,110] In one study of 11 patients who underwent the ligation procedure, the early mortality was 27%, and the late mortality, which was related to heart failure in all patients, was 25%.[15] Most survivors had late complications, including residual shunts through the anomalous coronary artery to the pulmonary artery, severe mitral regurgitation, and angina. In another study,[7] the mortality was 30%, which compared unfavorably with that of patients undergoing a two-coronary repair. Therefore, ligation of the anomalous artery is no longer recommended for patients with ALCAPA. Furthermore, patients who have had this procedure should undergo periodic Holter monitoring and stress studies. If objective evidence of ischemia is present, elective coronary revascularization should be considered.

Patients with ALCAPA commonly have enhanced ventricular irritability because of severe ongoing left ventricular ischemia. Therefore, the heart should be manipulated very carefully, especially when cardiopulmonary bypass is not available for hemodynamic support.

Establishment of a Two-Coronary System

Establishment of a two-coronary system is the optimum surgical treatment for ALCAPA if it can be performed with a low operative risk and a high probability of permanent patency. Techniques for achieving a two-vessel system include aortocoronary bypass[21] and subclavian[57] or internal mammary artery anastomosis,[20,56] direct reimplantation of the anomalous left coronary artery,[21,95,104] and intrapulmonary tunnel repair with either a pulmonary arterial flap or a free segment of the subclavian artery.[94]

Aortocoronary Bypass and Subclavian or Internal Mammary Artery to Coronary Anastomosis

In 1966, Cooley and associates[21] reported the first successful revascularization with a two-coronary system in two patients with ALCAPA. A Dacron graft was interposed between the aorta and the transected anomalous coronary artery in one patient, and a saphenous vein graft was used in the second patient. However, the potential for late fibrous changes and graft occlusion was a serious concern, especially in young children who would rely on coronary blood flow through the venous conduit for a lifetime.[9,30] Therefore, procedures using arterial conduits to revascularize the anomalous artery were developed. In 1968, Meyer and colleagues[70] reported successful anastomosis of the left subclavian artery to the anomalous artery in an infant. Although this technique can be performed in infants and should offer good long-term patency, kinking of the subclavian artery at its origin and inadequate vessel length are potential concerns.[72,82] Furthermore, stenosis at the site of the anastomosis has been reported.[7] In older patients, upper-extremity ischemia after distal ligation of the subclavian artery is a concern.[54] Anastomosis of the internal mammary artery to the anomalous artery has been performed in a few patients, but long-term follow-up data are not available.[20,56] Despite the small size of the artery, this procedure is technically feasible even in infants and small children.[104]

The mortality of bypass graft procedures ranges from 0 to 38% for saphenous vein bypass grafting[19,60,110] and from 0 to 29% for left subclavian artery to anomalous artery bypass.[72,92,114] These rates are similar to those reported for aortic reimplantation of the anomalous artery, but the rate of late stenosis or occlusion is significantly higher for saphenous bypass and subclavian artery grafts than for reimplantation procedures. In a long-term study of 10 patients who underwent saphenous vein bypass grafting, El-Said and coworkers[30] observed occlusion or stenosis in 30% of the grafts.

Saphenous vein bypass and subclavian artery grafting can be performed either with or without cardiopulmonary bypass. In the absence of cardiac arrest, the procedure is technically more difficult, but the already ischemic, compromised myocardium is spared additional insult. The anomalous artery is ligated to prevent a steal to the pulmonary artery.

Because the results of newer procedures (especially aortic reimplantation of the anomalous artery) are more encouraging, we believe that graft revascularization procedures should no longer be used to treat ALCAPA.

Reimplantation of the Anomalous Artery

In 1972, Tingelstad and associates[95] reported the first reimplantation of an anomalous right coronary artery into the aorta. A few years later, Neches and coworkers[77] and Cooley and colleagues[22] described the technically more complex procedure of reimplanting the left coronary artery. The initial drawbacks of this procedure were its level of difficulty and the possibility that the anomalous artery would not be lengthy enough for transplantation. However, experience, especially with the arterial switch operation, has shown these drawbacks to be insignificant. In most cases, the anomalous artery arises from the left coronary posterior sinus. The artery should be fully mobilized up to its bifurcation but can usually be transplanted without causing undue tension. When the anomalous artery arises from the anterior, nonfacing pulmonary sinus or from the most distal part of the pulmonary trunk, a different method of repair may be preferred, because the artery may be subjected to excessive tension if translocated.[104] In the unusual case in which the anomalous artery arises from the right-facing pulmonary sinus, reimplantation should be easily accomplished with minimal dissection.

For reimplantation of the left coronary artery, we prefer to make a transverse incision in the pulmonary artery and to evaluate the left coronary arterial ostium from within the pulmonary artery (Fig. 5.5, A and B). If the ostium seems to originate from the posterior aspect of the pulmonary trunk, the ostium is excised as a button, or the incision can be extended until the pulmonary trunk is completely transected (Fig. 5.5, C and D). Then the button is directly implanted into the aortic wall with the aid of a trapdoor flap (Fig. 5.5E). The pulmonary artery is reconstructed with a pericardial patch to avoid deforming the pulmonary artery (Fig. 5.5, F–I).

In a recent report, Laks and coauthors[61] used a technique described by Yacoub[112] in which the translocation is performed through an aortotomy from inside the aorta. This technique is performed under direct vision and allows the anomalous artery to be precisely implanted in the sinus, thereby avoiding the aortic valvular apparatus.

Experimental studies and clinical experience with the arterial switch operation have shown that the aortocoronary anastomoses will grow if an adequate cuff of tissue surrounding the coronary ostium is taken.[14] In addition, long-term patency rates are excellent.[7,25,105] For these reasons, reimplantation is considered the method of choice for most patients with ALCAPA.

Intrapulmonary Tunnel Repair With Either a Pulmonary Arterial Flap or a Free Segment of the Subclavian Artery

Described in 1979 by Takeuchi and associates,[94] before the translocation technique became widely performed, intrapulmonary tunnel repair is now used for patients in whom reimplantation of the anomalous artery would be technically difficult. For example, tunnel repair may be considered when the anomalous artery arises from the anterior nonfacing sinus of the pulmonary artery or when the tension on the translocated artery would be unacceptable.

The repair is performed with the aid of cardiopulmonary bypass. A transverse incision is made in the main pulmonary

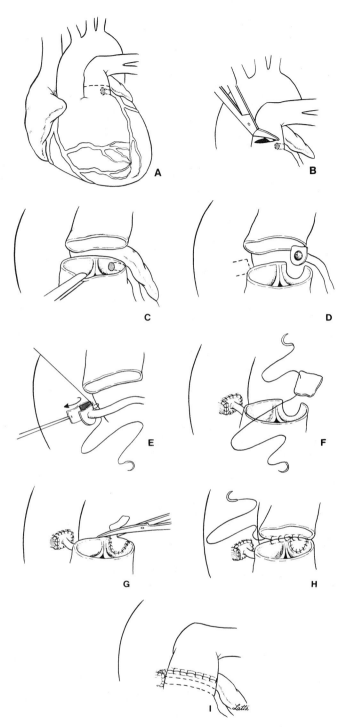

FIGURE 5.5. A and **B.** To reimplant the anomalous left coronary artery, the pulmonary artery is opened by means of a transverse incision above the sinuses of Valsalva. **C** and **D.** The coronary ostium is resected. **E.** A trap-door opening is created, and the coronary artery is reimplanted directly onto the aortic wall. **F** and **G.** A pericardial patch is used to repair the pulmonary artery. **H** and **I.** The ends of the pulmonary artery are anastomosed.

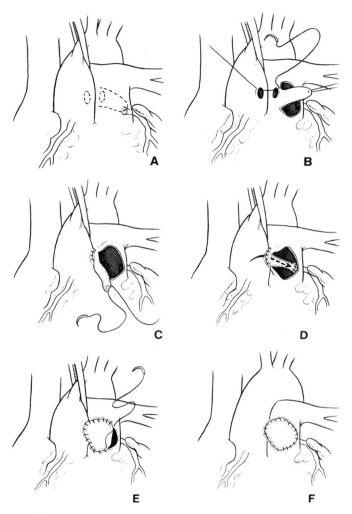

FIGURE 5.6. A and **B.** Intrapulmonary repair of anomalous origination of the left coronary artery. A flap is created from the pulmonary artery wall, and a communication is created between the aorta and the pulmonary artery. **C** and **D.** The flap is sutured to the internal wall of the pulmonary artery to create a coronary tunnel between the aorta and the anomalous coronary artery. **E** and **F.** The pulmonary artery is reconstructed with a pericardial patch.

artery. A flap from the pulmonary arterial wall or a pericardial flap is then used to construct a coronary tunnel inside the pulmonary trunk between a surgically created aortopulmonary window and the left coronary ostium (Fig. 5.6, A–D). The tunnel diverts the blood into the anomalous coronary orifice via the aortopulmonary window. The pulmonary artery is reconstructed with a pericardial patch (Fig. 5.6, E and F). The mortality is low and long-term patency is good, but late complications include supravalvar pulmonary stenosis and baffle obstruction.[7] Despite the risk of these complications, we believe that tunnel repair is the procedure of choice when translocation of the anomalous artery is unsafe.

Postoperative Management

Because myocardial function is usually impaired, often severely, in patients undergoing surgical correction of AL-CAPA, postoperative hemodynamic support is commonly required. In a study of 18 consecutive patients undergoing translocation of an anomalous left coronary artery, Vouhe and coworkers[104] reported that 64% of the patients required pharmacologic support for more than 48 hours because of a low cardiac output. In some cases, mechanical support with a centrifugal left ventricular assist device (LVAD) is necessary. If hemodynamic support is successful during the perioperative period, systolic and diastolic myocardial function should progressively improve, and mitral insufficiency should resolve.[18] If severe myocardial dysfunction persists after surgery, heart transplantation should be considered. All patients should undergo serial follow-up electrocardiographic and echocardiographic studies. Pulsed Doppler and color-flow mapping can be used to assess coronary blood flow perioperatively by means of transesophageal echocardiography. The electrocardiogram usually shows a gradual resolution of ischemic changes at rest, but T-wave inversion may persist in the aV_L lead.

CONGENITAL CORONARY ARTERY FISTULA

In the first report of a fistulous connection between the coronary arteries and the cardiac chambers, published in 1865, Krause[58] described an abnormal vessel that drained into the pulmonary arteries. In 1906, Abbott[2] detailed the pathology of these lesions. Forty years later, Bjork and Crafoord[10] reported the first surgical treatment of a coronary artery fistula. In 1963, Haller and Little[40] were the first to use preoperative angiography to diagnose coronary fistulas. Since then, many case reports and small studies have furthered our knowledge of the anatomy, physiology, and treatment of this anomaly.

Seen in 0.2% of patients referred for coronary angiography, coronary artery fistulas are the most common hemodynamically significant congenital defects of the coronary arteries,[44,62] being found in 1 of every 50,000 patients with congenital heart disease.[65]

Anatomy

Congenital coronary fistulas may arise from any major or minor coronary artery branch (Table 5.3). Single or multiple fistulas may be present. Multiple fistulas usually involve only one coronary system, either the right or the left; rarely are both systems involved.[69,87] In a review of 97 children with congenital coronary artery fistulas, McNamara and Gross[69] found that the site of origin was the right coronary artery in 59% of patients, the left coronary artery in 32%, a single coronary artery system in 7%, and both systems in 2%.

Fistulous connections may drain into any of the cardiac chambers, the pulmonary arteries, or the central veins. How-

TABLE 5.3. *Features of coronary fistulas*

Origin	Right coronary artery, 50–60% Left coronary artery, 30–40% Multiple coronary arteries, 2–5%

Termination	Right side of the heart in 90% of cases:
	  Right ventricle, 50–55%
	  Right atrium or vena cavas, 20–25%
	  Pulmonary arteries, 10–20%

Types	1. Simple fistula to chamber (side or end connection) 2. Multiple connection sites 3. Plexiform (or telangiectasia: to left ventricle or pulmonary artery) 4. Side-to-side
"Secondary fistulas" or coronary collaterals	In tetralogy of Fallot, pulmonary valve atresia With cardiac tumors, hemangiomas, hamartomas, myxomas

ever, the right side of the heart is the most common site of drainage; more than 90% of all coronary fistulas from both the right and left coronary artery systems drain into the right side of the heart.[29,69,98] The drainage site is the right ventricle in 52% of all patients (Fig. 5.7, *A* and *B*), the right atrium and central veins in 24% (Fig. 5.8, *A* and *B*), and the pulmonary arteries in 14% (Fig. 5.9, *A* and *B*).[69,87]

The fistula drains into left heart structures in less than 10% of patients.[81] In a comprehensive review of 171 cases of congenital coronary fistula, Rittenhouse and colleagues[87] reported that only 6% of the fistulas drained into the left side of the heart; 4% drained into the left atrium and 2% into the left ventricle. These percentages are consistent with others reported for pediatric patients.[69]

Although coronary artery fistulas sometimes occur as isolated lesions, they are more commonly seen in association with other congenital coronary malformations. Severe obstruction of the right and left ventricular outflow tracts predisposes patients to the development of fistulas.[69] Coronary artery fistulas that communicate with the right ventricle are often seen in patients who have critical pulmonary valve stenosis or pulmonary valve atresia with an intact ventricular septum (Fig. 5.10, *A* and *B*). In patients with pulmonary valve atresia, a coronary fistula, and proximal coronary artery stenosis, the primary blood supply to the ventricular myocardium may be derived from the right ventricle via the fistulous connection. This condition is referred to as "right ventricular dependent coronary artery circulation."[36,38] The

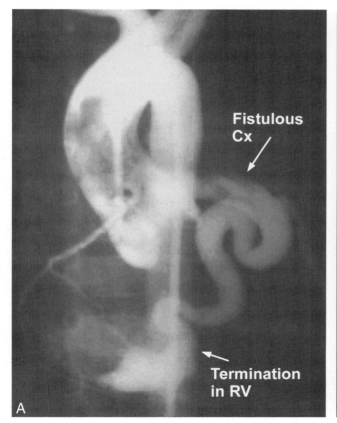
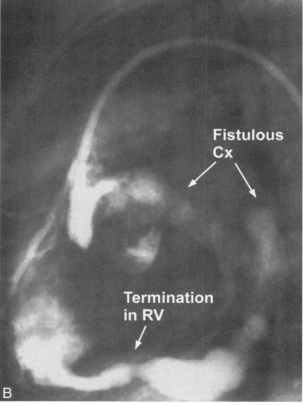

FIGURE 5.7. Aortic root injection in the anteroposterior **(A)** and lateral **(B)** projections, showing a fistulous circumflex coronary artery (Cx) terminating in the right ventricle (RV).

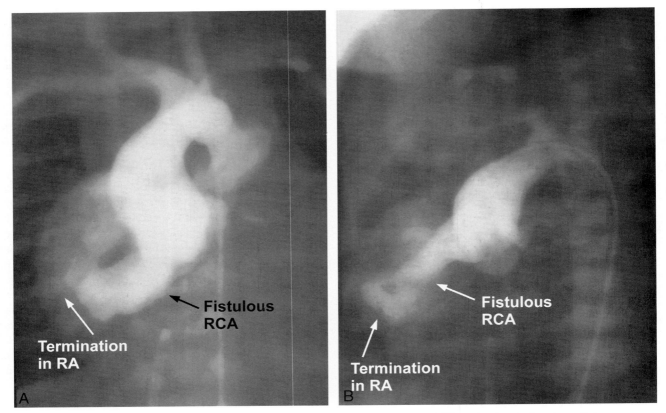

FIGURE 5.8. Aortic root injection in the anteroposterior **(A)** and lateral **(B)** projections, showing a fistulous right coronary artery (RCA) terminating in the right atrium (RA).

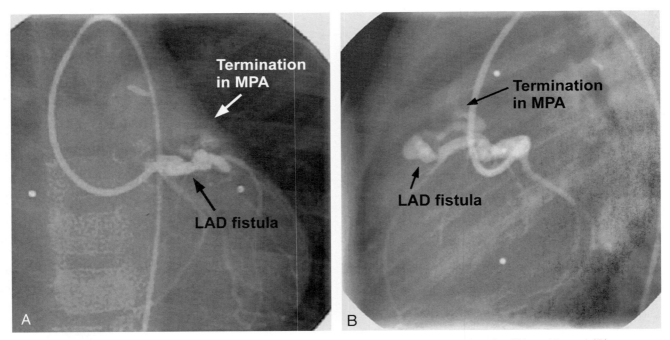

FIGURE 5.9. Selective injection into the left coronary artery in the anteroposterior **(A)** and lateral **(B)** projections, showing a fistula arising from the left anterior descending coronary artery (LAD) and terminating in the main pulmonary artery (MPA).

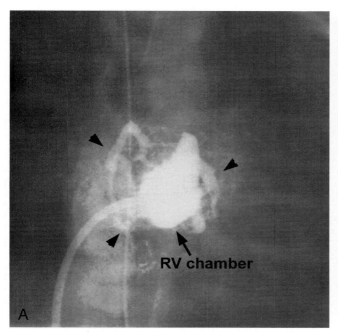 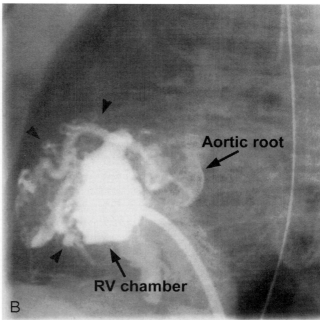

FIGURE 5.10. Right ventriculogram, performed in the anteroposterior **(A)** and lateral **(B)** projections, in a patient with pulmonary valve atresia and an intact ventricular septum. A diminutive right ventricular (RV) chamber with a blind-ending outflow tract is seen. Multiple right ventricular to coronary artery fistulas (arrowheads) fill in retrograde fashion with flow directed into the aortic root.

remainder of this chapter discusses isolated coronary artery to cardiac chamber fistulas.

Embryology (see Chapter 2)

During early embryonic development, the highly trabecular ventricular myocardium is perfused by blood from within the cardiac chambers. Endothelial outgrowths penetrate the myocardium, forming intertrabecular spaces that increase the endothelial surface area and improve myocardial perfusion.[106] The coronary arteries, which first appear as endothelial channels within the subepicardial space, eventually communicate with the intramyocardial capillary network.[97,103] As circulation through the coronary arteries increases, the intramyocardial sinusoids regress and become obliterated. If they do not regress, a fistulous communication persists between the coronary arteries and the cardiac chamber.[35] In congenital lesions such as pulmonary atresia with intact ventricular septum, the systemic or suprasystemic right ventricular pressure may impede normal regression of the sinusoids.

Pathophysiology

The hemodynamic effects of coronary artery fistulas depend on the fistula's termination site and the diameter and length of the fistulous connection. Fistulas that drain into the right side of the heart produce a left-to-right shunt and increase the volume of flow through the affected cardiac chambers. Large fistulas with low resistance can create a large left-to-right shunt (Qp:Qs >2:1),[64] producing a significant volume load on the pulmonary arteries and subsequently on the left ventricle. If the fistula drains into the right atrium, right ventricle, or systemic veins, volume overload of the right ventricle also occurs. The left-to-right shunt is obligatory and does not usually depend on pulmonary vascular resistance. The shunt may produce marked dilation of the right heart chambers. Pulmonary vascular resistance may increase because of the volume overload from the shunt, but Eisenmenger's complex has not been seen in patients with coronary artery fistulas.

Fistulas that drain into the left side of the heart produce a significant volume load only on the left ventricle. When the fistula drains into the left ventricle, the hemodynamic consequences are similar to those of aortic valve insufficiency, because the flow from the aorta into the left ventricle occurs during diastole.[87]

Coronary artery fistulas produce a pattern of coronary flow that may divert blood away from the myocardium, creating a "coronary steal." In this situation, myocardial perfusion decreases and ischemia may ensue. Even in the presence of large fistulas, however, ischemia is unusual in children.[68]

Clinical Manifestations

Most patients with a congenital coronary artery fistula are asymptomatic. Symptoms are usually related to ventricular volume overload resulting from large left-to-right shunts and may develop anytime from early infancy to the fourth to fifth decade of life.[87] Occasionally, infants may present with tachypnea, diaphoresis, increased irritability, and feeding intolerance. Older patients may have fatigue, dyspnea on exertion, edema, palpitations, and chest pain. Even when cardiomegaly is present, however, most patients thrive and remain active, with a normal exercise tolerance.[35,87]

Although complications related to a congenital coronary artery fistula are rare, they may cause patients to seek medical attention. Angina may occur on exertion, and this symptom has been observed in children, along with clinical evidence of myocardial infarction.[74] Ischemia during exercise testing is rare. Subacute bacterial endocarditis is encountered in about 10% of patients.[69,91] Rarely, the dilated fistula will rupture and result in hemopericardium. Thrombosis in the fistulous tract may lead to a reduction in fistulous flow or a myocardial infarction.

In most patients with a coronary artery fistula, a continuous murmur is heard on precordial auscultation.[6,8,35] Fistulas to the left ventricle produce only a diastolic murmur. Locating the maximal intensity of the murmur may help determine where the fistula drains.[78]

Signs related to a very large left-to-right shunt (cardiac enlargement, a ventricular heave, a gallop rhythm, hepatomegaly, and respiratory compromise) are rarely seen. Flow of blood away from the aorta to the low-pressure chambers during diastole may cause a widened pulse pressure.

Differential Diagnosis

Patients with a congenital coronary artery fistula usually present with a continuous murmur, with or without cardiomegaly. Locating the murmur may help exclude other forms of congenital heart disease. Other lesions with a clinical presentation similar to that of coronary fistula include patent ductus arteriosus, ventricular septal defect with aortic insufficiency, aortopulmonary window, and aortopulmonary collateral vessels. ALCAPA may mimic the clinical presentation of a coronary artery fistula, especially if evidence of ischemia or infarction is seen on electrocardiography (a rare event in cases of fistulas).

Diagnostic Evaluation

Radiographic findings in patients with a congenital coronary artery fistula are usually normal or nonspecific. If the fistula terminates in the right side of the heart and a small left-to-right shunt is present, chest films may be normal. In patients with larger shunts, nonspecific signs of cardiomegaly and increased pulmonary vascular markings may be seen. If the fistula terminates in the left side of the heart, the affected structures on that side may be enlarged. Older patients may develop calcific aneurysms of the involved coronary artery.

Electrocardiographic findings are usually normal or nonspecific. Approximately 60% of patients have right, left, or biventricular hypertrophy.[68,69] Electrocardiographic evidence of resting myocardial ischemia or myocardial infarction is unusual. If the fistula drains into the right atrium or

central veins, atrial fibrillation may develop as a late complication in adults.

Echocardiography was first used to evaluate patients with coronary artery fistulas in the mid 1970s.[102] In the first reported cases, the diagnosis was suggested by evidence of a large left-to-right shunt (right ventricular dilation and paradoxical interventricular septal motion) and by exclusion of other congenital heart lesions. As echocardiographic techniques improved, detection of proximal coronary artery dilation and visualization of the fistulous artery became more accurate. These improvements, combined with Doppler detection of turbulent flow patterns, increased the diagnostic capabilities of echocardiography.[34,59,113] With Doppler color-flow mapping, one can detect continuous flow within the fistula and a flow jet extending into the chamber of termination. Localizing the fistulous tract and the chamber of termination helps determine the appropriate therapy, which may be either medical or surgical.

Invasive forms of echocardiography may be used for diagnosing coronary artery fistulas and aiding in their treatment. Contrast echocardiography, performed during cardiac catheterization, may be used to identify the chamber in which the fistula terminates.[23,84] In this procedure, agitated saline solution (or indocyanine dye) is injected into the aortic root.

Transesophageal echocardiography (TEE) can aid in the diagnosis of coronary artery fistulas, especially in large patients who have a poor transthoracic window. Furthermore, TEE can be used perioperatively to evaluate the success of surgical correction.[24,37]

Magnetic resonance imaging (MRI) can be used to diagnose congenital coronary artery fistulas.[12,100] In this procedure, a large field is examined in multiple planes so as to obtain an optimal view of the lesion without the need for contrast material. The sensitivity of MRI can be increased by using spin "echo" and three-dimensional reconstruction.

Myocardial perfusion scans and stress tests can detect areas of decreased perfusion or ischemia in adults and older children but cannot usually be performed in infants and small children. Stress myocardial perfusion scans in older children or adults with an isolated coronary artery fistula may be useful to rule out ischemia. In patients who have cardiac structural abnormalities in addition to a coronary artery fistula, myocardial perfusion scans are abnormal, and the results are not specifically related to ischemia or decreased perfusion. This fact is especially pertinent for patients who have had cardiac surgery.

Cardiac catheterization is the most accurate procedure for defining the anatomy and hemodynamic status of patients with a congenital coronary artery fistula. Catheterization and cineangiography, the gold standards for diagnosis, should be performed if uncertainty about the anatomy or physiology of the lesion persists after noninvasive techniques have been used.

Hemodynamic assessment may show a step-up in oxygen saturation if the fistula drains into the right heart or a systemic or coronary vein. The chamber with the initial increase in oxygen saturation is usually the site of fistula termination.

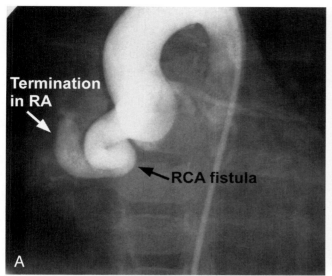 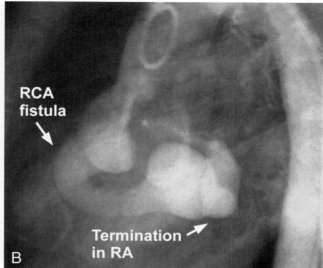

FIGURE 5.11. Aortic root injection, in the anteroposterior **(A)** and lateral **(B)** projections, showing a large, tortuous right coronary artery (RCA) fistula that terminates in the right atrium (RA). No other lesions involving a left-to-right shunt are present at the level of the great vessels.

Oxygen saturation data can be used to calculate the degree of left-to-right shunting and absolute flow through the fistula. Patients with large shunts may develop increased pulmonary vascular resistance. The pulse pressure is usually widened in those with a large coronary artery fistula, but pressure data can be normal.

The coronary anatomy, the fistula, and the fistula's site of termination are clearly visualized on cineangiography. Injection of contrast material into the aortic root will opacify both coronary arteries, allowing the fistula to be visualized and other lesions that cause left-to-right shunting (patent ductus arteriosus, aortopulmonary window, and aortopulmonary collaterals) to be excluded (Fig. 5.11, *A* and *B*). Aortic root angiography provides initial information about the number and distribution of coronary fistulas. Selective coronary angiography is essential to assess the individual coronary anatomy, including fistulous tracts, aneurysm formation, and the chamber involved in the fistulous connection.[33] In addition, nutrient branches arising from the fistulous coronary artery can be seen (Fig. 5.12). When a large fistula with significant flow (Qp:Qs >2:1) is present, manual injections through the coronary catheters may not adequately opacify the coronary artery or fistula; therefore, selective angiography, using side-hole angiographic catheters (NIH®) and mechanical injections, may be necessary. "Laid-back" (left posterior oblique-caudal) aortography may be used in children to improve visualization of the fistulous connection.[45]

Management

Most patients with a fistulous connection between a coronary artery and a cardiac chamber are asymptomatic. Patients who are symptomatic or have abnormal cardiac hemodynamics should undergo closure of the fistula, which usually alleviates symptoms and normalizes cardiac function. Some investigators recommend closure of the fistula in asymptomatic patients because of the risk of late complications, including myocardial ischemia, infarction, endocarditis, and rupture of coronary aneurysms.[64,71,81,87]

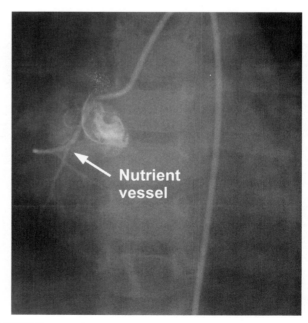

FIGURE 5.12. Selective injection of the right coronary artery fistula in the same patient as in Figure 5.11. Note the nutrient vessel arising from the fistula.

Elective closure of coronary artery fistulas in asymptomatic patients is not universally endorsed. In most pediatric patients with smaller fistulas (Qp:Qs <1.3:1), expectant management, with prophylaxis for endocarditis, is recommended.[17,46,68] In rare cases, spontaneous closure of a congenital coronary artery fistula has been reported.[17,67] If the patient becomes symptomatic or if blood flow through the fistula increases, the fistula should be closed.

Transcatheter Techniques

In the last 15 years, percutaneous transcatheter techniques have been used to occlude fistulous coronary communications. In 1983, Reidy and associates[86] reported the first transcatheter occlusion of a coronary artery fistula terminating in the pulmonary artery. They used a small, detachable balloon to occlude the fistulous branch. By the 1990s, other occlusive devices such as metallic detachable coils,[80,85] detachable coils,[42,107] double-umbrella devices,[80] and microparticles of polyvinyl alcohol foam[93] were being used. Occlusive devices have been placed via both the retrograde and the anterograde approach. Transcatheter occlusion is currently considered to be effective, with minimal morbidity and mortality.

At Texas Children's Hospital, we use Gianturco coils (Cook; Bloomington, Indiana, USA) and Target coils (Target Therapeutics; Fremont, California, USA) to occlude coronary artery fistulas (Fig. 5.13, A–J). Selective coronary angiography is initially performed to clarify the coronary anatomy, the site of fistulous termination, the presence of aneurysm formation, and the origin of nutrient branches. Intravenous heparin (50 to 100 units/kg) is given for anticoagulation during the procedure. In the retrograde approach,

a coaxial system [Fasttracker Infusion Catheter; Target Therapeutics, Fremont, California, USA] (Fig. 5.13, C–E) is used to position a small-diameter, end-hole catheter at the appropriate site of coil placement. In an anterograde approach, a coronary catheter can be inserted into the downstream fistulous ostium to deliver the coil. The coil size depends on the diameter and length of the vessel at the site of implantation. During coil delivery, the patient should be monitored by means of continuous electrocardiography. After coil delivery, coronary angiography is repeated to assess coronary artery perfusion and occlusion of the fistula.

Transcatheter occlusion is not suitable for all fistulous lesions. Occlusive devices cannot be used if the site cannot be properly cannulated, if multiple fistulas are present, or if the procedure could inadvertently occlude coronary nutrient branches. Furthermore, transcatheter occlusion cannot be performed if the fistulous communication is too short.

Surgical Treatment

Because of the anatomic variability of coronary artery fistulas, several surgical techniques have been developed.[17,68,97] The goal of surgery is to obliterate the fistula without reducing the flow of blood through the nutrient coronary artery branches. The appropriate technique depends on the coronary anatomy. If the fistula can be identified on the surface of the heart, simple ligation can be performed. To prevent myocardial ischemia, the vessel should be ligated at the point of entry into the cardiac chamber. If the fistula cannot be externally identified, it will have to be closed internally, from within the cavity where the fistula terminates. In patients with multiple lateral communications between the coronary artery and the cardiac chamber, a tangen-

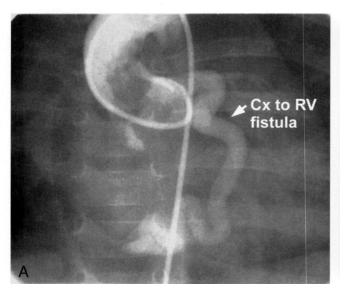

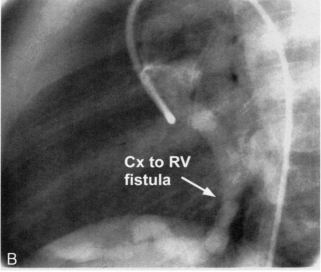

FIGURE 5.13. Delivery of a Target coil for occlusion of a coronary artery fistula. Selective coronary artery angiography in the anteroposterior **(A)** and lateral **(B)** projections shows a large, tortuous circumflex coronary artery to right ventricular (Cx to RV) fistula. (*continued*)

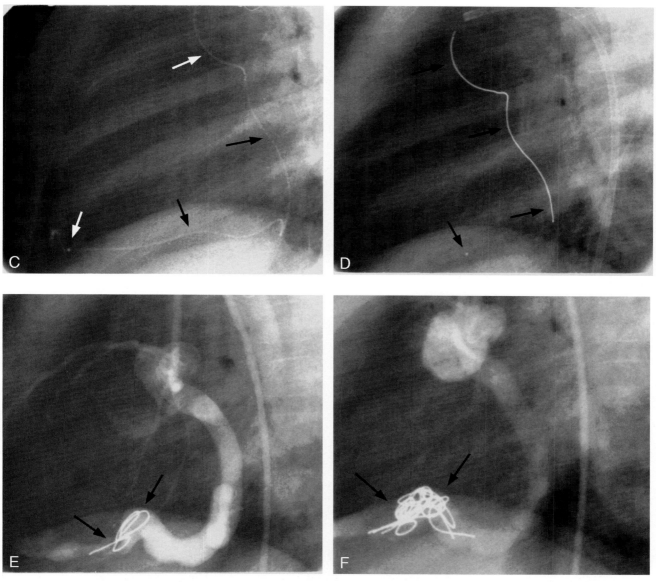

FIGURE 5.13. *continued.* A radiolucent Fasttracker infusion catheter (arrows) is placed in the fistula and filled with contrast material **(C)**. The Target coil is delivered through the infusion catheter. A radiopaque band is seen at the distal end of the catheter (arrowhead) **(D)**. Selective injection after delivery of a single coil shows that residual shunting is present (arrows) **(E)**. After placement of an additional coil, residual shunting is still present **(F)**. (*continued*)

tial arteriorrhaphy can be performed. In this technique, the fistula is located by palpating a thrill over the involved vessel and then placing multiple horizontal mattress sutures under the coronary artery. Complete obliteration of the fistula is indicated by disappearance of the thrill, reduction in the size of the recipient chamber, lack of an increase in oxygen saturation in the recipient chamber (on oximetry), and disappearance of Doppler evidence of residual fistulous flow on transesophageal echocardiography.[24] In treating 104 patients, as reported in 1992, surgeons at the Texas Heart Institute[31] used an internal closure in 46% of the cases, a tangential

arteriorrhaphy in 29%, distal ligation in 11%, proximal and distal ligation in 7%, ligation and bypass grafting in 4%, and closure from within a vessel dilated by an aneurysm in 3%.

When simple ligation is performed, cardiopulmonary bypass may not be necessary. However, when the fistula is closed from within the heart or when the route of exposure is difficult, cardiopulmonary bypass should be used. Exposure is often difficult if the fistula is located in the left atrioventricular groove, the distribution of the circumflex artery, or the distal right coronary artery. To prevent injury to the

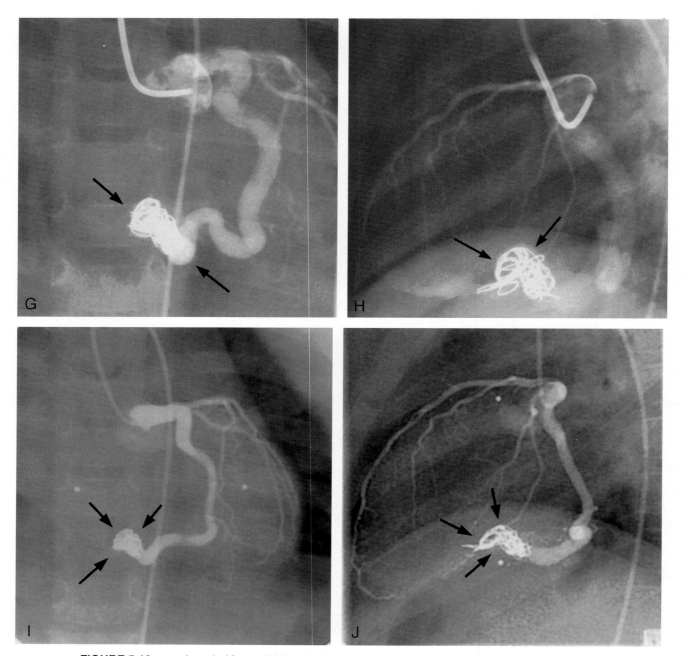

FIGURE 5.13. *continued.* After multiple coils have been delivered, only minimal shunting remains (**G**& **H**). A selective left coronary angiogram performed 1 year after coil delivery shows no residual shunting (**I**&**J**).

coronary artery, cardiopulmonary bypass is often used if the fistula is located in the course of the coronary artery rather than at its termination.

In a series of 174 patients who underwent surgical treatment of coronary fistulas,[87] the mortality was 4%; however, other series have had a mortality of 0%.[26,31,99] Associated cardiac defects may increase the risk of operative death. Complications usually result from ischemic events after ligation. The risk of complications is higher in patients who have a right coronary to left ventricular fistula or a large

aneurysm of the fistula.[55] In all series, the recurrence rate is low and the late outcome is good.[26,65]

REFERENCES

1. Abbott M. Anomalous origin from the pulmonary artery. In: Osler W, ed. Theory and practice. Vol 4. Philadelphia: Lea & Febiger, 1908: 420.
2. Abbott ME. Anomalies of the coronary arteries. In: McCrea T, ed. Osler's modern medicine. Philadelphia: Lea & Febiger, 1906:420.
3. Alexi-Meskishvili V, Hetzer R, Weng Y, et al. Anomalous origin of

the left coronary artery from the pulmonary artery. Early results with direct aortic reimplantation. J Thorac Cardiovasc Surg 1994;108:354.

4. Arciniegas E, Farooki ZQ, Hakimi M, et al. Management of anomalous left coronary artery from the pulmonary artery. Circulation 1980; 62:180.

5. Augustsson MH, Gasul BM, Fel EH, et al. Anomalous origin of left coronary artery from pulmonary artery. JAMA 1962;180:15.

6. Azcuna JE, Cabrera A, Arruza F, et al. Fistulae between the coronary arteries and the right cavities of the heart. Br Heart J 1971;33:451.

7. Backer CL, Stout MJ, Zales VR, et al. Anomalous origin of the left coronary artery: a twenty-year review of surgical management. J Thorac Cardiovasc Surg 1992;6:1049.

8. Baim DS, Kline H, Silverman JF. Bilateral coronary artery-pulmonary artery fistula: report of five cases and review of the literature. Circulation 1982;65:810.

9. Benrey J, Hallman GL, Cooley DA, et al. Origin of left coronary artery from the pulmonary artery: eight year follow-up after revascularization with a dacron tube graft. Cardiovasc Dis Bull Tex Heart Inst 1974;1:413.

10. Bjork G, Crafoord C. Arteriovenous aneurysm on the pulmonary artery simulating patent ductus arteriosus Botalli. Thorax 1947;2:65.

11. Bland EF, White PD, Garland J. Congenital anomalies of the coronary arteries: report of an unusual case associated with cardiac hypertrophy. Am Heart J 1933;8:787.

12. Boxer RA, LaCorte MA, Singh S, et al. Noninvasive diagnosis of congenital left coronary artery to right ventricle fistula by nuclear magnetic resonance imaging. Pediatr Cardiol 1989;10:45.

13. Brooks HSJ. Two cases of an abnormal coronary artery of the heart arising from the pulmonary artery: with some remarks upon the effect of this anomaly in producing cirsoid dilation of the vessels. J Anat Physiol 1886;20:26.

14. Brutel de la Riviere A, Quaegebeur JM, Hennis PI, et al. Growth of an aorto-coronary anastomosis. J Thorac Cardiovasc Surg 1983;86: 393.

15. Bunton R, Jonas RA, Lang P, et al. Anomalous origin of left coronary artery from pulmonary artery: ligation versus establishment of a two coronary artery system. J Thorac Cardiovasc Surg 1987;93:103.

16. Caldwell RL, Hurwitz RA, Girod DA, et al. Two-dimensional echocardiographic differentiation of anomalous left coronary artery from congestive cardiomyopathy. Am Heart J 1983;106:710.

17. Carrel T, Tkebuchava T, Jenni R, et al. Congenital coronary fistulas in children and adults: diagnosis, surgical technique and results. Cardiology 1996;87:325–330.

18. Carvalho JS, Redington AN, Oldershaw PJ, et al. Analysis of left ventricular wall movement before and after reimplantation of anomalous left coronary artery in infancy. Br Heart J 1991;65:218.

19. Chiariello L, Meyer J, Reul GJ, et al. Surgical treatment for anomalous origin of left coronary artery from pulmonary artery. Ann Thorac Surg 1975;19:443.

20. Cohen AJ, Grishkin BA, Helsel RA, et al. Surgical therapy in the management of coronary anomalies: emphasis on utility of internal mammary artery grafts. Ann Thorac Surg 1989;47:630.

21. Cooley DA, Hallman GL, Bloodwell RD. Definitive surgical treatment of anomalous origin of left coronary artery from pulmonary artery: indications and results. J Thorac Cardiovasc Surg 1966;52: 798.

22. Grace RR, Angelini P, Cooley DA. Aortic implantation of anomalous left coronary artery arising from pulmonary artery. Am J Cardiol 1977; 39:609.

23. Cooper MJ, Bernstein D, Silverman NH. Recognition of left coronary artery fistula to the left and right ventricles by contrast echocardiography. J Am Coll Cardiol 1985;6:923.

24. Cox ID, Murday AJ. Value of transoesophageal echocardiography in surgical ligation of coronary artery fistulas. Heart 1996;76:181.

25. Driscoll DJ, Nihill MR, Mullins CE, et al. Management of symptomatic infants with anomalous origin of the left coronary artery from the pulmonary artery. Am J Cardiol 1981;47:642.

26. Edis AJ, Schattenberg TT, Feldt RH, et al. Congenital coronary artery fistula. Surgical considerations and results of operation. Mayo Clin Proc 1972;47:567.

27. Edwards JE. Anomalous coronary arteries with special reference to arteriovenous-like communications. Circulation 1958;17:1001.

28. Edwards JE. The direction of blood flow in coronary arteries arising from the pulmonary trunk (editorial). Circulation 1964;29:163.

29. El-Said GM, Dawson JT, Sandiford FM, et al. Coronary artery anomalies: diagnosis, indications and results of surgical management. Eur J Cardiol 1973;1:63.

30. El-Said GM, Ruzyllo W, Williams RL. Early and late results of saphenous vein grafts for anomalous origin of left coronary artery from pulmonary artery. Ann Thorac Surg 1975;19:443.

31. Fernandes ED, Kadivar H, Hallman GL, et al. Congenital malformations of the coronary arteries: the Texas Heart Institute experience. Ann Thorac Surg 1992;54:732.

32. Fisher EA, Sepehri B, Lendrum B, et al. Two-dimensional echocardiographic visualization of the left coronary artery in anomalous origin of the left coronary artery from the pulmonary artery: pre and postoperative studies. Circulation 1981;63:698.

33. Formanek A, Nath PH, Zollikofer C, et al. Selective coronary arteriography in children. Circulation 1980;61:84.

34. Friedman DM, Rutkowski M. Coronary artery fistula: a pulsed Doppler/two-dimensional echocardiographic study. Am J Cardiol 1985;55: 1652.

35. Gasul BM, Arcilla RA, Fell EH, et al. Congenital coronary arteriovenous fistula. Pediatrics 1960;25:531.

36. Gentles TL, Colan SD, Giglia TM, et al. Right ventricular decompression and left ventricular function in pulmonary atresia with intact ventricular septum: the influence of less extensive coronary anomalies. Circulation 1993;88:183.

37. Giannoccaro PJ, Sochowski RA, Morton BC, et al. Complementary role of transesophageal echocardiography to coronary angiography in the assessment of coronary artery anomalies. Br Heart J 1993;70: 70.

38. Giglia TM, Mandell VS, Connor AR, et al. Diagnosis and management of right ventricle-dependent coronary circulation in pulmonary atresia with intact ventricular septum. Circulation 1992;86:1516.

39. Gouley BA. Anomalous left coronary artery arising from the pulmonary artery (adult type). Am Heart J 1950;40:630.

40. Haller JA, Little JA. Diagnosis and surgical correction of coronary artery-coronary sinus fistula. Circulation 1963;27:939.

41. Hallman GL, Cooley DA, Singer DB. Congenital anomalies of the coronary arteries: anatomy, pathology and surgical treatment. Surgery 1966;59:133.

42. Harris WO, Andrews JC, Nichols DA, et al. Percutaneous transcatheter embolization of coronary arteriovenous fistulas. Mayo Clin Proc 1996;71:37.

43. Heifetz S, Rabinowitz M, Mueller K, et al. Total anomalous origin of the coronary arteries from the pulmonary artery. Pediatr Cardiol 1986;7:11.

44. Hobbs RE, Millit HD, Raghavan PV, et al. Coronary artery fistulae: a 10-year review. Cleve Clin Q 1982;49:191.

45. Hofbeck M, Wild F, Singer H. Improved visualization of a coronary artery fistula by the ''laid-back'' aortogram. Br Heart J 1993;70:272.

46. Jaffe RB, Glancy DL, Epstein SE, et al. Coronary arterial-right heart fistulae: long-term observation in seven patients. Circulation 1973; 47:133.

47. Johnsrude CL, Perry JC, Cecchin F, et al. Differentiating anomalous left main coronary artery originating from the pulmonary artery in infants from myocarditis and dilated cardiomyopathy by electrocardiogram. Am J Cardiol 1995;75:71.

48. Jureidini SB, Nouri S, Crawford CJ, et al. Reliability of echocardiography in the diagnosis of anomalous origin of the left coronary artery from the pulmonary trunk. Am Heart J 1991;122:61.

49. Jureidini SB, Nouri S, Pennington DG. Anomalous origin of the left coronary artery from the pulmonary: repair after diagnostic cross-sectional echocardiography. Br Heart J 1987;58:173.

50. Karr SS, Parness IA, Spevak PJ, et al. Diagnosis of anomalous left coronary artery by Doppler color flow mapping: distinction from other causes of dilated cardiomyopathy. J Am Coll Cardiol 1992;19:1271.

51. Keith J. The anomalous origin of the left coronary artery from the pulmonary artery. Br Heart J 1959;21:149.

52. Kelly RA, Smith TW. Pharmacological treatment of heart failure In: Hardman JG, Limbird LE, eds. Goodman and Gilman's the pharmacological basis of therapeutics. 9th ed. New York: McGraw-Hill, Health Professions Division, 1996:806.

53. Kenakin TP. An in vitro quantitative analysis of the alpha-adrenoceptor partial agonist activity of dobutamine and its relevance to inotropic selectivity. J Pharmacol Exp Ther 1981;216:210.

54. Kesler KA, Pennington G, Nouri S, et al. Left subclavian–left coronary artery anastomosis for anomalous origin of the left coronary artery: long-term follow-up. J Thorac Cardiovasc Surg 1989;98:25.

55. Kirklin JW, Barratt-Boyes BG. Congenital anomalies of the coronary arteries. In: Kirklin JW, Barratt-Boyes BG, eds. Cardiac surgery. New York: Churchill Livingston, 1993:1179.

56. Kitamura S, Kawachi H, Nishii T, et al. Internal thoracic artery grafting for congenital coronary malformations. Ann Thorac Surg 1992; 53:513.

57. Kittle CF, Diehl AM, Heilbrunn A. Anomalous left coronary arising from the pulmonary artery: report of a case and surgical consideration. J Pediatr 1955;47:198.

58. Krause W. Uber den ursprung einer akzessorischen a. coronaria aus der a. pulmonalis. Z Ratl Med 1865;24:225.

59. Kronzon I, Winer HE, Cohen M. Noninvasive diagnosis of left coronary arteriovenous fistula communicating with the right ventricle. Am J Cardiol 1982;49:1811.

60. Laborde F, Marchan M, Leca F, et al. Surgical treatment of anomalous origin of the left coronary artery in infancy and childhood. Early and late results in 20 consecutive cases. J Thorac Cardiovasc Surg 1981; 82:423.

61. Laks H, Ardehali A, Grant PW, et al. Aortic implantation of anomalous left coronary artery. J Thorac Cardiovasc Surg 1995;109:519.

62. Levin DC, Fellows KE, Abrams HL. Hemodynamically significant primary anomalies of the coronary arteries. Angiographic aspects. Circulation 1978;58:25.

63. Levitsky S, van der Horst RL, Hastreiter AR, et al. Anomalous left coronary artery in the infant: recovery of ventricular function following early direct aortic implantation. J Thorac Cardiovasc Surg 1980; 79:598.

64. Liberthson RR, Sagar K, Berkoben JP, et al. Congenital coronary arteriovenous fistula: report of 13 patients, review of the literature and delineation of management. Circulation 1979;59:849.

65. Lowe JE, Oldham HN, Sabiston DC Jr. Surgical management of coronary artery fistula. Ann Surg 1981;194:373.

66. Maccarone C, Malta E, Raper C. Beta-adrenoceptor selectivity of dobutamine: in vivo and in vitro studies. J Cardiovasc Phamacol 1984; 6:132.

67. Mahoney LT, Schieken RM, Lauer RM. Spontaneous closure of a coronary artery fistula in childhood. Pediatr Cardiol 1982;2:311.

68. Mavroudis C, Backer CL, Rocchini AP, et al. Coronary artery fistula in infants and children: a surgical review and discussion of coil embolization. Ann Thorac Surg 1997;63:1235.

69. McNamara JJ, Gross RE. Congenital coronary artery fistula. Surgery 1969;65:59.

70. Meyer BW, Stefanik G, Stiles QR, et al. A method of definitive treatment of anomalous origin of the left coronary artery. J Thorac Cardiovasc Surg 1968;56:104.

71. Midell AI, Bermudez GA, Replogle R. Surgical closure of left coronary artery–left ventricular fistula: the second case report in the literature and a review of the five previously reported cases of coronary artery fistula terminating in the left ventricle. J Thorac Cardiovasc Surg 1977;74:199.

72. Montigny M, Stanley P, Chartrand C, et al. Postoperative evaluation after end-to-end subclavian–left coronary artery anastomosis in anomalous left coronary artery. J Thorac Cardiovasc Surg 1990;100:270.

73. Moodie DS, Fyfe D, Gill CC, et al. Anomalous origin of the coronary artery from the pulmonary artery (Bland-White-Garland syndrome) in adult patients: long-term follow-up after surgery. Am Heart J 1983; 106:381.

74. Morgan JR, Forker AD, O'Sullivan MJ, et al. Coronary arterial fistulas. Am J Cardiol 1972;30:432.

75. Mustard WT. In: Pediatric surgery, Vol. 1. Chicago: Mosby–Year Book, 1953:433–440.

76. Nadas AS, Gamboa R, Hugenholtz PG. Anomalous left coronary artery originating from the pulmonary artery. Report of two surgically treated cases with a proposal of hemodynamic and therapeutic classification. Circulation 1964;24:167.

77. Neches WH, Mathews RA, Park SC, et al. Anomalous origin of the left coronary artery from the pulmonary artery. Circulation 1974;50: 582.

78. Neufeld HN, Lester RG, Adams P Jr, et al. Congenital communication of a coronary artery with a cardiac chamber or the pulmonary trunk. Circulation 1961;24:171.

79. Paul RN, Robbins SG. Surgical treatment proposed for either endocardial fibroelastosis or anomalous left coronary artery. Pediatrics 1955; 16:147.

80. Perry SB, Rome J, Keane JF, et al. Transcatheter closure of coronary artery fistulas. J Am Coll Cardiol 1992;20:205.

81. Pezzella AT, Falaschi G, Ott DA, et al. Congenital coronary artery–left heart fistulas: report of three cases. Cardiovasc Dis, Bull Tex Heart Inst 1981;8:355.

82. Pinsky WW, Fagan LR, Mudd JFG, et al. Subclavian-coronary artery anastomosis in infancy for the Bland-Garland-White syndrome. J Thorac Cardiovasc Surg 1976;72:15.

83. Rao BN, Lucas RV Jr, Edwards JE. Anomalous origin of the left coronary artery from the right pulmonary artery associated with ventricular septal defect. Chest 1970;58:616.

84. Reeder GS, Tajik AJ, Smith HC. Visualization of coronary artery fistula by two-dimensional echocardiography. Mayo Clin Proc 1980; 55:185.

85. Reidy JF, Anjos RT, Qureshi SA, et al. Transcatheter embolization in the treatment of coronary artery fistulas. J Am Coll Cardiol 1991; 18:187.

86. Reidy JF, Sowton E, Ross DN. Transcatheter occlusion of coronary to bronchial anastomosis by detachable balloon combined with coronary angioplasty at same procedure. Br Heart J 1983;49:284.

87. Rittenhouse EA, Doty DB, Ehrenhaft JL. Congenital coronary–cardiac chamber fistula: review of operative management. Ann Thorac Surg 1975;20:468.

88. Robinson PJ, Sullivan ID, Kumpeng V, et al. Anomalous origin of the left coronary artery from the pulmonary trunk: potential for false negative diagnosis with cross sectional echocardiography. Br Heart J 1984;52:272.

89. Sabiston DC Jr, Neill CA, Taussig HB. The direction of blood flow in anomalous left coronary artery arising from the pulmonary artery. Circulation 1960;22:591.

90. Sabiston DC, Pelargonio S, Taussig HB. Myocardial infarction in infancy: the surgical management of a complication of congenital origin of the left coronary artery from the pulmonary artery. Circulation 1960;22:591.

91. Spaedy TJ, Wilensky RL. Coronary artery fistulas: clinical implications. ACC Curr J Rev 1994;24.

92. Stephenson LW, Edmunds LH Jr, Friedman S, et al. Subclavian–left coronary artery anastomosis (Meyer operation) for anomalous origin of the left coronary artery from the pulmonary artery. Circulation 1981;64:II130.

93. Strunk BL, Hieshima GB, Shafton EP. Treatment of congenital coronary arteriovenous malformations with micro-particle embolization. Cathet Cardiovasc Diagn 1991;22:133.

94. Takeuchi S, Imamura H, Katsumoto K, et al. New surgical method for repair of anomalous left coronary artery from pulmonary artery. J Thorac Cardiovasc Surg 1979;78:7.

95. Tingelstad JB, Lower RR, Eldredge WJ, et al. Anomalous origin of the right coronary artery from the main pulmonary artery. Am J Cardiol 1972;30:670.

96. Tokahashi M, Turie P. Abnormalities and diseases of the coronary vessels. In: Adams FH, Emmonouilides GC, Reinerschenerder TA, eds. Moss' heart diseases in infants, children and adolescents. Baltimore: Williams & Wilkins, 1992:627.

97. Tokuyasu KT. Development of myocardial circulation. In: Ferrans VJ, Rosenquist G, Weinstein C, eds. Cardiac morphogenesis. Amsterdam: Elsevier, 1985:226.

98. Upshaw CB. Congenital coronary arteriovenous fistula: report of a case with an analysis of 73 reported cases. Am Heart J 1962;63:399.

99. Urrutia-S CO, Falaschi G, Ott DA, et al. Surgical management of 56 patients with congenital coronary artery fistulas. Ann Thorac Surg 1983;35:300.

100. Vanderbossche JL, Felice H, Grivegnee A, et al. Noninvasive imaging of left coronary arteriovenous fistula. Chest 1988;93:885.

101. Vargo TA. Cardiac catheterization: hemodynamic measurements. In: Garson A Jr, Bricker JT, Fisher DJ, et al., eds. The science and practice of pediatric cardiology. 2nd ed. Baltimore: Williams & Wilkins, 1998: 961–994.

102. Verani MS, Lauer RM. Echocardiographic findings in right coronary arterial–right ventricular fistula: report of a neonate with fatal congestive heart failure. Am J Cardiol 1975;35:444.

103. Viragh S, Gittenberger-de Groot AC, Poelmann RE, et al. Early development of quail heart epicardium and associated vascular and glandular structures. Anat Embryol 1993;188:381.

104. Vouhe PR, Baillot-Vernant F, Trinquet F, et al. Anomalous left coronary artery from the pulmonary artery in infants. Which operation? When? J Thorac Cardiovasc Surg 1987;94:192.

105. Vouhe PR, Tamisier D, Sidi D, et al. Anomalous left coronary artery from the pulmonary artery: results of isolated aortic re-implantation. Ann Thorac Surg 1992;54:621.

106. Waldo KL, Willner W, Kirby ML. Origin of the proximal coronary artery stems and a review of ventricular vascularization in the chick embryo. Am J Anat 1990;188:109.

107. Wax DF, MaGee AG, Nykanen D, et al. Coil embolization of a coronary artery to pulmonary artery fistula from an antegrade approach. Cathet Cardiovasc Diagn 1997;42:68.

108. Wesselhoeft H, Fawcett JS, Johnson AL. Anomalous origin of the left coronary artery from the pulmonary trunk: its clinical spectrum, pathology and pathophysiology, based on a review of 140 cases with seven further cases. Circulation 1968;38:403.

109. Wilcox WD, Hagler DJ, Lie JT. Anomalous origin of left coronary artery from pulmonary artery in association with intracardiac lesions: report of two cases. J Thorac Cardiovasc Surg 1979;78:12.

110. Wilson CL, Dlabal PW, McGuire SA. Surgical treatment of anomalous left coronary artery from pulmonary artery: follow-up in teenagers and adults. Am Heart J 1977;98:440.

111. Wright NL, Baue AE, Baum S, et al. Coronary artery steal due to an anomalous left coronary artery originating from the pulmonary artery. J Thorac Cardiovasc Surg 1970;59:461.

112. Yacoub MH, Radley-Smith R, Hilton CJ. Anatomical correction of complete transposition of the great arteries and ventricular septal defect in infancy. Br Med J 1976;1(6018):1112.

113. Yoshikawa J, Katao H, Yanagihara K, et al. Noninvasive visualization of the dilated main coronary arteries in coronary artery fistulas by cross-sectional echocardiography. Circulation 1982;65:600.

114. Zannini L, Iorio FS, Ghiselli A, et al. Surgical treatment of anomalous origin of the left coronary artery in infancy. J Cardiovasc Surg (Torino) 1989;30:706.

Coronary Artery Anomalies: A Comprehensive Approach, edited by P. Angelini.
Lippincott Williams & Wilkins, Philadelphia © 1999.

CHAPTER 6

The Relationship Between the Coronary Arteries and Congenital Heart Disease

Paolo Angelini and María V. de la Cruz

Congenital heart defects may be thought of as a series of naturally occurring experiments (which would be quite difficult to recreate artificially in animal models), whereby one original, essential change (developmental error) in the normal embryogenetic sequence leads to secondary changes during later phases of development. Researchers who focus on the coronary arteries are especially interested in developmental errors that arise before aortic origination of the coronary arteries occurs. Initially, at least, these researchers are concerned with formation of the aortic root and development of the compact myocardium.

The study of the relationship between the coronary arteries and congenital heart disease is important for two basic reasons: first, because it provides potentially relevant clinical information, and second, because it may provide important clues about the interplay between coronary artery patterns and related cardiac structures during embryonic development. Information about the coronary arteries is not usually of clinical relevance in cases of congenital heart disease. Indeed, most patients with congenital heart defects have an adequate coronary circulation and do not develop coronary artery obstructive disease; moreover, surgical correction of the defects does not generally interfere with the coronary arteries. In some congenital coronary artery diseases, however, the coronary circulation pattern is clinically and developmentally important. These diseases include common truncus arteriosus, transposition of the great arteries (TGA), pulmonary valve atresia with intact ventricular septum, double-outlet right ventricle (DORV), isolated aortic valve intrinsic anomalies, and tetralogy of Fallot. This chapter will focus on these conditions.

For the purposes of this discussion, we assumed the nature and nomenclature of each major coronary artery (right, left main, circumflex, and left anterior descending) was assumed to be determined by the intrinsic anatomic characteristics and dependent myocardial areas of the involved vessel, not necessarily by the aortic sinus of origin or its location. For example, as proposed in Chapter 4 of this book, the right coronary artery was defined as the artery that lies in the anatomic right atrioventricular groove (at the upper edge of the anatomic right ventricle) and that reaches at least the acute margin of the heart. In ventricular inversion in situs solitus, the anatomic right ventricle is the left-sided one, and the right coronary artery is the vessel that provides blood flow to the free wall of the left-sided ventricle, which has the intrinsic anatomy of a right ventricle.

Illustrative Case (Figs. 6.1 through 6.8)

The case presented here illustrates situs solitus with ventricular inversion and TGA. Because of an associated ventricular septal defect and severe pulmonary valve stenosis, the patient had previously undergone a modified Rastelli repair, with insertion of a valved conduit (containing a Bjork-Shiley prosthesis) from the right-sided left ventricle to the pulmonary artery. The left ventricular angiogram, in the posteroanterior (Fig. 6.1) and lateral (Fig. 6.2) projections, shows the typical features of an anatomic left ventricle, including a native posterior outlet, an ovoidal shape, and two papillary muscles. In Figure 6.1, the surgically created outlet for the valved conduit may be clearly seen. The coronary arterial pattern (Figs. 6.3 to 6.5) features a single coronary ostium, positioned in the anterior-right aortic sinus (Fig. 6.6). The main, mixed coronary trunk (Figs. 6.3 and 6.4) is short; it gives rise to the circumflex and left anterior descending arteries (to the right and anteriorly) and to the right coronary artery. The latter vessel is the dominant coronary artery, almost reaching the obtuse margin of the heart (right-sided), beyond the posterior descending and arteriovenous nodal branches (Figs. 6.3 and 6.5). A typical variant of coronary origination commonly seen in TGA (single coronary artery)

173

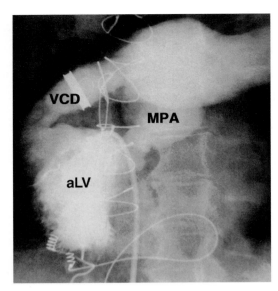

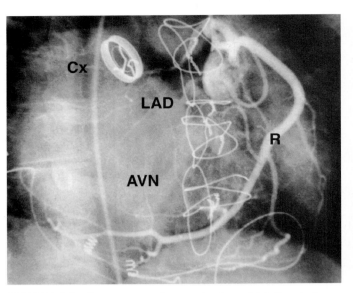

FIGURE 6.1. Illustrative case (see text). Left ventricular angiogram in the posteroanterior projection, showing the typical features of an anatomic left ventricle (aLV), with a native posterior outlet, ovoidal shape, and two papillary muscles. The surgically created valved conduit (VCD) outlet is clearly seen. MPA = main pulmonary artery.

FIGURE 6.3. Coronary angiogram in the mid left anterior oblique projection. The main, mixed trunk is short; it gives rise to the circumflex (Cx) and left anterior descending (LAD) arteries (to the right and anteriorly) and to the right coronary artery (R). The latter vessel is the dominant coronary artery, almost reaching the obtuse margin of the heart (right-sided). AVN = atrioventricular node artery.

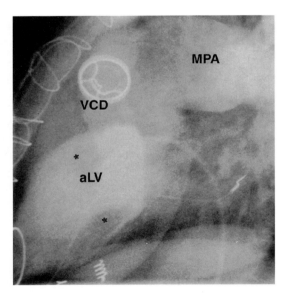

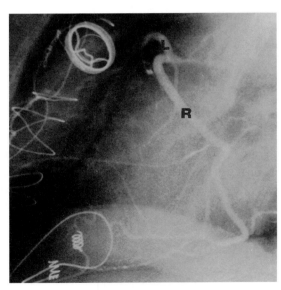

FIGURE 6.2. Same as Figure 6.1, except that this angiogram is in the lateral projection. Abbreviations as in Figure 6.1. The asterisks indicate the two papillary muscles.

FIGURE 6.4. Coronary angiogram in the lateral projection. R = right coronary artery.

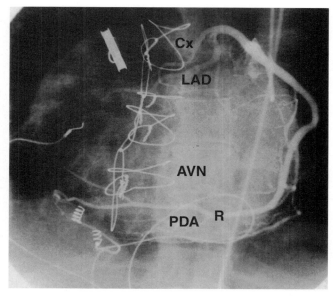

FIGURE 6.5. Coronary angiogram in the mild left anterior oblique projection. AVN = atrioventricular node artery; Cx = circumflex artery; LAD = left anterior descending artery; PDA = posterior descending artery; R = right coronary artery.

is associated with the distal coronary pattern expected in the presence of ventricular inversion (the coronary arteries essentially follow the ventricles).

COMMON TRUNCUS ARTERIOSUS

As pointed out in Chapter 2 of this book, septation of the primitive common truncus arteriosus has an important influ-

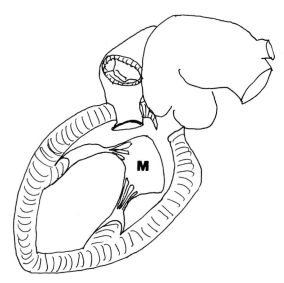

FIGURE 6.7. Diagrammatic representation of the illustrative case in the lateral plane (cf. Fig. 6.2). M = mitral valve.

ence on coronary artery origination. The naturally occurring phenomenon represented by persistence of the common truncus arteriosus implies the embryologic error of total absence of septation of the root of the primitive common truncus. Whatever type of common truncus is involved,[7] the basic anatomic feature of this anomaly remains the same: a single semilunar outlet valve and root, in the absence of an atretic valve as seen in pulmonary or aortic atresia. In a recent review of a large series of patients with common truncus, de la Cruz and colleagues[21] used the number of truncal valve cusps as the basic reference parameter for describing the coronary anatomy. An essential feature used for defining the aortic root architecture in that series was the location of the

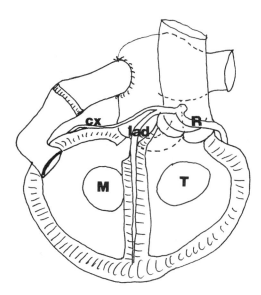

FIGURE 6.6. Diagrammatic representation of the illustrative case in the frontal plane (cf. Fig. 6.1). cx = circumflex artery; lad = left anterior descending artery; M = mitral; R = right coronary artery; T = tricuspid.

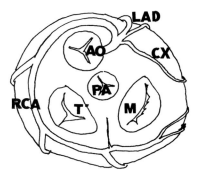

FIGURE 6.8. Representative case. The single coronary artery is shown in the coronal plane to better visualize its relationships with the atrioventricular and semilunar valves. The single coronary ostium is situated in the anterior-right sinus of the aorta. AO = aorta; CX = circumflex artery; LAD = left anterior descending artery; PA = pulmonary artery; M = mitral; T = tricuspid.

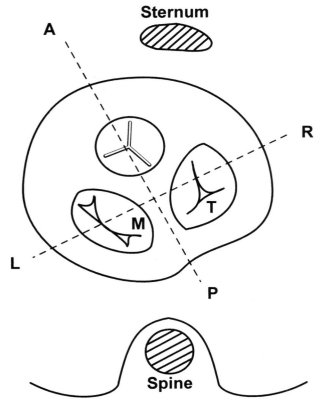

Sternum

A

R

L

M

T

P

Spine

FIGURE 6.9. Schematic representation of the heart (coronal plane) as related to the essential skeletal structures (sternum and dorsal spine) in a case of persistent common truncus arteriosus. The reference axes suggested for the description of cardiac structures are intrinsic to the cardiac anatomy, not necessarily to the body axis. The axis that connects the centers of the atrioventricular valves is used as the "left-right" one, and its perpendicular axis is assumed to be the "anteroposterior" one. M = mitral; T = tricuspid. (Modified from de la Cruz et al. Coronary arteries in truncus arteriosus. Am J Cardiol 1990;66:1482–1486. Reprinted with permission from Excerpta Medica, Inc.)

truncal leaflets with respect to other intracardiac structures. The terms "anterior," "posterior," "right," and "left," were related to the atrioventricular valves (Fig. 6.9). The line connecting the centers of the right and left atrioventricular valves (tricuspid and mitral, respectively) defined the intrinsic right-to-left axis at its two extremes. The orthogonal line (in the coronal plane) corresponding to that right-to-left axis defined an intrinsic anteroposterior axis. (This axis is not necessarily identical with the dorsoventral axis of the body as a whole but is a useful descriptive device that provides a reliable intrinsic reference, especially for anatomic and echocardiographic studies.)

Figures 6.10 through 6.13 summarize the results of the investigation by de la Cruz and coauthors[21] involving 39 autopsy specimens of common truncus arteriosus. The data point to several important features of the coronary anatomy in common truncus arteriosus:

1. Forty-four percent (17/39) of the specimens had either two cusps (8/39) or four cusps (9/39), versus 56% (22/39) that had tricuspid truncal valves. To further complicate this fundamental reference parameter for describing coronary ostial location, the orientation of the leaflets and sinuses was not consistent for specimens with the same number of cusps. For example, in cases involving quadricuspid truncal valves, the two cusps were either side-to-side or anteroposterior (Figs. 6.10 to 6.13).

2. The coronary ostia were located either in the middle third of a given aortic sinus (the most frequent pattern, as in the normal heart) or in a juxta-commissural position next to an aortic valve commissure (30%; 9/39). The literature reports occasional cases of coronary origination from the divided pulmonary trunk.[9]

3. The coronary patterns were quite variable, 17 different ones being observed in the 39 specimens. The incidence of single coronary artery was high (18%; 7/39).

4. The distal coronary anatomy was relatively unaffected by the obvious inconsistency in coronary origination. In only one case was a double (split) left anterior descending artery observed. In all cases, the left anterior descending and circumflex arteries originated with a common left trunk.

5. Independently of the truncal cusp location in the truncal root circumference, there tended to be a clustering of the right coronary ostia in the right side of the truncus and of the left coronary ostia in the left side, although the area of distribution was wide (Fig. 6.13). The predominant location for single coronary ostia was posterior.

Studies of the coronary arteries in common truncus arteriosus have been published by a few authors,[9,11,59] but each study used different descriptive criteria, so the results are hard to compare, and the only consistent, reliable data refer to the high incidence (4 to 19%) of single coronary artery. Bogers and associates[11] (Fig. 6.14) reported a high incidence of juxta-commissural location of the coronary ostia (56%, left coronary artery; 61%, right coronary artery; 40%, single coronary artery). For reporting the location of the ostia (Fig. 6.15), these authors used a circumferential scheme like that of de la Cruz, but Bogers' laterality axis was less strictly defined and apparently did not correspond to that of de la Cruz. Bogers suggested that the anterior-left side of the truncal wall is the only segment devoid of coronary ostia, but this finding was not confirmed by de la Cruz, probably because of the different definition of "anterior" and "left."

Two specific findings were surgically relevant and should be borne in mind during correction of common truncus arteriosus by means of the Rastelli procedure (using a right ventricle-to-pulmonary artery conduit)[1]:

1. The incidence of an anterior coronary trunk crossing the outflow tract of the right ventricle was 13% in de la Cruz's series.

2. The incidence of high origination of a coronary ostium

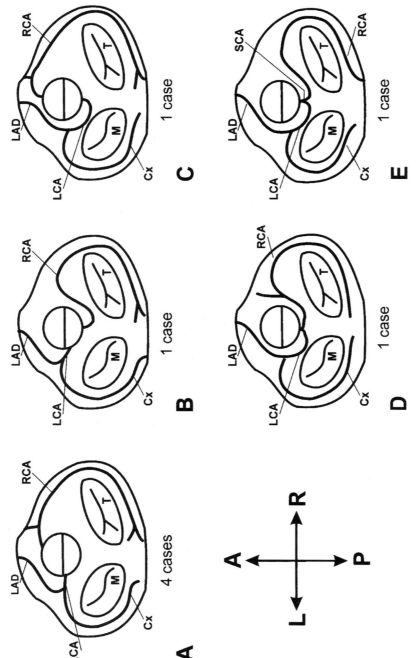

FIGURE 6.10. Diagrammatic representation of the origin and distribution of the coronary arteries in truncus arteriosus with bicuspid valve. **A** and **B.** Right and left cusps. **C–E.** Anterior and posterior cusps. ANT = anterior; Cx = circumflex; LAD = left anterior descending artery; LCA = left coronary artery; M = mitral; POST = posterior; SCA = single coronary artery; T = tricuspid. (Modified from de la Cruz et al. Coronary arteries in truncus arteriosus. Am J Cardiol 1990;66:1482–1486. Reprinted with permission from Excerpta Medica, Inc. and modified for consistency of style.)

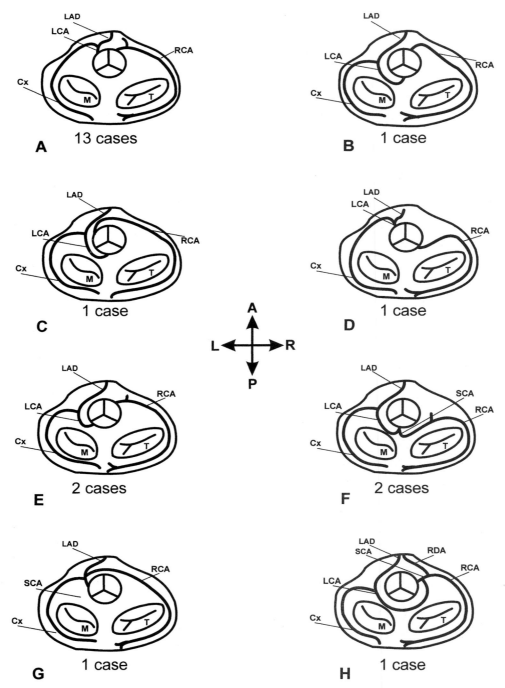

FIGURE 6.11. Diagrammatic representation of the origin and distribution of the coronary arteries in truncus arteriosus with tricuspid valve, with two anterior cusps and one posterior cusp. Abbreviations as in Figure 6.10. (Modified from de la Cruz et al. Coronary arteries in truncus arteriosus. Am J Cardiol 1990;66:1482–1486. Reprinted with permission from Excerpta Medica, Inc., and modified for consistency of style.)

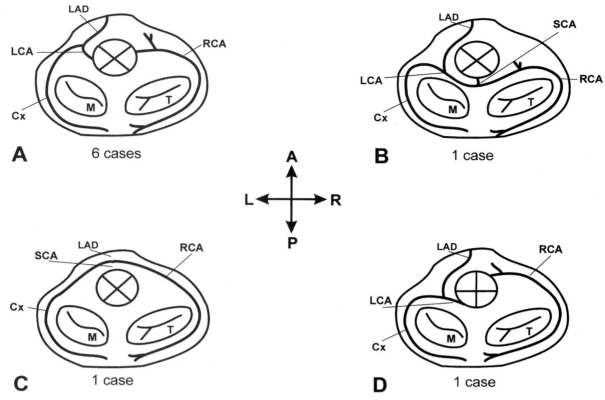

FIGURE 6.12. Diagrammatic representation of the origin and distribution of the coronary arteries in truncus arteriosus with quadricuspid valve. **A–C.** Oblique commissures. **D.** Anteroposterior cusps, with two posterior and two anterior cusps (right and left). Abbreviations as in Figure 6.10. (Modified from de la Cruz et al. Coronary arteries in truncus arteriosus. Am J Cardiol 1990;66:1482–1486. Reprinted with permission from Excerpta Medica, Inc., and modified for consistency of style.)

(above the sinotubular junction or truncal commissures) was reported as 60% by Bogers and coworkers. This parameter was not quantified by Bogers or in the series reported by Bharati,[9] who cited a 28% incidence of this anomaly.

All authors agree that variation in the truncal type, according to origination of the pulmonary circulation from the common truncus, does not affect the coronary pattern.

The absence of truncal septation implies an absence of those organizing factors that, in a normal heart, make origination of a coronary artery from the noncoronary aortic sinus or from the pulmonary sinuses such a rare finding. This observation may lend further credence to the theory that the neural crest is, indeed, critically involved in both formation of the truncal septum and determination of coronary origination (as also indicated by experiments involving neural crest ablation, as discussed in Chapter 2 of this book).

TRANSPOSITION OF THE GREAT ARTERIES

In TGA, according to a widely accepted definition, the aortic and pulmonary roots are exchanged with respect to those of a normal heart. This condition involves a variable intrinsic relationship between the great arteries, but also a necessary continuity (anatomic connection) between the right ventricle and the aorta, as well as the left ventricle and the pulmonary artery. In uncomplicated TGA, the ventricles are normally aligned with their respective atria. Development of the coronary arteries is severely affected by the anomalous connection between the ventricles and great arteries.

In a recent review,[5] we concluded, in accordance with other investigators,[53,60] that, in classifying transposition complexes, the essential factor is the intrinsic relationship between aortic and pulmonary root. When the atria are positioned normally (situs solitus), transposition may occur:

1. With an anterior aorta (which is usually anterior and to the right of the pulmonary artery). This is the most frequent, typical variant (Fig. 6.16).
2. With side-by-side great arteries (right laterality of the aorta) (Fig. 6.17).
3. With a posterior aorta (right laterality of the aorta).

''Anterior'' and ''posterior'' were assumed[5] to depend on the relationship to the atrioventricular valves (rather than the ventral/dorsal axis of the body): this relationship is an

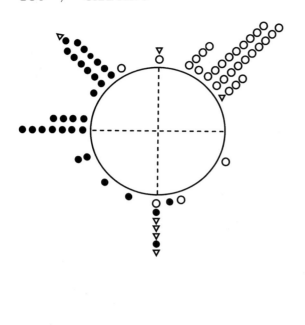

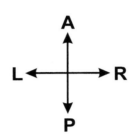

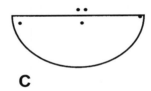

FIGURE 6.13. Diagrammatic representation of the origin of the coronary arteries in de la Cruz's series of 39 cases. The truncal wall is subdivided into conventional quadrants. Abbreviations as in Figure 6.10. Solid circles = left coronary ostia; open circles = right coronary artery ostia; triangles = ostia of single coronary arteries. (Modified from de la Cruz et al. Coronary arteries in truncus arteriosus. Am J Cardiol 1990;66:1482–1486. Reprinted with permission from Excerpta Medica, Inc., and modified for consistency of style.)

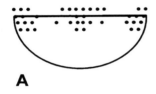
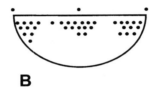

A   **B**   **C**

FIGURE 6.14. Schematic representation of the position of the coronary orifices in relation to the valvular sinuses, according to Bogers et al[11] (see text). **A.** Orifices of the left coronary artery. **B.** Orifices of the right coronary artery. **C.** Orifices of a single coronary artery. (From Bogers et al. cf. earlier figs, which state article title. J Thorac Cardiovasc Surg 1993;106:1133–1137. Reprinted with permission, as modified for consistency of style.)

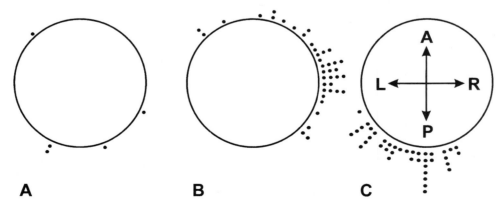

A   **B**   **C**

FIGURE 6.15. Schematic representation of the position of the coronary orifices, as projected on the truncal valve circumference, according to Bogers et al[11] (see text). **A.** Orifices of a single coronary artery. **B.** Orifices of the right coronary artery. **C.** Orifices of the left coronary artery. (From Bogers et al. cf. earlier figures, which state article title. J Thorac Cardiovasc Surg 1993;106:1133–1137. Reprinted with permission, as modified for consistency of style.)

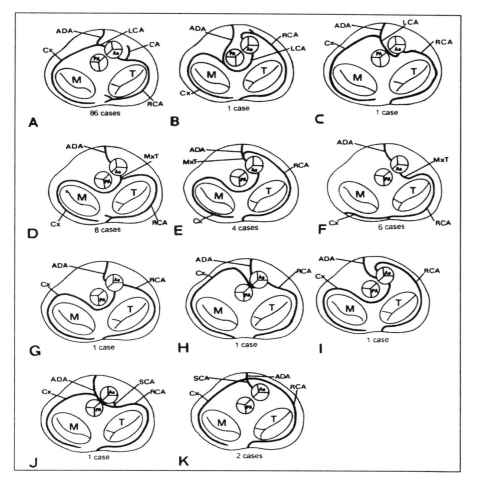

FIGURE 6.16. Schematic representation, with frequency of observed variants of coronary patterns in cases of anterior aorta (total, 112 cases), according to Angelini et al[5] (see text). The most frequent pattern was that shown in **A:** 86 cases, 76%. ADA = anterior descending artery; Ao = aortic valve; Cx = circumflex artery; LCA = left coronary artery (common trunk of the Cx and ADA); M = mitral valve; MxT = mixed trunk (either ADA + RCA or Cx + RCA); PA = pulmonary valve; RCA = right coronary artery; SCA = single coronary artery; T = tricuspid valve. (Reprinted from Angelini et al. Coronary arteries in transposition of the great arteries. Am J Cardiol 1994;74:1037–1041. Reprinted with permission from Excerpta Medica, Inc.)

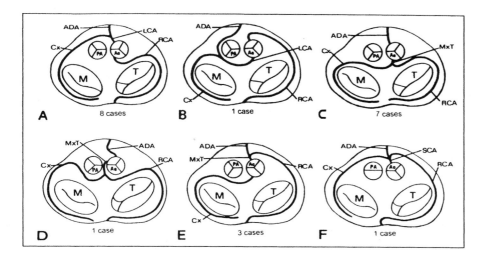

FIGURE 6.17. Schematic representation, with frequency of coronary patterns observed in side-by-side TGA, according to Angelini et al[5] (see text). No single coronary pattern seems to be clearly predominant. Abbreviations as in Figure 6.16. (Reprinted from Angelini et al. Coronary arteries in transposition of the great arteries. Am J Cardiol 1994;74:1037–1041. Reprinted with permission from Excerpta Medica, Inc.)

intrinsic one that is not altered by changes in the position of the cardiac apex (as in dextroversion) or made dubious by an unclear relationship to the body axis (as in examination of autopsy specimens or in echocardiography).

Whereas the intrinsic anatomy of the aortic valve is usually normal (tricuspid, semilunar) in TGA, the nomenclature used to identify each sinus is not yet uniform. We used the term ''facing'' for the two sinuses adjacent to the pulmonary valve and ''nonfacing'' for the sinus opposite the pulmonary valve, as well as anatomically correct nomenclature for each sinus.[5] Other authors follow either the Leiden convention[32] (designating sinus-1 and sinus-2 as the left and right sinuses, respectively, for an observer looking from the pulmonary artery toward the aorta) or the terminology used by the Mayo Clinic[60] (sinus-1, right; sinus-2, left).

In TGA, a great number of coronary patterns have been described by various authors.[17,25,57,58,60,61,65,69] In two recent extensive anatomic series, Sim and colleagues[60] observed 13 different patterns in 255 autopsy specimens (Fig. 6.18), and we[5] encountered 17 different patterns in 133 specimens. Six of the patterns described by Sim were not found in our specimens, and 11 of the patterns that we encountered were not found by Sim (Fig. 6.18). With respect to the frequency of specific coronary patterns in association with the various aortopulmonary relationships, we and Sim observed similar findings. In both studies, side-by-side transposition was associated with a particularly inconsistent coronary anatomy, similar to that observed with side-by-side great vessels in DORV.[34] In the typical form of TGA, in which the aorta is located anteriorly and to the right, the most common pattern (a single trunk for both the left anterior descending and the circumflex artery, originating from the anterior left-facing cusp, and a right coronary artery originating from the posterior right-facing cusp) was present in only about 60% of cases.[5,53,60]

The different coronary artery patterns observed in TGA point to one common rule, which also applies to the normal heart: the distal coronary branches are remarkably consistent. It is the proximal origination that may vary greatly. In TGA—as in the normal heart—the right, circumflex, and anterior descending arteries uniformly supply the right ventricular free wall and posterior left ventricle (right coronary artery), the posterolateral free wall of the left ventricle (circumflex artery), and the ventricular septum and anterolateral free wall of the left ventricle (anterior descending artery). In transposed hearts, the term ''left'' anterior descending loses its validity because, in a large percentage of cases, the anterior descending artery does not originate from the left sinus or from a left coronary trunk, in conjunction with the circumflex artery. Also, in a large percentage of TGA cases, the proximal trunk that joins two or three arteries is neither a right nor a left one, but a mixed trunk (anterior descending/right coronary artery; anterior descending/right coronary artery/circumflex; or right coronary artery/circumflex, etc.).[55]

Variations in the relationship between the coronary ostial location and the sinuses of Valsalva have acquired great

Diagram	Pattern	No.	%
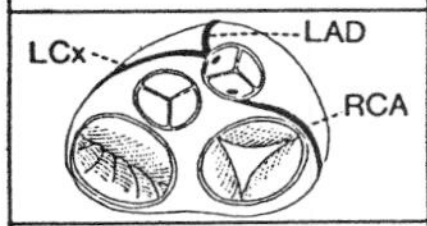	Usual	184	72
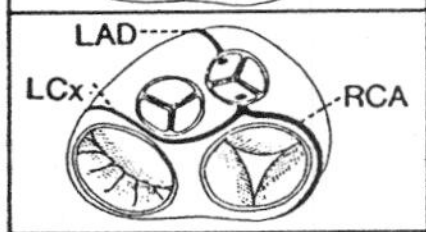	LCx from RCA	46	18
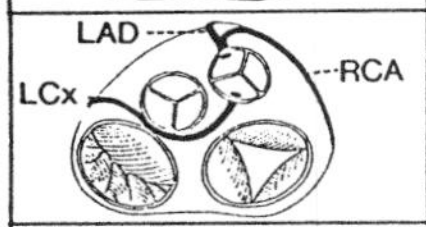	Inverted LCx and RCA	6	2
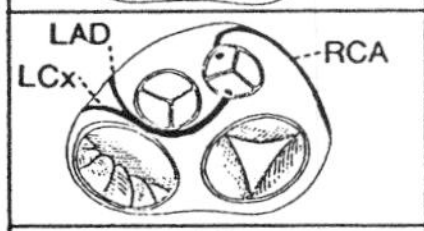	Inverted coronary arteries	4	2
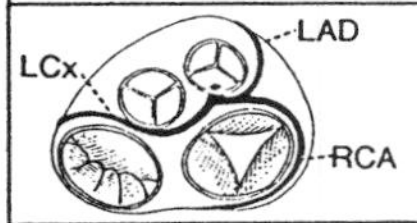	Single RCA	3	1
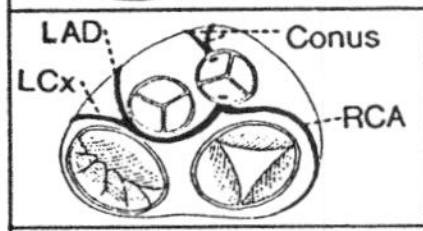	Single RCA	3	1
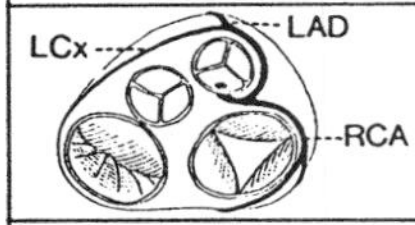	Single RCA	2	1
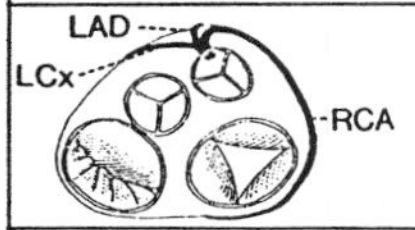	Single LCA	2	1
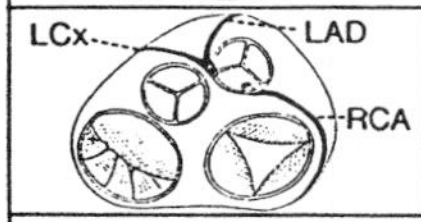	Commissural origin of intramural LCA	1	<1
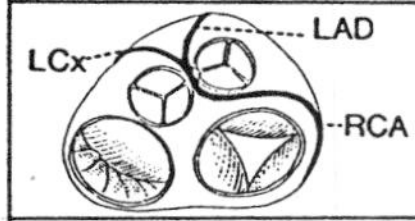	Commissural origin of both coronary arteries	1	<1
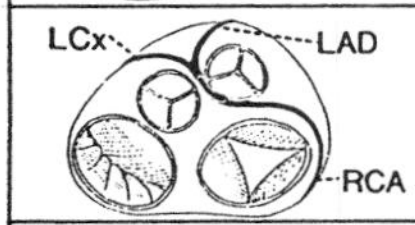	Single ostium of both coronary arteries distal to right sinotubular junction; intramural LCA	1	<1
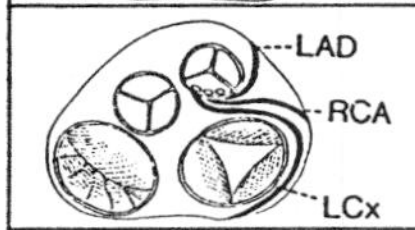	3 separate origins of coronary arteries from right sinus	1	<1
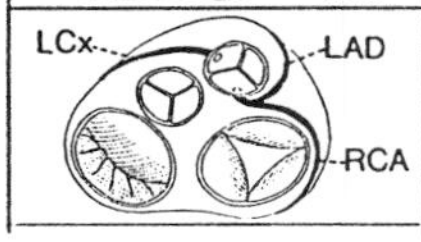	LAD from RCA; LCx from left sinus	1	<1

FIGURE 6.18. Thirteen patterns of origin and proximal epicardial course of the coronary arteries in 255 hearts with complete transposition of the great arteries, according to Sim et al[60] (see text). LAD = left anterior descending coronary artery; LCA = left coronary artery; LCx = left circumflex coronary artery; RCA = right coronary artery. (From Sim et al. Coronary artery anatomy in complete transposition of the great arteries. Ann Thorac Surg 1994;57:890–894. Reprinted with permission from Excerpta Medica, Inc.)

clinical relevance since the introduction of the switch procedure for correcting TGA.[17,37,39] In patients with this condition, more frequently than in normal hearts, coronary ostia are located eccentrically—arising away from the middle third of the aortic sinuses, next to the commissures, or high in the ascending aorta.[25,26,32,33,65,69] This type of coronary ectopia is associated with increased occurrence of an intramural proximal segment (coursing within the aortic wall) and acute proximal angulation from the aortic wall, as extensively reported in the literature.[17,33,39,45,53] Even more than by the atypical coronary patterns themselves, surgical switching of the great arteries is complicated technically or even precluded by some forms of ectopic coronary origination with an intramural course (marked intussusception or commissural ostial location) and by a coronary artery coursing between the great arteries (Figs. 6.2, C–J, 6.3D, and 6.4D).

Even on the basis of a relatively small number of cases, one can conclude that, in TGA, despite the fact that the coronary patterns show great anatomic inconsistency, the nonfacing aortic sinus almost never gives rise to a coronary ostium. (A few early authors[58,65] reported this exceptional event, but their description was imprecise and therefore dubious.) Origination of a coronary artery from the nonfacing aortic sinus should be considered a rare anomaly and a contraindication for the switch procedure.

Because, in any given case of TGA, the first goal of anatomic or angiographic studies should be to provide a correct anatomic description of the aortic sinuses, the great vessels' reciprocal relationships are a particularly useful descriptor: as in a normal heart, the point of contact between the root of the aorta and the pulmonary artery corresponds to the aortic commissure between the two facing sinuses, and the opposite sinus is the nonfacing one (Figs. 6.16 to 6.18). Because of the unpredictability of the coronary patterns in TGA, biplane aortography is frequently a useful preliminary method for guiding selective coronary angiography. The caudal (''laid-back'') projection, in the posteroanterior view, is frequently assumed to be adequate for describing coronary patterns in newborns.[53] Because preformed catheters are designed for normal aortic roots and normal coronary ostia, TGA poses special challenges for the angiographer. The ascending aorta is shorter and straighter than in normal hearts, and, in the most frequent variety of TGA (anterior-right aorta), the facing aortic sinuses are posterior. Shorter, curved Judkins catheters (3.5-cm) are useful in most older patients with TGA, as these devices have a good chance of selectively cannulating coronary ostia located in the concavity of the aorta. If attempts with Judkins catheters are unsuccessful, the angiographer should resort to a moderate-sized Amplatz curve (right-1; left-2).

PULMONARY VALVE ATRESIA WITH INTACT VENTRICULAR SEPTUM

Most congenital malformations of the pulmonary valve are potentially associated with coronary anomalies, because abnormal development of this valve is probably influenced by abnormal behavior of the cardiac neural crest, which also affects formation of the coronary ostia. More specifically and importantly, however, pulmonary atresia with intact ventricular septum (PA-IVS) creates a dysfunctional physiology during embryonic and postnatal life, which can affect the morphogenesis and later evolution of the coronary arteries. As has been well described in the literature,[13,27,31,49,66] the basic pathology of this malformation involves atresia of the pulmonary valve, with an intact ventricular septum and a peculiar right ventricular anatomy, generally entailing a small cavity and severe wall hypertrophy. PA-IVS is associated with the following findings, as documented by pathologists and clinicians:

1. Coronary origination and patterns of dominance are only slightly affected by this anomaly, with the possible exception of an increased incidence of single coronary artery.

2. For several years, right ventricular-to-coronary communications have been recognized anatomically[27,35] and angiographically,[15,16,31,49,66,71] as manifested by systolic filling of the right coronary artery and the left anterior descending artery during right ventricular angiography and by filling of the right ventricle at end-diastole during coronary angiography (see Chapter 5, Fig. 5.10, A and B). Seventy-five percent of patients with PA-IVS have large abnormal communications, which have walls that include all three arterial layers (intima, media, and adventitia). Affected vessels include the left anterior descending artery, the right coronary artery, and less frequently the distal portion of the circumflex artery.[14] Only a small percentage of patients (especially those who die during infancy) have no ventriculo-coronary communications; anatomically, however, they still have large numbers of prominent sinusoidal, intertrabecular spaces, which are frequently covered by a thick, fibrous layer but lack a tunica media.[31] These spaces communicate with the intramyocardial capillary vessels and (via these vessels alone) with the coronary arteries.

3. Severe intimal thickening has been observed in 70% of these ventriculo-coronary communications and in the affected epicardial coronary arteries.[10,68] Occlusions or interruptions of the epicardial coronary arteries (especially the left anterior descending and right coronary artery but also the circumflex) are frequently encountered at the level of the ostium or proximal or even distal to the ventriculo-coronary communication (the incidence was reported as 44% in one series[31] and 35% in another[14]). The severity of the intimal proliferative process seems to increase with the extent of the ventriculo-coronary communication and with the patient's age. Only in the absence of such communications can one find coronary arteries free of intimal thickening. Occasional cases of absent aortic origination of the coronary circulation have been reported.[10,40]

4. Endocardial fibroelastosis, myocardial fibrosis, and acute myocardial infarction (with associated ischemic damage) are observed in the great majority of cases.[27,29,31,35]

5. Functionally, it is apparent that, in some cases (38% in one series[31]), coronary steal occurs during diastole, allowing coronary arterial blood to be shunted to the right ventricular cavity.[71] More importantly, the suprasystemic right ventricular cavity is vented through the ventriculo-coronary communications.[71] These defects also cause unoxygenated blood to be delivered to the myocardium. Myocardial fibrosis of the free wall of the right ventricle and of the ventricular septum is consistently observed, to varying degrees. Endocardial fibroelastosis of the diminutive right ventricular cavity is usually seen, but it is independent of the degree of tricuspid insufficiency or the extent of the ventriculo-coronary communication.[31]

Coronary communications and obstructions have important prognostic and surgical implications,[14,49] and coronary angiography has become the standard for their preoperative evaluation. The consistent pathologic coronary findings in PA-IVS suggests that the suprasystemic right ventricular pressure interferes with normal maturation of the coronary arteries of aortic origin. During the early embryonic stage, the intertrabecular spaces communicate normally with the developing coronary subepicardial arteries and veins. At the onset of suprasystemic right ventricular pressure after closure of the ventricular septum, a hemodynamic gradient is created that fosters the progressive enlargement of ventriculo-coronary communications. It is worth noting that, in pulmonary atresia with a ventricular septal defect (extreme tetralogy of Fallot), coronary arterial development does not appear to be affected, except for the occasional presence of coronary-to-pulmonary collateral circulation.

DOUBLE-OUTLET RIGHT VENTRICLE

Double-outlet right ventricle is generally defined as origination of both (or most) of the great arteries from the anatomic right ventricle.[3,6,22] Most authors agree that, in DORV, the great-vessel relationships can vary from normal (anterior pulmonary infundibulum situated to the left of the aortic root, or normally crossed great arteries), to a side-by-side pattern (aorta to the right of the pulmonary artery, both vessels having the same anteroposterior position and a similar infundibular size) or transposed great arteries (aortic root anterior to, and to the right of, the pulmonary artery).[3,6,22]

According to the few published studies,[9,12,34,53,62] the coronary patterns seen in DORV seem to depend more on the great vessels' relationships than on the mere common denominator of DORV (Fig. 6.19). In DORV with normally crossed great vessels, the coronary patterns resemble those of the normal heart.[9,34] When DORV is associated with an anterior right-sided aorta, the coronary patterns have greater variability, but some 73% of the cases[34] involve the pattern most frequently observed in TGA without DORV,[5] in which the right coronary artery originates from the right posterior sinus and the left main artery arises from the left posterior sinus. In DORV with side-by-side great vessels, the variability of coronary origination reaches its highest level, no individual pattern being encountered in more than 33% of the cases.[34]

ISOLATED AORTIC VALVE ANOMALIES

As anticipated in Chapter 3 of this book, which discussed bicuspid aortic valve in a hamster model, intrinsic aortic valve anomalies may entail an increased variability in coronary artery origination. In the same animal model, the incidence of coronary anomalies was greatly increased even in the absence of bicuspid aortic valve; this finding points to a common genetic influence, with variable expression in the animal world.

Few researchers have prospectively addressed the issue of coronary origination in human congenital aortic valve defects, and published reports have been substantially limited to bicuspid aortic valve. In our own clinical experience, many cases of coronary ectopic origination have been associated with definite, but frequently minor, asymmetry of the aortic valve sinuses, as occasionally mentioned in the literature.[9] To investigate this issue, specific prospective studies should be carried out, probably in autopsy specimens or by means of echocardiography or special angiographic techniques designed to describe the aortic valve morphology (Fig. 6.20). In cases of bicuspid aortic valve, coronary origination must be affected, because one or both of the facing ''coronary'' cusps is always abnormal[4,64] (Fig. 6.21). Bicuspid aortic valve is encountered in about 1% of autopsy series.[36,46,52,63,64,67] Figure 6.21 shows the expected site of origination of the coronary arteries in the various types of bicuspid aortic valve. According to the limited literature on the subject, bicuspid aortic valve is associated with an increased frequency of mildly ectopic coronary arterial origination,[9,41] especially left coronary artery dominance,[41,56] high origination of the left coronary artery,[9,41] and shortening of the left main trunk.[41,51]

Because the aortic sinuses are the basic reference structure for defining normal origination of the coronary arteries, the criteria for coronary normality must be adapted in this condition. Most of the literature about bicuspid aortic valve refers to the two aortic cusps as ''right and left'' or ''anterior and posterior,'' but these terms are approximate and imprecise (Fig. 6.21). First, the facing sinus(es) should be identified and interpreted. The site of contact (adjacency) between the aortic and pulmonary valvular annuli is still the basic reference point, as in most other hearts. This site is identified easily in autopsy specimens but not so easily on coronary angiograms. Ideally, the angiographer should identify the exact right anterior oblique projection in which the ascending aorta and pulmonary main trunk are not superimposed

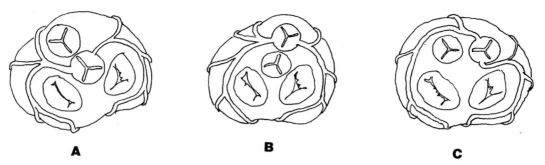

FIGURE 6.19. The most common coronary artery anatomic patterns in 44 cases of double-outlet right ventricle. **A.** All 17 cases with normally related great vessels (39%) had normal coronary origination. **B.** Coronary artery pattern seen in 11 (73%) of the 15 patients with transposition of the great arteries (34% of the overall 44 cases). **C.** Coronary artery pattern seen in four (33%) of the 12 cases with side-by-side arrangement of the great arteries. Five other coronary patterns were less frequently observed. (Modified from Gordillo L, Faye-Petersen O, de la Cruz MV, et al. Coronary arterial patterns in double-outlet right ventricle. Am J Cardiol 1993;71(12):1108–1110.)

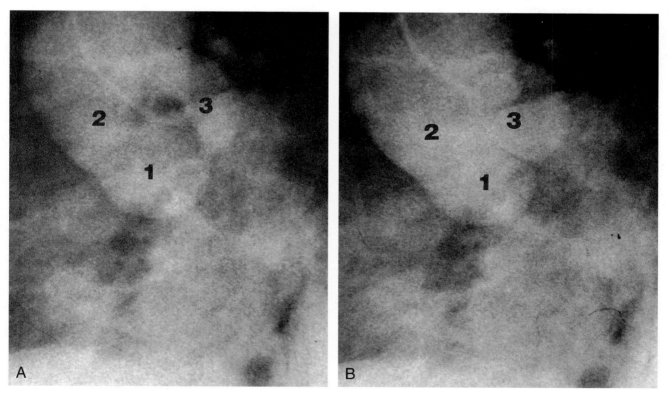

FIGURE 6.20. Systolic **(A)** and diastolic **(B)** frames of an aortic root angiogram, in the caudal left anterior oblique projection, which optimally shows the three aortic cusps/sinuses. This projection is grossly perpendicular to the normal aortic annulus plane. This view may also be valuable for visualizing ectopic coronary ostia and the functional aortic opening in systole. 1 = noncoronary sinus; 2 = right anterior sinus; 3 = left anterior sinus.

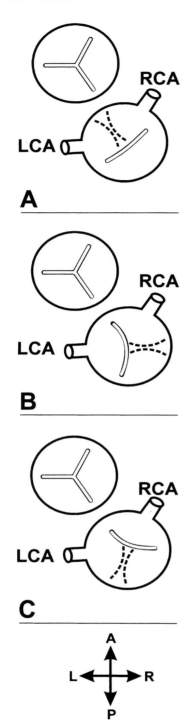

FIGURE 6.21. Schematic representation of the three fundamental types of bicuspid aortic valves, with typical sites of origination of the coronary arteries. **Type A:** "Anteroposterior" type, interpreted as resulting from fusion of the right and left anterior (coronary) cusps. The RCA and LCA originate at sites opposite the raphe (dotted lines). **Type B:** "Side-by-side type with a left tilt," interpreted as resulting from fusion of the right anterior and posterior cusps. **Type C:** "Side-by-side type with a right tilt," interpreted as resulting from fusion of the left anterior and posterior cusps. A = anterior; L = left; P = posterior; R = right.

(see Chapter 4 of this book). In otherwise normal hearts, this is approximately the right anterior oblique 60° projection, which indicates the aortopulmonary contact point at about 30° in the aortic valve annulus. This contact point should be used to further define the aortic sinuses according to their relative location (Fig. 4.5). In bicuspid aortic valve, each cusp should also be identified as a single versus a double, fused, or mixed cusp (the latter type results from embryologic fusion of two cusps). The literature contains no evidence to indicate that the two cusps of a bicuspid aortic valve have an identical embryologic origin (corresponding to one-and-a-half of the normal three cusps); on the contrary, substantial evidence points to the fact that one of the two cusps is analogous to a single normal one, while the other cusp corresponds embryologically to two normal ones, although the size of the two cusps may be similar. The raphe that is sometimes observed in the middle of the aortic side of a fused cusp[24,46,51,67] points to the morphogenetic mechanism of bicuspid aortic valve.

The coronary arterial orifices are the most consistent, readily available reference points for identifying the cusps (Fig. 6.21), but their use for this purpose involves the caveat that anomalous origination of the coronary arteries may exist in a given case. The individual sinus size and the presence of a raphe (as seen on only some 15% of bicuspid aortic valves) are variables of great importance to the anatomist but are essentially undeterminable by the angiographer. Even with autopsy materials, the differential diagnosis of right-noncoronary (R-NC) versus left-noncoronary (L-NC) bicuspid valve must be based only on the tenuous criterion of the location of the posterior commissure (Fig. 6.21): a right-left bicuspid valve would be called R-NC when the commissure is tilted to the left and L-NC when it is tilted to the right. A raphe (when present) may be a more reliable means of identifying a double fused, mixed cusp.

Identification of the cusps is essential for labeling the ostial location with respect to normality. In cases of bicuspid aortic valve with a right-left mixed cusp, the two coronary arteries are expected to be situated on opposite sides of the aortopulmonary contact point (the adjacent point of the anterior sinuses). In cases of bicuspid aortic valve with an R-NC mixed cusp, the right coronary artery is expected to arise from the anterior segment of such cusp (Fig. 6.21). Specific prospective studies, based on proper identification of the aortic cusps, must be performed before valid conclusions can be drawn in regard to a supposed increase in coronary anomalies in humans with bicuspid aortic valve.

Supraaortic stenosis, involving abnormalities of both luminal size (hypoplasia) and wall thickness (fibrotic ingrowth) at the aortic sinotubular segment, has been associated with ostial coronary stenosis or atresia. The extreme degree of aortic stenosis, aortic atresia, is a dominant, defining feature of hypoplastic left heart syndrome. Coronary arteries are frequently affected by the presence of such defects.[27,30,43,48,50,54] The coronary patterns are not greatly disturbed, except that left coronary dominance is found in about 56% of cases.[54]

Intimal thickening, stenotic lesions, and ventriculo-coronary communications have been observed, both angiographically and anatomically, in cases of hypoplastic left heart syndrome without mitral atresia.[8]

TETRALOGY OF FALLOT

For several years, investigators have recognized that tetralogy of Fallot entails an increased incidence of coronary anomalies and that these anomalies have important implications during the surgical repair of this anomaly. Tetralogy of Fallot is characterized by four features: right ventricular hypertrophy, a ventricular septal defect (nonobstructive), juxtaposition of the aortic valve (overriding the ventricular septum), and pulmonary infundibular hypoplasia with valve stenosis or atresia. The basic embryologic defect seems to be related to uneven septation of the conus and the common truncus arteriosus, leading to both pulmonary stenosis and primary ectasia of the aortic annulus.[18] It is most likely the latter defect which creates the primary condition that leads to an increased frequency of coronary anomalies of origination. After extensively studying the coronary arteries in tetralogy of Fallot by means of selective coronary angiography, Dabizzi and collaborators[19,20] reported a series of 181 such cases in 1990. Twenty-four cases (about 13%) involved ectopic coronary origination, and 72 cases (about 39%) involved a coronary-to-pulmonary fistula. Similar data have been presented by other authors.[28,47,65,70]

CONCLUSION

In reviewing several forms of congenital heart defects, we have presented evidence to support a few important general concepts:

1. Coronary arteries show a distal ramification pattern that is intrinsically related to the anatomic features of each ventricle,[2,23,38,42,44] independent of that ventricle's spatial location and connections with the great vessels. The blood supply of the ventricular septum is consistently provided by epicardial coronary arteries (anterior and posterior) that course in the interventricular grooves.

2. The proximal coronary patterns of origin and course are variably affected by different heart defects. The presence of a single, common truncus arteriosus leads to the greatest instability in the proximal coronary anatomy.

3. Coronary arterial origination is not related either to increased oxygen saturation (see Transposition of the Great Arteries) or to increased pressures (see Pulmonary and Aortic Valve Atresia or to origination of the aorta from the right ventricle (see Transposition of the Great Arteries; Double-Outlet Right Ventricle; and Taussig-Bing malformation). The coronary arteries' consistent connection with the facing cusps is probably due to the fact that cardiac neural crest cells are present in those cusps (and not in the nonfacing cusp, which is embryologically derived from the intercalated swellings of the common truncus).

4. The two facing aortic cusps, next to the pulmonary artery, are the site of origination for coronary arteries in the great majority of cases involving a congenital anomaly.

5. During embryonic or fetal life, the onset of suprasystemic pressure in the left or right ventricle leads to the development of abnormal ventriculo-coronary communications. Although these communications allow some venting of the affected ventricular cavity, they also cause obstructive changes in the affected coronary artery.

6. Intrinsic aortic valve anomalies may affect coronary origination, as in bicuspid aortic valve or tetralogy of Fallot.

Larger, detailed studies of coronary morphology in congenital heart disease have considerable potential for establishing firm correlations between cardiac defects and coronary morphogenesis.

REFERENCES

1. Anderson KR, McGoon DC, Lie JT. Surgical significance of the coronary arterial anatomy in truncus arteriosus communis. Am J Cardiol 1978;41:76.
2. Anderson RH, Becker AE. Coronary arterial pattern: a guide to identification of congenital heart disease. In: Becker AE, Losekoot G, Marcelletti C, Anderson RH, eds. Pediatric cardiology. Edinburgh: Churchill Livingston, 1981:251–262.
3. Anderson RH, Becker AE, Wilcox BR, et al. Surgical anatomy of double-outlet right ventricle—a reappraisal. Am J Cardiol 1983;52:555.
4. Angelini A, Ho SY, Anderson RH, et al. The morphology of the normal aortic valve as compared with the aortic valve having two leaflets. J Thorac Cardiovasc Surg 1989;98:362.
5. Angelini P, de la Cruz MV, Valencia AM, et al. Coronary arteries in transposition of the great arteries. Am J Cardiol 1994;74:1037.
6. Angelini P, Leachman RD. The spectrum of double outlet right ventricle: an embryologic interpretation. Cardiovasc Dis, Bull Tex Heart Inst 1976;3:2.
7. Angelini P, Leachman RD. Trunco-conal defects. An anatomic and embryologic discussion of common truncus and related malformations. Eur J Cardiol 1974;2:11.
8. Baffa JM, Chen SL, Guttenberg ME, et al. Coronary artery abnormalities and right ventricular histology in hypoplastic left heart syndrome. J Am Coll Cardiol 1992;20:350.
9. Bharati S, Lev M. The pathology of congenital heart disease: a personal experience with more than 6,300 congenitally malformed hearts. Armonk, NY: Futura, 1996:207.
10. Blackman MS, Schneider B, Sondheimer HM. Absent proximal left main coronary in association with pulmonary atresia. Br Heart J 1981;46:449.
11. Bogers AJ, Bartelings MM, Bokenkamp R, et al. Common arterial trunk, uncommon coronary arterial anatomy. J Thorac Cardiovasc Surg 1993;106:1133.
12. Bomex MMR, Weidman WH, McGoon DC, et al. Double outlet right ventricle with pulmonary stenosis. Surgical consideration and result of operation. Circulation 1971;43:889.
13. Bull C, de Leval MR, Mercanti C, et al. Pulmonary atresia and intact ventricular septum: a revised classification. Circulation 1982;66:266.
14. Burrows PE, Benson LN, Freedom RM. Coronary angiography in pulmonary atresia with intact ventricular septum. In: Freedom RM, ed. Pulmonary atresia with intact ventricular septum. Mount Kisko, NY: Futura, 1989:207–228.

15. Burrows PE, Freedom RM, Benson LN, et al. Coronary angiography of pulmonary atresia, hypoplastic right ventricle, and ventriculocoronary communications. Am J Roent 1990;154:789.

16. Calder AL, Co EE, Sage MD. Coronary arterial abnormalities in pulmonary atresia with intact ventricular septum. Am J Cardiol 1987;59:436.

17. Castaneda AR. Arterial switch operation for simple and complex TGA: indication, criteria, and limitations relevant to surgery. Thorac Cardiovasc Surg 1991;39:151.

18. Clancy DL, Morrow AG, Roberts WC. Malformations of the aortic valve in patients with the tetralogy of Fallot. Am Heart J 1968;76:755.

19. Dabizzi RP, Caprioli G, Aiazzi L, et al. Distribution and anomalies of coronary arteries in tetralogy of Fallot. Circulation 1980;61:95.

20. Dabizzi RP, Teodori G, Barletta GA, et al. Associated coronary and cardiac anomalies in tetralogy of Fallot. An angiographic study. Euro Heart J 1990;11:692.

21. De la Cruz MV, Cayre R, Angelini P, et al. Coronary arteries in truncus arteriosus. Am J Cardiol 1990;66:1482.

22. De la Cruz MV, Cayre R, Arista-Salado Martinez O, et al. The infundibular interrelationships and the ventriculoarterial connection in double outlet right ventricle. Clinical and surgical implications. Int J Cardiol 1992;35:153.

23. Deanfield JE, Tommasini G, Anderson RH, et al. Tricuspid atresia: analysis of coronary artery distribution and ventricular morphology. Br Heart J 1982;48:485.

24. Edwards JE. The congenital bicuspid aortic valve. Circulation 1961; 23:485.

25. Elliott LP, Amplatz K, Edwards JE. Coronary arterial patterns in transposition complexes. Anatomic and angiocardiographic studies. Am J Cardiol 1966;17:362.

26. Elliott LP, Neufeld HN, Anderson RC, et al. Complete transposition of the great vessels: I. An anatomic study of sixty cases. Circulation 1963;27:1105.

27. Essed CE, Klein HW, Krediet P. Coronary and endocardial fibroelastosis of the ventricles in the hypoplastic left and right heart syndromes. Virchows Arch 1975;368:87.

28. Fellows KE, Freed MD, Keane JF, et al. Results of routine preoperative coronary angiography in tetralogy of Fallot. Circulation 1975;51:561.

29. Freedom RM, Benson L, Wilson GJ. The coronary circulation and myocardium in pulmonary and aortic atresia with an intact ventricular septum. In: Marcelletti C, Anderson RH, Becker AE, et al., eds. Paediatric cardiology. Vol. 6. Edinburgh: Churchill-Livingstone, 1986:78–96.

30. Freedom RM, Culham JA, Moes CA, et al. Selective aortic root angiography in the hypoplastic left heart syndrome. Eur J Cardiol 1976;4:25.

31. Gittenberger-de Groot AC, Sauer U, Bindl L, et al. Competition of coronary arteries and ventriculo-coronary arterial communications in pulmonary atresia with intact ventricular septum. Int J Cardiol 1988;18:243.

32. Gittenberger-de Groot AC, Sauer U, Oppenheimer-Dekker A, et al. Coronary arterial anatomy in transposition of the great arteries: a morphological study. Pediatr Cardiol 1983;4(Suppl 1):15.

33. Gittenberger-de Groot AC, Sauer U, Quaegebeur J. Aortic intramural coronary artery in three hearts with transposition of the great arteries. J Thorac Cardiovasc Surg 1986;91:566.

34. Gordillo L, Faye-Petersen O, de la Cruz MV, et al. Coronary arterial patterns in double-outlet right ventricle. Am J Cardiol 1993;71(12):1108–1110.

35. Hubbard JF, Girod DA, Caldwell RL, et al. Right ventricular infarction with cardiac rupture in an infant with pulmonary valve atresia with intact ventricular septum. J Am Coll Cardiol 1983;2:363.

36. Hutchins GM, Nazarian IH, Bulkley BH. Association of left dominant coronary arterial system with congenital bicuspid aortic valve. Am J Cardiol 1978;42:57.

37. Jatene AD, Fontes VF, Paulista PP, et al. Anatomic correction of transposition of the great vessels. J Thorac Cardiovasc Surg 1976;72:364.

38. Keeton BR, Lie JT, McGoon DC, et al. Anatomy of coronary arteries in univentricular hearts and its surgical implications. Am J Cardiol 1979;43:569.

39. Kurosawa H, Imai Y, Kawada M. Coronary arterial anatomy in regard to the arterial switch procedure. Cardiol Young 1991;1:54.

40. Lenox CC, Briner J. Absent proximal coronary arteries associated with pulmonic atresia. Am J Cardiol 1972;30:666.

41. Lerer PK, Edwards WD. Coronary arterial anatomy in bicuspid aortic valve. Necropsy study of 100 hearts. Br Heart J 1981;45:142.

42. Lev M, Liberthson RR, Kirkpatrick JR, et al. Single (primitive) ventricle. Circulation 1969;39:577.

43. Lloyd TR, Evans TC, Marvin WJ. Morphologic determinants of coronary blood flow in the hypoplastic left heart syndrome. Am Heart J 1986;112:666.

44. Macartney FJ, Partridge JB, Scott O, et al. Common or single ventricle. An angiocardiographic and hemodynamic study of 42 patients. Circulation 1976;53:543.

45. Mayer JE Jr, Sanders SP, Jonas RA, et al. Coronary artery pattern and outcome of arterial switch operation for transposition of the great arteries. Circulation 1990;82:IV139.

46. Moore GW, Hutchins GM, Brito JC, et al. Congenital malformations of the semilunar valves. Human Pathol 1980;11:367.

47. Moss RL, Backer CL, Zales VR, et al. Tetralogy of Fallot with anomalous origin of the right coronary artery. Ann Thorac Surg 1995;59:229.

48. O'Connor WN, Cash JB, Cottrill CM, et al. Ventriculocoronary connections in hypoplastic left hearts: an autopsy microscopic study. Circulation 1982;66:1078.

49. O'Connor WN, Cottrill CM, Johnson GL, et al. Pulmonary atresia with intact ventricular septum and ventriculocoronary communications: surgical significance. Circulation 1982;65:805.

50. Raghib G, Bloemendaal RD, Kanjuh VI, et al. Aortic atresia and premature closure of foramen ovale. Myocardial sinusoids and coronary arteriovenous fistula serving as outflow channel. Am Heart J 1965;70:476.

51. Roberts WC. The congenitally bicuspid aortic valve. A study of 85 autopsy cases. Am J Cardiol 1970;26:72.

52. Roberts WC. The structure of the aortic valve in clinically isolated aortic stenosis. An autopsy study of 162 patients over 15 years of age. Circulation 1970;42:91.

53. Sauer U. Cineangiographic diagnosis of coronary artery anatomy in transposition of the great arteries and double outlet right ventricle: significance of aortic intramural coronary arteries. A study of 103 patients undergoing arterial switch operation and 16 neonates with elective Senning-Brom operation. In: Vogel M, Buhlmeyer K, eds. Transposition of the great arteries 25 years after Rashkind balloon septostomy. Heidelberg: Steinkopff, 1992:97–112.

54. Sauer U, Gittenberger-de Groot AC, Geishauser M, et al. Coronary arteries in the hypoplastic left heart syndrome. Histopathologic and histometrical studies and implications for surgery. Circulation 1989;80:I168.

55. Sauer U, Gittenberger-de-Groot AC, Peters DR, et al. Cineangiography of the coronary arteries in transposition of the great arteries. Pediatr Cardiol 1983;4:25.

56. Scholz DG, Lynch JA, Willerscheidt AB, et al. Coronary arterial dominance associated with congenital bicuspid aortic valve. Arch Pathol Lab Med 1980;104:417.

57. Shaher RM. Complete transposition of the great arteries. New York: Academic Press, 1973:138–151.

58. Shaher RM, Puddu GC. Coronary arterial anatomy in complete transposition of the great vessels. Am J Cardiol 1966;17:355.

59. Shrivastava S, Edwards JE. Coronary arterial origin in persistent truncus arteriosus. Circulation 1977;55:551.

60. Sim EK, van Son JA, Edwards WD, et al. Coronary artery anatomy in complete transposition of the great arteries. Ann Thorac Surg 1994;57(4):890–894.

61. Smith A, Arnold R, Wilkinson JL, et al. An anatomical study of the patterns of the coronary arteries and sinus nodal artery in complete transposition. Int J Cardiology 1986;12:295.

62. Spidardmont S, Ritter DG, Feldt RH, et al. Double-outlet right ventricle: anatomic and angiocardiographic correlations. Mayo Clinic Proc 1978;53:555.

63. Subramanian R, Olson LJ, Edwards WD. Surgical pathology of pure aortic stenosis: a study of 374 cases. Mayo Clin Proc 1984;59:683.

64. Turri M, Thiene G, Bortolotti U, et al. Surgical pathology of aortic valve disease: a study based on 602 specimens. Eur J Cardiothorac Surg 1990;4:556.

65. Vlodaver Z, Neufeld HN, Edwards JE, eds. Patterns of origin and distribution of coronary arteries in transposition complexes and tetralogy of Fallot. In: Coronary arterial variations in the normal heart and in congenital heart disease. New York: Academic Press, 1975:109–134.

66. Waldman JD, Lamberti JJ, Mathewson JW, et al. Surgical closure of the tricuspid valve for pulmonary atresia, intact ventricular septum and right ventricle-to-coronary artery communications. Pediatr Cardiol 1984;5:221.

67. Waller BF, Carter JB, Williams HJ Jr, et al. Bicuspid aortic valve. Comparison of congenital and acquired types. Circulation 1973;48:1140.
68. Wilson GJ, Freedom RM, Koike K, et al. The coronary arteries: anatomy and histopathology. In: Freedom RM, ed. Pulmonary atresia with intact ventricular septum. Mount Kisko, NY: Futura, 1989:75–88.
69. Yacoub MH, Radley-Smith R. Anatomy of the coronary arteries in transposition of the great arteries and methods for their transfer in anatomical correction. Thorax 1978;33:418.
70. Yoshigi M, Momma K, Imai Y. Coronary artery-pulmonary artery fistula in pulmonary atresia with ventricular septal defect. Heart & Vessels 1995;10:163.
71. Giglia TM, Mandell VS, Connor AR, et al. Diagnosis and management of right ventricle-dependent coronary circulation in pulmonary atresia with intact ventricular septum. Circulation. 1992;86:1516.

Coronary Artery Anomalies: A Comprehensive Approach, edited by P. Angelini.
Lippincott Williams & Wilkins, Philadelphia © 1999.

CHAPTER 7

Coronary Artery Anomalies: More Work is Needed

James T. Willerson

In this book, Dr. Angelini and his colleagues have reviewed the important, but often neglected, subject of coronary artery anomalies and have provided detailed descriptions of the embryology relative to coronary artery formation and development. The book includes in-depth discussions of normal and variant coronary artery origination, myocardial course, and connection. It also describes the clinical complications of malformations, anomalous origins, and fistulas involving the coronary arteries. The authors remind us that anomalies of the coronary arteries sometimes coexist with other developmental abnormalities of the heart, including selected forms of congenital heart disease and abnormalities of the cardiac valves.

Although we recognize the existence of coronary artery anomalies, we know relatively little about them. Figure 7.1 lists the causes of sudden death in competitive athletes with a median age of 17 years, based on systematic tracking of 158 athletes in the United States, primarily from 1985 to 1995. These data suggest that 19% of sudden deaths in this select and relatively small group of competitive athletes are related to congenital coronary artery anomalies and that another 5% of sudden deaths may be caused by a tunneled left anterior descending coronary artery.

Unfortunately, we know relatively little about the frequency of coronary anomalies and the clinical consequences of such anomalies in a large population of patients with varying backgrounds. We also have very little information about the specific genetic mechanisms involved in the development of individual coronary anomalies or the genetic relationship of these anomalies to other forms of congenital heart disease. Clearly, we need more epidemiologic information and focused research at the molecular genetic level to elucidate the basic mechanisms involved in the development of coronary anomalies. From such information, we should gain a far better ability to predict the consequences of specific anomalies in individual patients and, ultimately, the ability to prevent these anomalies with specific therapy, possibly including gene or gene-product therapy.

We also need to develop relatively noninvasive imaging techniques that will allow the identification of coronary artery anomalies and their origins, courses, and connections in the presence or absence of other forms of congenital heart disease. Today, coronary anomalies are usually recognized by means of coronary arteriography. In the future, however, we may be able to recognize these anomalies with echocardiography, magnetic resonance imaging, rapid computer tomography, and similar noninvasive methodologies. This will be a major step forward.

To address the need for better epidemiologic, molecular genetic, and noninvasive detection methods, I have several suggestions. First, I believe that it would be very useful for the American Heart Association's Council for Cardiovascular Diseases in the Young to develop an international registry of specific coronary artery anomalies. Physicians worldwide would be encouraged to enter their patients with coronary anomalies in this registry, allowing follow-up and elucidation of these patients' morbidity and mortality. It would be important to enlist the support of the European Society of Cardiology and the Pacific Rim Cardiovascular Society in this endeavor. The resulting international database could prove extremely valuable in identifying the frequency of coronary artery anomalies, as well as their consequences, their modes of therapy in different countries, and the possible genetic or environmental influences on these anomalies.

Second, it is necessary to focus molecular genetic research on these problems by developing appropriate experimental animal models and using tissue from humans with these abnormalities whenever feasible. Financial support should be made available to help develop the noninvasive imaging methods necessary for progress in this field. A commitment

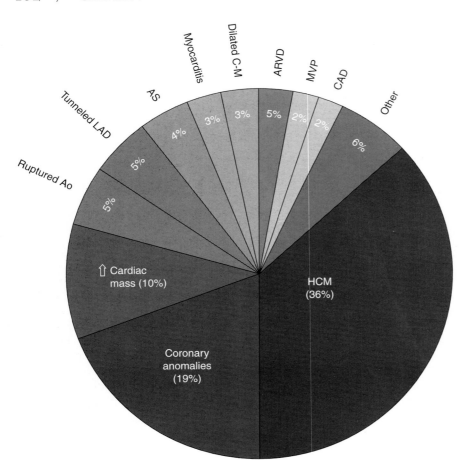

FIGURE 7.1. Causes of sudden cardiac death in young competitive athletes (median age, 17 years), based on systematic tracking of 158 athletes in the United States, primarily from 1985 to 1995. Ao = aorta; ARVD = arrhythmogenic right ventricular dysplasia; AS = aortic stenosis; CAD = coronary artery disease; C-M = cardiomyopathy; HCM = hypertrophic cardiomyopathy; LAD = left anterior descending coronary artery; MVP = mitral valve prolapse; ↑ = increased. (Adapted from Maron BJ, Thompson PD, Puffer JC, et al. Cardiovascular preparticipation screening of competitive athletes: a statement for health professionals from the Sudden Death Committee [Clinical Cardiology] and Congenital Cardiac Defects Committee [Cardiovascular Disease in the Young], American Heart Association. Circulation 1996;94:850 with permission of the American Heart Association.)

from the American Heart Association and the National Institutes of Health, in the United States, to providing dedicated research support would hasten progress toward the necessary biologic understanding. Philanthropic support could surely also be gained from families and institutions whose members have suffered from a coronary artery anomaly.

Third, greater attention must be devoted to teaching cardiologists in training about coronary artery anomalies. This topic is rarely given adequate attention by current training programs in cardiovascular medicine, and it needs to be strengthened for both pediatric and adult cardiologists in training. Dr. Angelini's book is a very positive step in that direction.

REFERENCE

1. Maron BJ, Thompson PD, Puffer JC, et al. Cardiovascular preparticipation screening of competitive athletes: a statement for health professionals from the Sudden Death Committee (Clinical Cardiology) and Congenital Cardiac Defects Committee (Cardiovascular Disease in the Young), American Heart Association. Circulation 1996;94:850.

Subject Index

Pages numbers in *italics* denote figures; those followed by a "t" denote tables.